A CULTURAL HISTORY OF THE SENSES

VOLUME 3

A CULTURAL HISTORY OF THE SENSES
IN THE RENAISSANCE

Edited by Herman Roodenburg

BLOOMSBURY ACADEMIC
LONDON • NEW YORK • OXFORD • NEW DELHI • SYDNEY

BLOOMSBURY ACADEMIC
Bloomsbury Publishing Plc
50 Bedford Square, London, WC1B 3DP, UK

BLOOMSBURY, BLOOMSBURY ACADEMIC and the Diana logo are trademarks of
Bloomsbury Publishing Plc

First published in Great Britain 2014
This edition published 2019
Reprinted 2019

Copyright © Bloomsbury Publishing, 2014, 2019

Herman Roodenburg has asserted his right under the Copyright, Designs and Patents Act, 1988,
to be identified as Editor of this work.

For legal purposes the Acknowledgments on p.xi constitute an extension of this copyright page.

Cover image: Detail from *Egg Dance*, Pieter Aertsen, 1552 © Rijksmuseum, Amsterdam

All rights reserved. No part of this publication may be reproduced or transmitted in any form or
by any means, electronic or mechanical, including photocopying, recording, or any information
storage or retrieval system, without prior permission in writing from the publishers.

Bloomsbury Publishing Plc does not have any control over, or responsibility for, any third-party
websites referred to or in this book. All internet addresses given in this book were correct at the
time of going to press. The author and publisher regret any inconvenience caused if addresses
have changed or sites have ceased to exist, but can accept no responsibility for any such changes.

A catalogue record for this book is available from the British Library.

Library of Congress Cataloging-in-Publication Data.
A cultural history of the senses in the Renaissance, 1450–1650 / edited by Herman Roodenburg.
    pages cm
Includes bibliographical references and index.
ISBN 978-0-85785-341-7 (hardback)
1. Senses and sensation—History 2. Renaissance. I. Roodenburg, Herman.
    BF233.C856 2014
    152.1094'09031–dc23
    2014005064

ISBN:	HB:	978-0-8578-5341-7
	PB:	978-1-3500-7790-4
	ePDF:	978-1-4742-3319-4
	eBook:	978-1-4742-3320-0
	HB Set:	978-0-8578-5338-7
	PB Set:	978-1-3500-7783-6

Series: The Cultural Histories Series

Typeset by RefineCatch Limited, Bungay, Suffolk

To find out more about our authors and books visit www.bloomsbury.com
and sign up for our newsletters.

CONTENTS

LIST OF ILLUSTRATIONS — vii

SERIES PREFACE — x

EDITOR'S ACKNOWLEDGMENTS — xi

Introduction: Entering the Sensory Worlds of the Renaissance — 1
Herman Roodenburg

1 The Social Life of the Senses: Architecture, Food, and Manners — 19
Niall Atkinson

2 Urban Sensations: Attractive and Repulsive — 43
Peter Burke

3 The Senses in the Marketplace: Sensory Knowledge in a Material World — 61
Evelyn Welch

4 The Senses in Religion: Towards the Reformation of the Senses — 87
Matthew Milner

5 The Senses in Philosophy and Science: From the Nobility of Sight to the Materialism of Touch — 107
Danijela Kambaskovic and Charles T. Wolfe

6 Medicine and the Senses: Physicians, Sensation, and the Soul — 127
Stephen Pender

7	The Senses in Literature: Renaissance Poetry and the Paradox of Perception *Holly Dugan*	149
8	Art and the Senses: Representation and Reception of Renaissance Sensations *François Quiviger*	169
9	Sensory Media: The Circular Links between Orality and Writing *Federico Barbierato*	203
	NOTES	221
	BIBLIOGRAPHY	225
	NOTES ON CONTRIBUTORS	261
	INDEX	265

LIST OF ILLUSTRATIONS

CHAPTER ONE

1.1	Vincenzo Campi, *Fish Vendors*, 1580s.	31
1.2	Pieter Aertsen, *Market Stallholder*, 1567.	32
1.3	Pieter Aersten, *Christ in the House of Mary and Martha*, 1553.	33
1.4	Dining *loggia* of the Villa Farnese with fresco cycle of Cupid and Psyche by Raphael and his workshop, 1517–19.	35
1.5	Illustration of the provisioning of the papal conclave, from Bartolomeo Scappi, *Opera*, 1596.	36

CHAPTER THREE

3.1	Abraham Bosse, *La Galerie du Palais*, etching, c. 1637–40.	63
3.2	The Antwerp Exchange, engraved illustration in Ludovico Guicciardini's *Commentarii di Lodovico Guicciardini delle cose più memorabili* (Venice, 1565).	70
3.3	Joachim Beuckelar, *The Four Elements: Water. A Fish Market with the Miraculous Draught of Fishes in the Background*, oil on canvas, 1569.	73
3.4	*Vende agli e cipolle*, after Annibale Carracci, engraving, 1646.	74
3.5	"Intartenimento che dano ogni giorno li Ciarlatani in Piazza di S. Marco al populo d'ogni natione che mattina e sera ordinariamente ui concore," engraved illustration from Giacomo Franco, *Habiti d'huomini et donne Venetiane* (Venice, 1610).	77

3.6 Ambrogio Brambilla, *Ritrato de quelli che vano vendendo et lavorando per Roma*, etching, 1582.   79
3.7 "Oderatus," engraving after George Glover, *c.* 1640.   81
3.8 "Gustus," engraving after George Glover, *c.* 1640.   83

CHAPTER EIGHT

8.1 Maerten de Vos, *The Five Senses*, Antwerp, 1570s.   171
8.2 Anatomical cut of the head from L. Dolce, *Dialogo . . . nel quale si ragiona del modo di accrescere e conseruar la memoria* (Venice, 1562).   174
8.3 Magdalene Master, *Virgin and Child*, tempera and guilding on panel, *c.* 1260–70.   177
8.4 Anonymous early sixteenth-century Italian, *Madonna and Child*.   177
8.5 Michael Pacher, *Flagellation*, *c.* 1495.   178
8.6 Sodoma, *Flagellation*, *c.* 1510.   179
8.7 Diego Velazquez, *Christ at the Column after the Flagellation*, *c.* 1628, oil on canvas.   180
8.8 Gian Lorenzo Bernini, *Ecstasy of Saint Theresa*, 1647–52, marble.   182
8.9 Scene of iconoclasm from a Catholic pamphlet: *Eyn Warhafftig erschrölich Histori von der Bewrischen uffrur so sich durch Martin Luthers leer in Teutscher nation . . .*, *c.* 1525–7.   183
8.10 The Joyful Mysteries of the Rosary, from *Unser Lieben Frauen Psalter* (Ulm, 1483).   186
8.11 *Virgin of the Rosary*, German, late fifteenth century.   187
8.12 Agnolo Bronzino, *Allegory*, *c.* 1545.   189
8.13 *The Laocoon*. Vatican Museum, Museo Pio Clementino.   192
8.14 Agostino Veneziano, ornamental panel, engraving, 199 × 135 mm, *The Illustrated Bartsch*.   193
8.15 Nicoletto da Modena, ornamental panel with the stories of Apollo, *c.* 1507.   195
8.16 Frontispiece of Enea Vico, *Ex Gemmis et Cameis Antiquorum Aliquot Monumenta ab Aenea Vico Parmensi incisa* (Paris, n.d.).   196
8.17 *Bacchanal of Children*, Ferrarese print, late fifteenth century.   197
8.18 Andrea Mantegna, *Bacchanal*, *c.* 1470.   198
8.19 Michelangelo, *Bacchus*, *c.* 1496–8.   199
8.20 Sandro Botticelli, Detail of *The Birth of Venus*, *c.* 1485.   202

LIST OF ILLUSTRATIONS

CHAPTER NINE

9.1 Giuseppe Maria Mitelli, *Agl'appassionati per le guerre*, etched
   engraving.   212
9.2 *Le crieur de gazette*, engraving.   214

Every effort has been made to trace copyright holders and to obtain their permission for the use of copyright material. The publisher apologizes for any errors or omissions there may be in the credits for the illustrations and would be grateful if notified of any corrections that should be incorporated in future editions of this book.

SERIES PREFACE

GENERAL EDITOR, CONSTANCE CLASSEN

A Cultural History of the Senses is an authoritative six-volume series investigating sensory values and experiences throughout Western history and presenting a vital new way of understanding the past. Each volume follows the same basic structure and begins with an overview of the cultural life of the senses in the period under consideration. Experts examine important aspects of sensory culture under nine major headings: social life, urban sensations, the marketplace, religion, philosophy and science, medicine, literature, art, and media. A single volume can be read to obtain a thorough knowledge of the life of the senses in a given period, or one of the nine themes can be followed through history by reading the relevant chapters of all six volumes, providing a thematic understanding of changes and developments over the long term. The six volumes divide the history of the senses as follows:

Volume 1. A Cultural History of the Senses in Antiquity (500 BCE–500 CE)
Volume 2. A Cultural History of the Senses in the Middle Ages (500–1450)
Volume 3. A Cultural History of the Senses in the Renaissance (1450–1650)
Volume 4. A Cultural History of the Senses in the Age of Enlightenment (1650–1800)
Volume 5. A Cultural History of the Senses in the Age of Empire (1800–1920)
Volume 6. A Cultural History of the Senses in the Modern Age (1920–2000)

EDITOR'S ACKNOWLEDGMENTS

One of the pleasures of editing volumes is the social adventures involved: discovering new colleagues and their writings and renewing the acquaintance of other colleagues whose work I have been following and admiring for many years. Reading and discussing their chapters, I learned much from all of them, as I also profited greatly from Constance Classen's excellent guidance and comments. I also learned from the conversations as well as from the writings of a number of other scholars, including Wietse de Boer, Mickaël Bouffard-Veilleux, Reindert Falkenburg, Christine Göttler, Daniela Hacke, Yannis Hadjinicolau, Philip Hahn, David Howes, Ulrike Krampl, Birgit Meyer, Jan-Friedrich Missfelder, Monique Scheer, Frits Scholten and Jojada Verrips. A special thanks goes to Alessandro Arcangeli, who kindly translated Federico Barbierato's chapter into English.

Introduction: Entering the Sensory Worlds of the Renaissance

HERMAN ROODENBURG

Let us start with a remarkable letter written in 1640 by a lover of the lute, a Frenchman who lived for some twenty years in the Dutch Republic. In it, he professed his belief that "all our nerves and muscles" serve the memory. He continued, "so that a lute player, for instance, has a part of his memory in his hands; for the ease of bending and positioning his fingers in various ways, which he has acquired by practice, helps him to remember the passages which need these positions when they are placed." The letter, addressed to the French mathematician Marin Mersenne, was written by no less a figure than René Descartes. In an earlier letter to the physician Lazare Meyssonnier he had expressed a similar idea, stating his conviction that "some of the species which serve the memory can be in various other parts of the body, for instance the skill of a lute player is not only in his head, but also partly in the muscles of his hands, and so on" (Descartes 1991: 143–6; Reiss 1996: 598–9; cf. Roodenburg 2004: 13–14).

Descartes was apparently intrigued by issues of sensory memory—not so much, like Marcel Proust, by the mnemonic workings of taste and smell (the famous *madeleine* dipped in limeblossom tea, taking "Marcel" back to his childhood years in Combray), as by those of touch and hearing. He considers the lute-player's fingers brushing the strings and, implicitly, his ears picking up the sounds. Of course, such observations may be expected from a musician, perhaps especially a lutenist or, in our own times, a jazz pianist (Sudnow 1978). But to encounter such a "thinking hand" (cf. Bredekamp 2005; Pallasmaa 2009; Roberts *et al.* 2007) in the writings of a philosopher noted first and foremost for his "Cartesian dualism" comes as something of a surprise. As Timothy Reiss observed, "Descartes was here expressing a sense of his own body, his very feel of memory under the skin, as it were, on the sinews of the body" (Reiss 1996: 599). Indeed, modern neuroscientists, all keen now to dismiss "Descartes' error," might well concur. To paraphrase Descartes, the mind is "also partly" in the skin (Damasio 1994; cf. Montagu 1986: 3–46).

Descartes' surprising, almost phenomenological observations may caution us to tread carefully before entering the captivating but often also confusing sensory worlds of Renaissance Europe. As Reiss and other scholars have argued, we have to realize that Descartes' paternity of "Cartesian dualism" is a fairly misleading (and at the earliest a late eighteenth-century) impression of things (Gaukroger 1995, 2002; Reiss 1996: 589 n. 9). Descartes never claimed such radical dualism and his musings on sensory memory, on the mnemonic workings of the hand, only confirm that conclusion. Despite the strict distinctions he sought to draw, his was still a basically psychophysiological (cf. Paster 2004: 11–12) and multisensory universe. In his philosophical quest, aiming "to be a spectator rather than an actor," as he put it himself, he certainly elevated the spectatorial, disembodied eye. But his quest was open enough to also reflect on two of the "lower" senses, those of hearing and touch, and their distinct role in uniting body and mind (see also Chapter 5).

Historians of the senses have a habit of apologizing to their audience that the field is young and that a lot of work remains to be done. That may still be true for some of the periods discussed in the five other volumes of this series, but it clearly holds less so for the two centuries investigated here, those between roughly 1450 and 1650. Some of the senses, those of smell and taste and also the various "inner senses" distinguished in the period, have received appreciably less scholarly attention than those of sight, hearing, and touch (but see for instance on smell, Classen *et al.* 1994; Dugan 2011; Jenner 2011; Le Guérer 1990a, 1990b). Due to a remarkable flowering of sensory history among English-speaking scholars we also know more about the sensory worlds of Tudor and Stuart England than about those elsewhere in Europe (Cahill 2009; Dugan 2009, 2011). But we can certainly say that over the last ten years or so many historians (art historians, cultural historians, intellectual, literary, or medical historians) all "discovered" the sensescapes of the Renaissance. This volume offers a first panorama on those scapes: on *what* people may have sensed but, in particular, on *how* they may have sensed, to how their acts of sensation informed both their bodies and the objects being sensed (Dugan 2009: 727). As Martin Jay has written, "Meaning comes to a great extent through the senses, while the senses filter the world through the prior cultural meanings in which we are immersed" (Jay 2011: 307; cf. Dugan 2009: 722; Krampl and Beck 2013: 22–3). In the following pages, ten prominent scholars, representing various generations, nationalities, and disciplinary fields, will take the reader back to these two centuries, which in their sensory complexity (or rather their "promise" of a more wholesome, richer sensory universe than ours), already fascinated Johan Huizinga, Lucien Febvre, and Norbert Elias, the first explorers of a cultural history of the senses.

To just speak of the "Renaissance" may cause some confusion, as the term may either denote the movement or the period (cf. Gombrich 1969: 35–8). In this volume it only occasionally refers to the movement, the great flowering of the arts and sciences, inspired in so many ways but certainly not exclusively by the classical tradition. Here the term generally denotes the period and alternates with another somewhat awkward notion, that of "early modernity." The latter has the disadvantage that its beginnings are often situated around 1500 rather than around 1450. Moreover, like the "Renaissance" concept, it has its teleological connotations. If not taken neutrally, as just a convenient shorthand, both terms may easily tempt the sensory historian to approach the age not on its own but on merely transitional terms—an age lined by major sensory ruptures just paving the way for "modernity," for the ascendancy of Descartes' disembodied eye and the ensuing denigration of all the other senses, those of taste, smell, and touch in particular.

Obviously, the history of the senses, like that of the emotions to which it is so closely related, follows its own rhythm, it does not care about any of the standard periodizations deriving from political, economic, or social history. Accordingly, modern sensory historians have grown critical, not only of the "grand narratives" sketched by Huizinga, Febvre, or Elias, but also those of media theorists Marshall McLuhan and Walter Ong.[1] In the present exoticised view, all these earlier and later pioneers portrayed the Middle Ages as a "lost world of synaesthetic complexity" in which the "lower" senses still held sway over the sense of sight (Missfelder 2012: 30). Indeed, similar objections have been raised to the nuanced and innovating interpretations of Alain Corbin and Martin Jay. Even they, it is argued, sketched the late Middle Ages as just a foil to modernity, thereby defining the early modern period once more in terms of major sensory transitions, what Mark Smith ironically summarized as the "great divide" (Le Guérer 1990; Missfelder 2012: 30–1; M. Smith 2007b: 8–13).

SOME HISTORIOGRAPHY

Of course, the Renaissance did see important changes. It witnessed the spread and increasing societal impact of court and urban cultures, just as it witnessed the first global voyages of discovery—three essential developments which in themselves resulted in there being much more to sense in towns (Peter Burke speaks of a "hyperstimulation of the senses") than would have been possible in the centuries before (see Chapter 2). Closely related to this urban growth, the Renaissance also saw the rise of new religious cultures. One of these was the "affective piety" of the fourteenth and fifteenth centuries, focusing on the humanity of Christ and surprisingly (at least to defenders of the "great divide") promoting inwardness through both the senses of touch and sight. In the sixteenth century the new devotional cultures of the Reformation and the Counter Reformation emerged, each with its own varieties of religious sensing and increasing anxieties about the trustworthiness of the senses (for a fine recent study, see de Boer and Göttler 2012). Other essential moments within any sensory history of the Renaissance are the outbreak of witchcraft prosecutions (the *Malleus Maleficarum* was published in 1487), the new interest in such fields as alchemy or anatomy, and the simultaneous revaluation of all artisanal knowledge (which still encompassed that of painters, sculptors, and architects). Finally, the period saw a range of technological innovations, from the "inventions" of oil painting (*c.* 1410), linear perspective (*c.* 1435) and moveable type (*c.* 1450) to those of the telescope (*c.* 1608), the compound microscope (*c.* 1620) and, slightly beyond our time frame, the spring balance watch (1660). The development of movable type print was especially emphasized by McLuhan and Ong (drawing on Febvre), convinced as they were that it isolated reading and writing from speech, thus helping Cartesian ocularcentrism to the throne (McLuhan 1962; Ong 1982).

All these key moments figure prominently in the writings of sensory historians today, but their approaches are decidedly different. They tend to emphasize not the sensory ruptures but the many sensory continuities, whether in the period's concrete devotional practices or in its philosophical, religious, and medical reasoning, with its continuing interest in Aristotelian, Galenic, or other traditional theories on body, mind, and soul. That does not mean that these historians are no longer interested in any sensory breaks or shifts. Rather, they like to focus on how people sensed, including how they perceived and experienced possible ruptures. In addition, they are starting to augment the many sense-by-sense investigations (already more and more devoted to the non-visual senses) with other research thematizing the cross-modality of the senses, their intersensoriality, and relating its study to that of human perception in general, including aspects of embodiment and material culture. Art historians and literary historians may have written the most innovating investigations here.

Though the popular pictures of the five senses seem to suggest otherwise (Ferino-Pagden 1996), early modern men and women distinguished more than these senses alone. They did not always have a distinct term for them, nor did they always use the same terms as we do now. But when Rembrandt, at the end of our period, explains about his striving for *die meeste en de naetureelste beweechgelickheit* ("the greatest and most natural motion"—"motion" both in the sense of the motion of the figures depicted and the figures' power to move the beholder), we may certainly conclude that he related the rousing of the viewers' emotions to what we would now describe as the kinesthetic sense, to the viewers' and his own proprioception. So did Leone Battista Alberti two centuries earlier, when he wrote about the movements of the soul made known by the movements of the body as they may be represented by painters. As François Quiviger has noted, sensory perceptions now labeled as proprioception, mechanoreception, nociception, and thermoreception were all part of the Renaissance sense of touch. They were a kind of "inner touch," not unlike our own notions of a body image or internal bodily awareness (Quiviger 2010: 105; see also Chapter 8).

To complicate things, Renaissance sensory theory still included the three (or four) "inner senses" distinguished in the Middle Ages: the common sense, the phantasy (or also the imagination), and memory. Aristotle located the common sense (*koine aisthesis*; Lat. *sensus communis*) in the heart. But since Avicenna it was generally situated in Galen's front ventricle of the brain, close to the phantasy and imagination, both situated in the second ventricle and comprising the cogitative and estimative faculties. Artists like Leonardo, eager to raise the intellectual and social status of their craft, also stressed its nearness to the eye (Summers 1987: 71–109). Basically, as also summarized in the following chapters by Matthew Milner, Stephen Pender, and Quiviger, the common sense was believed to distinguish, coordinate and unify all the sense data coming through the five outer senses, thus transforming them into mental images. In Aristotle's view, it enabled humans to perceive such "common sensibles" as movement, rest, shape, or magnitude—qualities typically perceived by two or more senses at once. In fact, through this master sense, the "sense of sensing," humans could integrate various senses into a single mental image. To use the classic example here, what is simultaneously white and sweet becomes sugar, what is simultaneously bitter and yellow becomes gall. But the common sense may always err, hence its close cooperation with phantasy and imagination, which assess all mental images before storing them in the memory at the back of the brain, situated in Galen's third ventricle (Heller-Roazen 2007: 31–45; Howes 2009: 16–20; Quiviger 2010: 17–19).

In his striving to root knowledge as much as possible in cognition rather than sensation, Descartes abandoned the notion of a common sense (Heller-Roazen 2007: 163–8). But most other Renaissance thinkers did not, just as many of them may still have accepted some variety of the Aristotelian notion of *aesthesis*, which refers to our total sensorial experience of the world, our knowing through the body (Meyer and Verrips 2008). For example, as Holly Dugan reminds us in her chapter, for Michel de Montaigne (to whom the common sense was still a familiar notion), to feel was to know (see Chapter 7; cf. Chapter 1).

In the remainder of this introduction I would like to broach a couple of issues presently informing the study of the sensory worlds of the Renaissance and accordingly informing the chapters to follow. I do not intend to cover all the relevant issues of the moment. But it may be helpful to discuss at least some of them, to present them as it were to the reader's "common sense" and thus to the cogitative and estimative faculties located in their "phantasy" and "imagination." These faculties may then decide what from this volume should be stored in their "memory" and what should not.

INTERSENSORIALITY

A first interesting feature emerging in this volume is the issue of "synaesthesia" or rather, allowing for various forms of the interrelation or transmutation of the senses, of "intersensoriality" (Connor 2001; Howes 2005a: 9–10, 2006: 164–5, 2013; M. Smith 2012). People in early modern Europe, writes Sophia Rosenfeld, "generally conceived of the body's senses in interconnected, networked terms," quite in line, one might add, with the coordinating and unifying functions ascribed to the common sense (Connor 2004: 154–6; Rosenfeld 2011b: 319; M. Smith 2007b: 125–6). As we saw above, even Descartes acknowledged the senses' interactivity. As he knew from his own playing, a lutenist's perception unifies the senses of touch and hearing. He might have mentioned sight as well: when playing *prima vista*—with the graphemes functioning as indices of the musician's somatic experience (B. Smith 1999: 129)—or just having the eyes control the fingers plucking the strings. Of course, what Descartes did not bring up were the equally intersensorial qualities of listening to music (Johnson 1995). Nor did he mention the therapeutic effects realized through these qualities (for instance, dispelling melancholia), discussed by contemporary physicians (Gouk 2004).

Of course, painters also reflected on intersensory relations, especially those of sight and touch. Describing a contest between the landscape painters François Knipbergen (1570–1655), Jan Porcellis (*c.* 1584–1632), and Jan van Goyen (1596–1656), their younger colleague Samuel van Hoogstraten praised the last of these three. Unlike his competitors, van Goyen had not devised his images in advance (the prevailing painterly code of *disegno interno*), but had allowed them to emerge in the process of painting "as though the mind and the eye were placed in his hand." If van Hoogstraten, one of Rembrandt's pupils, was lyrical, not so the sixteenth-century writer Anton Francesco Doni, who just scoffed at all these Netherlandish artists "who have the brain in their hands" (Hadjinicolau 2012: 244–7; Kemp 1974; Van de Wetering 2004: 85–6). Van Goyen, like Rembrandt, Frans Hals, and many others, liked to use *impasto*, working if need be with his fingers and letting brush, knife, or fingers devise the images from the paint—a fine instance of an early modern painter's haptic visuality and, through such interconnectedness, of directly enhancing the viewer's sensory and emotional engagement.

Traveling two centuries back, we might take Michael Baxandall's concept of the "period eye" as our point of departure (Baxandall 1972: 29–108). Through this notion, which he first developed in his research on fifteenth-century Italy, Baxandall sought to capture how the habitual visual practices of contemporary merchants could inform the painting of their day and vice versa. A perfect alliance of art history and cultural history, Baxandall's investigations even made Pierre Bourdieu rethink his notion of the habitus (Langdale 1999).

But as various sensory historians suggested, why merely distinguish a "period eye"? Looking at the many recent studies on the non-visual senses of the Renaissance, why not also trace a "period ear," a "period nose," a "period tongue," or—answering to the ubiquity of touch, its being dispersed throughout the body—even a "period skin"? Interestingly, not only the blind John Milton but many early modern authors (philosophers, poets, artists, anatomists) all stressed this unique quality of touch, its "being simultaneously everywhere and nowhere" (Classen 2012: 55; Harvey 2002: 4–5, 2011: 386, 390). However, such a "division of labor" might easily neglect the common sense's coordinating functions and thus unwittingly adopt Descartes' conceptual breaking up of the senses, as already criticized by Michel Foucault (Rosenfeld 2011b: 321). Nor would it do justice to the intersensoriality already addressed in Baxandall's "period eye." Among his merchants' visual practices he discussed various cases in which sight and touch closely interact, for instance where he relates the merchants' visual understanding of volume in a picture to their daily gauging the volumes of barrels, a mathematical skill acquired in secondary education by painters and merchants alike. Baxandall also presented cases of kinesthetic empathy. One of them connects the merchants' (and painters') dancing practices to their visual comprehension of figure patterns, for instance in Botticelli's art. Sight and hearing's interconnectedness (in this volume, see especially Chapter 9) was discussed as well: when the merchants heard and saw the preachers preach.

For a third example we might have a look at the period's religious developments, how perhaps very different varieties of intersensoriality may be traced in how Catholics and how Protestants sensed. As Matthew Milner writes, Renaissance Christianity "revolved around what religious sensing meant" (see Chapter 4). Focusing on the widespread affective piety of the fifteenth century, we might ask whether the believers' devotional practices did not display a different, more visceral or proximate, visuality than the practices of sixteenth- or seventeenth-century Protestants. Though both attending to inwardness, the incorporating practices to construct the inner person may have differed substantially in the way the outer and inner senses interconnected.

The concept of "affective piety" is a fairly recent coinage. Introduced by medievalist Caroline Walker Bynum to describe the new, sentiment-laden devotion of the twelfth century, it was eagerly adopted by her colleagues studying the fourteenth and fifteenth centuries in which they noticed a veritable wave of affective piety (Walker Bynum 1982: 82–109; cf. Karant-Nunn 2010: 63–4, 275 n. 1). No longer construing God as a harsh and distant judge, the new devotion centered on the humanity and vulnerability of Christ. It developed an intense interest in the particulars of his life, especially the Passion, all the bodily violence done to him from his arrest in the Garden of Gethsemane to his horrifying death on the cross. It was this sensuous, emotion-drenched devotion to God incarnate—this "touchable God," in Constance Classen's felicitous phrase (Classen 2012: 27–46; cf. Quiviger 2010: 47–51, 67–9, 110–16)—that from the mid-fourteenth century onward came to be reflected in numerous passion narratives, passion sermons, passion plays, and passion paintings. Among the most influential narratives, those most translated (or rather adapted) into the vernacular, were the anonymous *Meditationes Vitae Christi*, dated *c.* 1300, and Ludolph von Sachsen's *Vita Christi*, dated some fifty years later (Bestul 1996; Marrow 1979; Merback 1999).

Most scholars have stressed the devotion's mental visualization. To quote Jeffrey Hamburger, this was "a culture in which sight had come to complement contemplation as an accepted avenue of insight and access to the divine" (Hamburger 1997: 217). First emerging as a monastic, mainly Franciscan and

Cistercian devotion, it was strongly oriented on rumination: on the ruminative hearing, reading, or copying of the many narratives and sermons and, with the same goal of gazing on Christ, on taking in his image as intensely as possible, on the ruminative viewing and hearing of the passion plays and the ruminative viewing of more and more devotional artifacts (the host, relics, sacramentals, sculptures, images, and so on). Yet all this visuality was also highly haptic, grafted onto the believers' tactile empathy with all the bloody and cruel acts of violence done to Christ's innocent body. This was not a Cartesian visuality based on "distance, mastery and objectification," as Suzannah Biernoff observed, but one which historians had better define "in terms of physical and affective proximity"—one might think of lovers looking each other in the eye (Biernoff 2002: 134). It was also supported by the proper meditational postures and gestures, including the handling of rosaries with their beads of amber and pomanders: believers could already "savour" the soul of God in the fragrances set free (Falkenburg 1994, 1999; Quiviger 2010: 44–7). Until at least the Devotio Moderna, concluded Thomas Lentes, the believers' bodily practices were the main instrument in their imaginative participation in the life of Christ, in imagining to be there themselves and thus suffer with all their senses the sufferings of Christ (Lentes 1999: 54–9).

In contrast, Rembrandt's Passion cycle, five paintings commissioned in the 1630s by the Calvinist courtier and poet Constantijn Huygens for his master, the Calvinist Prince of Orange Frederic Henry, hardly appeals to the beholder's tactile empathy. First, Rembrandt substantially reduced the "events" of the Passion. Those who had the privilege to view the cycle in the prince's private gallery were spared all the gory scenes so often depicted by fifteenth-century German and Netherlandish painters. They did not see Christ insulted, mocked, or his face being spat at, nor did they see his bleeding body being beaten, scourged, or crowned with thorns or his hands and feet pierced by blunt nails. The first of the five scenes shows already the raising of the cross. Indeed, the visitors to the gallery could hardly identify with Christ or his mother, as their faces do not emotionally reach out—no "affective proximity" here. Rembrandt made it even difficult to trace Mary, whose face remains in the dark or covered under her hood.

Yet the paintings' emotional hold may have been as powerful as that of the late medieval Passion paintings. Of course, the affective piety of seventeenth-century Protestants was different. Calvin and his followers no longer believed in Christ's or Mary's proximity. As Susan Karant-Nunn put it in her admirable study on the "reformation of feeling," the God of Calvin was again a distant and righteous God, separated by an unbridgeable metaphorical space from his children, though he could occasionally reach down to test them or assuage their fears. These fears were considerable. The minds of Calvinists in particular were bent on regret and self-abasement, for they had been taught that it was not the Jews but their own sinful lives which caused Christ to suffer and suffer again. If they were horrified about what the villains did to Christ, they should be as horrified about their own villainy, their own permanent state of corruption (Karant-Nunn 2010: 252).

SENSORY ANXIETY

In her most recent book, *Christian Materiality*, Bynum returns to some of her earlier insights. Though she fully agrees with the present scholarly interest in both visuality and inward piety, she asks her audience to consider another, contradictory, tendency of late medieval devotion. As she tells us, believers also had an intense interest in materiality, in all such "living holy matter" as animated hosts, relics, statues, images, and so on. They never experienced matter as mere dead stuff. Instead, it was felt to be dynamic and vital, filled with creative potential (Bynum 2011: 19–25). Like other scholars, Bynum thus raises issues of sensory anxiety, of good versus bad sensing: how were the faithful to distinguish such miracles?

For all these men and women, objects had agency but not, as Alfred Gell or Bruno Latour might have argued, because of their naturalism or similitude. Objects were not felt to come alive, to start bleeding, weeping, moving, or speaking (to only mention the more "daily" miracles), the closer they resembled the living. What in Bynum's view lent them agency was their lability. Within the period's incarnational piety, matter was by definition "labile, changeable, and capable of act." "To oversimplify a bit," as Bynum sums up, "one might say that to a modern theorist, the problem is to explain how things 'talk'; to a medieval theorist, it was to get them to shut up" (Bynum 2011: 280–4). Matter, especially numinous matter, never was inert, a conviction that both fascinated and disturbed the people of the fourteenth and fifteenth centuries. These were the same centuries developing an interest in all kinds of metamorphosis, from "spontaneous generation" (insects, reptiles, or other creatures emerging from putrefying matter; indeed, for the sixteenth-century miller Menocchio even God and the angels first emerged as worms), to the more disturbing "miracles" of alchemy, demonology, or witchcraft. Naturally, if both the sacred and the devil may erupt in matter, if its vitality may also seriously delude the senses, believers had to control their sensing. There was already a widespread anxiety over all sensory perception, long before the Reformers would voice their louder distrust of the senses (Bynum 2011: 25, 269–73; Ginzburg 1980: 53).

The historian Stuart Clark may have been the first to discuss such sensory anxiety. Wishing to develop another, more nuanced, perspective on Descartes and Thomas Hobbes as the famed "revolutionaries of the cognitive process," he focused on a range of problems defining Renaissance visuality from the start, those "that made their revolution something of a necessity" (Clark 2007: 6). As he argued, both the fifteenth and sixteenth centuries were already highly ocularcentric, making his investigations directly fit in with the recent research on late medieval visuality. But he also observed a long period of "viewerly confusion." Sight was increasingly experienced as imbued with uncertainty and unreliability, all too susceptible to delusions, misapprehensions, and moral corruption. Physicians, for example, blamed the four humors or, in discussing melancholy or lycanthropy, the workings of the imagination. Both one's bodily and mental states could distort one's visual perceptions and even cause purely imagined perceptions. Alarming also were the apparitions and illusions effected by demons and witches in those they possessed. In addition, there was the Renaissance vogue for all visual artifice, for the optical illusions created by painters, magicians, and jugglers alike. Most importantly, visual uncertainty played a major role in the period's religious controversies, the fiery debates on mass, images, or miracles, while the Pyrrhonian skeptics, emerging around the middle of the sixteenth century, doubted the human ability to ever discern true from false visual experience. The visual culture traced by Clark was very different from the pre-Cartesian "enchanted whole" that never was (Reiss 1996: 592–3).

In this volume, Matthew Milner, drawing on his own investigations on the English Reformation, extends Clark's picture of a viewerly confusion to a sensory confusion *tout court*. To quote Galileo (here quoted by Evelyn Welch, see Chapter 3), "any one of the senses is fallacious." But like Clark, Milner emphasizes the—largely Galenic and Aristotelian—lines of continuity: "the fundamentals of traditional medieval sensory culture did not change ... If anything they intensified" (Milner 2011: 4).

One of those fundamentals was the need to govern the senses, to subject them to reason, for it was only if managed properly that they could perform their God-given task of discerning virtue from evil. That was a complex one. It urged the faithful to shun sensory enticements as much as possible but also, when called for (and just as in the affective piety of the centuries before), to immerse themselves in sensory sacred affect. Good sensing "literally shaped believers" (Milner 2011: 53), whether Catholic or Protestant, but how were they to distinguish good from bad religious sensing? And how could the new liturgies arrange that bad things would not continue to enter the senses?

Various Lutheran liturgies, writes Milner, still accepted the elevation of the host until 1542. Similarly, the Reformer himself still used an amber rosary with all its religious scenting in 1531 (King 2012: 155). More typically, English ministers were not so sure whether the faithful came to hear the sermon for comprehending the Word or for its sensory pleasures, "its experience as a transient, lively, sensible manifestation" (Milner 2011: 310; cf. Chapter 9). All these issues were deemed so important, because contemporary theories continued to lend matter agency (see also Chapter 4).

Sensory governance (or rather the lack of it) was also a major polemical argument in the great religious debates. Protestants accused Catholics of "idolatry," the reproach so often swallowed whole in older historical accounts of the Reformation, those contrasting the late medieval "enchanted whole" to the self-ascribed sensory self-discipline of Protestants. Inversely, Catholics accused the Protestants of "heresy," which in its contemporary meanings could only mean that their opponents were guilty of sensory misgovernance and even deviancy. Were Luther's senses functioning properly, asked Thomas More, was he not deluded in his senses (Milner 2011: 193)?

In foregrounding the period's sensory anxiety, historians like Bynum, Clark, and Milner have opened up an absorbing and important perspective on the sensory worlds of the Renaissance. But as Welch reminds us in her chapter, sensory uncertainty governed life outside the town or village churches as well (see Chapter 3). Visiting the markets, knowing they may be deceived by frauds and mountebanks, early modern men and women needed all their senses to discern the good from the bad on offer and the true from the false—Francis Bacon aptly referred to the "idols of the marketplace." In Welch's own words, "being able to separate out the true from the false was a constant marketplace dilemma." Buyers should know how to gauge the volumes of barrels, as described by Baxandall, but also how to use their eyes in testing the color of salt and the tips of their fingers in feeling its structure. They also had to use their ears in judging glass, metalwork, or minerals, their nose in controlling perfumes and drugs, and of course both their nose and their tongue in trying wines and oils.

Thanks to a growing number of studies on the "urban senses," here also represented by Niall Atkinson, Federico Barbierato, and Peter Burke (for some earlier studies, see Beck and Krampl 2013; Cockayne 2007; Cowan and Steward 2007), we are now increasingly informed on how also ordinary men and women had to cope with the "hyperstimulation of the urban environment" (see Chapter 2). Like towns today, early modern towns had their own sensory identities. The authorities could take different measures to control or even remove the sources of filth, noise, or stench. In addition, in its physical structures (flat or hilly, having spacious or narrow streets and plazas, few or many waterways) each town had its own auditory, olfactory, or tactile identity, often already varying from neighborhood to neighborhood, even from street to street (Alazard 2013; cf. Atkinson 2012). But as the "anonymous city" developed, with more and more travelers and immigrants crowding the streets and houses, people's appearances and identities, the town's social structures, created further sources of sensory anxiety (cf. Burke 1995, 2006).

The classic example used to illustrate these developments is *La Vida de Lazarillo de Tormes* (1554), the famous "autobiographical" bestseller telling the tale of the servant Lazarillo and his master. The latter may have been grand and impressive in appearance, looking "pretty well-off" and "quite well-dressed," but as Lazarillo soon found out, he had no money whatsoever, not even some furniture in his house. The novel struck a chord all over Europe. As Ulinka Rublack writes, "The whole plot brought into question the relationship of dress to reality in a much larger and dynamic urban world where one could not trust appearances and yet had few means to gather secure knowledge about newcomers" (Rublack 2010: 25–6). Another well-known picaresque tale is that of the painter Adriaen Brouwer, who was rumored to have cut a sackcloth into a suit and then, to the jealousy of all the fashionable ladies of Amsterdam, to have painted it into the "best and most expensive material in the world" (B. Smith 1999: 432–3). Such tall stories ridiculed the "new money," but also thematized the old and new elite's play with appearances, the dissimulatory practices inherent to the codes of civility (Castiglione [1528] 1959; cf. Chapter 1; Burke 1995) and bringing their own sensory uncertainties.

Perhaps Renaissance artisans worried the least about the senses, working with matter every day. Interestingly, in her fine study, *The Body of the Artisan*, Pamela Smith already referred to Bynum's views on materiality (P. Smith 2004: 117). She addressed the world of artisans before the Scientific Revolution and investigated their own artisanal epistemology and experience. Her sources were the materials they selected, the objects they made from these materials, and the striking manuals and other texts they produced. The latter have often been interpreted as illustrating their authors' strategy to climb the social and intellectual ladders. But as Smith puts it elsewhere, the texts convey a far more interesting idea—the artisans' conviction "that matter was like a living being one had to come to know through intimate and bodily acquaintance" (P. Smith 2010: 45). They articulate the artisans' sensory and embodied cognition as opposed to the "scientia" of their day.

One of the most influential manuals was written by Paracelsus, the German medical and religious reformer, a text also mined by Baxandall in his study of the "period eye" characterizing the art of the limewood sculptors in fifteenth-century Germany (Baxandall 1980). Moving from fifteenth-century Flanders to sixteenth-century Germany and from there to the seventeenth-century Dutch Republic, Smith devotes the central chapters of her book not only to Paracelsus but also to the works and writings of Benvenuto Cellini, Cennino Cennini, and Bernard Palissy, who all defended an alchemical epistemology grafted onto the generative power of nature and the artisan's bodily and sensory cognition of that power, acquired by "practice over and over again." The texts, writes Smith, "are full of directives about this type of discernment by listening, tasting and smelling, which is very hard to describe in words, but instead is known in the body" (P. Smith 2010: 45).

In their striving to sense the vitality of matter, artisanal and alchemical practices obviously intersected. In the eighteenth century, with the "death of the sensuous chemist," instruments eventually replaced the former tasting and smelling (Roberts 1995). Alchemy and chemistry came to be separated from each other. That Isaac Newton, Robert Boyle, and many other well-known figures of the Scientific Revolution never made that distinction was conveniently forgotten. It is only recently that historians of science again recognize the dynamics and diversity of early modern alchemy and even replicate its experiments: seeing, smelling (but not yet, as Lawrence Principe confesses, also tasting) the materials for themselves (Principe 2011: 310). Of course, as Smith and many other scholars have pointed out, not only alchemy but artisanal knowledge in general, with all its sensory implications, played a major role in the Scientific Revolution, thus counterbalancing Descartes' objectifying eye (e.g. Dupré and Lüthy 2011; Harkness 2007; Roberts *et al.* 2007; see also Chapters 5 and 6).

AESTHESIS

To return once more to Descartes, as we saw he also noticed that the lutenist's "ease of bending and positioning his fingers" on the strings of his instrument was "acquired by practice." In other words, he seems to construe sensory memory in terms of what the anthropologist Paul Connerton describes as "incorporating practices." Drawing on notions of "habitus" and "hexis" as already integrated in Marcel Mauss' *techniques du corps* but much more fully developed by Bourdieu, Connerton sees such practices as integral to all bodily memory (Connerton 1989). Like Bourdieu he emphasizes the practices' acquired and socialized nature: we often start incorporating them from childhood on. He also agrees with Bourdieu that the practices, once incorporated, are largely pre-reflective. Through practicing "over and over again," to quote Pamela Smith, postures, gestures, and all sorts of practices become bodily automatisms: awareness retreats, as all artisans, artists and, for instance, football players know (Bourdieu 1977: 93–4; Roodenburg 2004).

Of course, not everybody possessed a lute, let alone learned to brush the strings as a child. It is no coincidence that Huygens, a close friend of Descartes, played the lute as well or that Descartes in some other letters to Mersenne brought up the subject of fencing (Briost *et al.* 2002: 164), like dancing and making music, another cherished exercise among the elite. Already lauded by Baldassare Castiglione in his *Libro del Cortegiano* (1528), the lute became the elite's favorite instrument, especially after the improvements introduced *c.* 1600 by Bolognese and Venetian lute-makers and, a few decades later, the adding of bass strings requiring its famous enlarged neck. Well-suited to accompany a single voice, as Castiglione recorded, the Renaissance lute provides a perfect example of how in these centuries "sonic discretion became attached to social distinction" (Rosenfeld 2011b: 322). In social terms it was far superior to all the fiddles, bagpipes, or hurdy-gurdies depicted in so many Netherlandish peasant scenes (who could afford the instrument and all the lessons to finally display one's Castiglionian *sprezzatura* brushing the strings?). It was the absolute acoustic antipole to the horribly squeaking *rommelpot* as recalled by Peter Burke in his chapter.

Social distinctions clearly sharpened in this period, not only in the Low Countries but in most parts of Europe, and the people's perceptual boundaries, their "distributions of the sensible" (Rancière 2004), changed along with them. But as Niall Atkinson cautions (see Chapter 1), we should certainly not construe these developments as if "the hierarchy of social groups was simply grafted onto a hierarchy of the senses." What he sees instead, reminding us of Bourdieu's writings on social distinction, is "that the senses were redefined to comprise a social hierarchy within themselves." Indeed, Baldassare Pisanelli's observations that fowl and fish befitted the elite, while the red meat of cows and pigs befitted all the other classes, would have pleased Bourdieu's bourgeoisie. In reconfiguring the existing sensorial regime the Renaissance elites sought to separate themselves from the "sensual promiscuity" that in the process would come to define the lower classes. This redefining, already starting with inculcating the proper bodily and sensory practices in childhood, ranged from courtiers and gentlemen adopting the last codes of Castiglionian *savoir faire* to Erasmus advising schoolboys, tomorrow's elite, to better mask their farting by coughing or to better not fart in company when standing on a mound. Of course, as various chapters in this volume show, a certain redefining of the senses could be found among all classes, even in the most crowded, noisy, and smelly of urban neighborhoods.

If Descartes' lute reminds us of the elite's sensory capital acquired through sustained and often wholly exclusive incorporating practices (as in the arts of dancing, fencing, or horse-riding), it also points once more to a definitely un-Cartesian experience of body and mind. To most early men and women body and mind were hardly separated. Instead, notions of an Aristotelian aesthesis seem to have dominated the Renaissance, forcing sensory historians to reflect not only on the views, attitudes, and theories of the people investigated but also on their own assumptions. Such reflection should not have some universalizing theory as its aim, but it may certainly help to grasp the sensory worlds of the Renaissance in all their complexity and perhaps cast some doubt on some of the generalizing that has already been done (cf. Bynum 2011: 30–1; also Howes 2009, 2011).

One such universalizing approach has been suggested by the art historian David Freedberg, who draws on the well-known investigations of Vittorio Gallese and Giacomo Rizzolatti on mirror neurons (Freedberg and Gallese 2007). His investigations are interesting, as he relates our mirror neurons to emotions and kinesthetic empathy. But he also seems to assume that human bodies hardly change through history or, to give a more concrete example, that the mirror neurons of seventeenth-century viewers facing Rubens' *A Peasant Dance* (c. 1636–40) responded quite like ours. But did they really? (cf. Roodenburg 2011).

Two other approaches look more promising. In her chapter, Dugan defends a "historical phenomenology," proposed some ten years ago by Shakespeare scholar Bruce Smith (2000). Critical of any view that bodies hardly have a history, she argues instead that all our acts of sensation (and they change all the time) inform both our bodies and the environment (both people and objects) that our bodies sense. Accordingly, it is the complex relationships between ideas, bodies, and objects which form the core of historical phenomenology, uniting cultural histories of perception, material culture, and embodiment (see Chapter 7; cf. Curran and Kearney 2012). Of course, bringing in materiality offers space for Bynum's and Pamela Smith's emphasis on the animated nature of matter. Danijela Kambaskovic and Charles Wolfe, drawing on the philosopher John Sutton, obviously move in a similar direction.

Recently, the art historian Horst Bredekamp coined the concept of "picture act" (*Bildakt*), which helpfully refers to the power of pictures to directly work the beholders' feelings, thoughts, and actions, and how these effects interact with their sense of sight, touch, and hearing (Bredekamp 2010; cf. Feist and Rath 2012). The research of Bredekamp and his team of scholars clearly intersects with recent theories that have been summarized under the heading of "situated cognition": embedded cognition, embodied cognition, enactivism, and the extended mind hypothesis (see Robbins and Ayede 2009). As Monique Scheer, a cultural historian of the emotions, summarizes such work, "The socially and environmentally contextualized body thinks along with the brain" (Scheer 2012: 197). Thinking is achieved not only conceptually but also in the body's sensorimotor systems. Perhaps, learning from these recent theories and looking not only at the senses but also at the emotions, we may gradually grasp how people in the Renaissance lived and sensed.

CHAPTER ONE

The Social Life of the Senses: Architecture, Food, and Manners

NIALL ATKINSON

In a story recounted by Franco Sacchetti (*c.* 1330–1400) around the turn of the fifteenth century, the wife of a Florentine wool worker would rise from bed on winter nights to spin thread (Sacchetti 1996: 655–60). Next door, the painter Buonamico Buffalmacco was having trouble sleeping. Separated only by a simple brick partition wall, the noise of her labor kept him awake all night, so he decided to teach her a lesson. By making a hole in the wall he was able to watch her movements as he poured salt through a slender hollow reed into the evening meal that simmered by the fire. At the taste of it, her husband flew into a rage. So Buonamico put even more salt in the next day's meal, which led to a beating so loud that the whole neighborhood heard her shrieks. Rushing in as a good neighbor, Buonamico tried to convince them, in vain, that their saline problem resulted from the wife's weariness from producing nighttime piecework. But several evenings of variously over and under salted meals later, the confused husband finally agreed to stop his wife's nighttime spinning and Buonamico was finally able to get a good night's sleep.

The dynamic interplay of the senses that drives this narrative reveals a great deal about social life in the Renaissance. It demonstrates how the senses could both hinder and facilitate the formation of social relationships, a topic that was at the heart of larger debates about how such relationships should be organized. Any straightforward appeal Buonamico might have made to his neighbor would likely have fallen on deaf ears unless he was able to show how the wife's nocturnal aural assault was directly connected to her husband's offended taste buds. And in order to do so, he secretly watched her while ruining the taste of the dish with a spice that she could not smell. He then relied on the husband's full access to and control of how his wife's body could be touched.

That all the senses were inextricably intertwined in social relations seems a far cry from the hierarchy of the senses that occupied the intellectual discussions of Renaissance humanists. This hierarchy has, in turn, dominated academic discussions about how the Renaissance paved the way for the ocular-centrism that pervaded Enlightenment discourses of knowledge. In the debate about the perception and understanding of truth and beauty, Renaissance theorists had to contend with Plato's insistence that sight was the noblest and most accurate sense and Aristotle's contention that learning was primarily an acoustic experience (Panofsky 1969: 120). Taste, touch, and smell, however, were usually understood as the baser elements of human experience. Although such arguments concerned the potential transcendence of human perception from the materiality of the world, they should not be misrecognized as the only pronouncement of how the senses were understood or experienced. For those hopelessly bound to the material world, the senses were a much more integrated system that needed to be both disciplined and celebrated in the formation of what we recognize as modern civil society.

Even in the most mundane domestic conditions, there existed an implied sensorial hierarchy. As a painter, Buonamico produced objects for purely visual consumption. His neighbor, however, was engaged in a practice whose tactile nature was considered appropriate for women. In her study on the sense of touch, Constance Classen quotes two texts, one from the fourteenth and one from the seventeenth century, that describe the arduous tasks and drudgery of female domestic labor common to both poor and middle-class women. In both texts, textile work constitutes an important wifely duty (Classen 2012: 78). The association of certain tactile forms of labor with the bodies of women, which moralists assumed were more "naturally" connected to the lower senses, is a common theme throughout the period (Classen 2012: 77–85).

However, Sacchetti's story also points to the complicated ways in which gendered sensual hierarchies were never fully fixed. Although Buonamico produced objects for visual and intellectual contemplation by others, his own immediate experience of painting was profoundly tactile, from the grinding and mixing of pigments to the application of color with brushes, knives, and hands. Similarly, the wife's tactile investment in the wool industry placed her within the complex production of fine cloth that caressed the bodies of the upper classes and marked them as objects of visual consumption in an emerging market of sartorial style. Painter and spinner were caught within a similar sensorial nexus.

In the Renaissance, elite society was beginning to distinguish itself from what Classen calls the sensual promiscuity that would come to define lower-class sensibilities. This did not mean that the hierarchy of social groups was simply grafted onto a hierarchy of the senses, but that the senses were redefined to comprise a social hierarchy within themselves. Everyone listened and ate, but they did not hear or taste in the same way.

THE RENAISSANCE OF THE SENSES

Buonamico's story sets out, presciently and ironically, important ways in which sensorial relations were mediated in Renaissance social life. Walls were never absolute barriers so the noise of the woman's spinning problematizes the degree to which architecture ought to function as an acoustic barrier, as well as the need to design dedicated spaces for human domestic and commercial activity. Teaching one's neighbors about how certain behavior was disrespectful to the sensibilities of others was emblematic, therefore, of a growing concern about the need to enforce manners generally throughout society as a remedy to less-than-ideal living conditions. Unsurprisingly, the Renaissance witnessed a proliferation of treatises that dealt with all manner of subjects that were supposed to mediate social interaction, not least among them architecture, food, and manners. These works reveal an increasing self-consciousness, on the part of elites, of their relationship to style in all aspects of social life, and the senses, therefore, would be at the center of this refashioning of the body and its surroundings.

The emerging Renaissance palace provided the setting for an ever more sophisticated culture of social interaction, where an increasingly choreographed social life was transformed into a performative event. François Quiviger has shown, for example, how the Renaissance banquet aestheticized taste and smell, the lower and more intimate senses, by integrating them into the visual and aural dimensions of the larger socially disciplined sensorial apparatus (Quiviger 2010: 153–65). As a result, the three thematic pillars of this chapter—architecture, food, and manners—present fertile ground for exploring the multiplicity of the sensory worlds of Renaissance culture. All three were critical parts of the material substructure of social relations that defined such divisions as class, age, and gender.

BODIES, BARRIERS, AND THRESHOLDS: THE SPATIALIZATION OF THE SENSES

Recent theoretical writing has made the case for the way in which architecture is always experienced by the body's entire sensorial matrix and ought to be designed in accordance with general rules that enhance rather than restrict or overwhelm that experience (see, for example, Pallasmaa 2005). However, less attention has been paid to the degree to which people in Renaissance Europe were intimately aware of how the spaces they inhabited affected their sensual well-being. Regulating excess in the realm of the senses was already considered a fundamental function of architecture as it organized and regulated domestic life. Such regulation was rendered in dramatically sharp relief when such functions collapsed completely during the Black Death of 1348. In Giovanni Boccaccio's eye-witness description of the devastation suffered by his native Florence, he outlines two different reactions to the plague that emphatically deploy the architectural metaphor (Boccaccio 1993: 6–14). His text pressed readers to think about their own physical, moral, social, and political relationships to the walls that enclosed them, the barriers that protected them, and the thresholds that connected them. In the first instance, people locked themselves up within houses that were plague-free and lived a moderate, elegant, but closeted lifestyle to protect them from infection. They partook of the "daintiest fare and the choicest of wines—all in strict moderation." They hoped that depriving themselves of seeing the horror first-hand or even *hearing* stories about the world of terror that lay beyond would protect them from getting sick (Boccaccio 1993: 8–9).

"Others found the contrary view more enticing . . . that the surest remedy was to drink their fill, have a good time, sing to their hearts' content, live it up, give free rein to their appetites . . . day and night would find them in one tavern or another, soaking up the booze like sponges, and carousing all the more in other people's houses," now abandoned by ruined families (Boccaccio 1993: 9). These reactions reveal how a decimated architecture no longer facilitated the proper interaction of the social body through the proper regulation of the senses. Instead, homes were either transformed into sensory deprivation chambers or spaces of unrestrained and distorted sensual excess.

In these two examples, opposing rituals of eating are the fulcrum around which a dysfunctional sensorial world was negotiated. The Swiss humanist

Johann Wilhelm Stuckius, in his encyclopedia of banquets (*Antiquitatum convivialium*, 1597), notes that meals pervade the entire range of human activities so that practically nothing happens in public or private, religious or secular life, without one (Jeanneret 1991: 37). What was particular to this period was the more concentrated attention to the spaces dedicated to such social activities.

Most domestic residences in an Italian city, but throughout Europe as well, would have contained multiple dwellings, where several family groups would have shared things such as front doors, staircases, and landings, a situation that provided the setting for Buonamico's restless nights (Dennis 2008b: 9). In a letter dated March 1550, the writer Anton Francesco Doni gives a vivid sense of what it was like to live in the tenements of Venice, the crowded blocks that housed the vast majority of the city's poorer and transient population. He heard one neighbor successively play the lute, the harp, the flute, and the bagpipes. His room was so small that he could at the same time be "writing, at table, in bed, or sitting in front of the fire, not to mention in the shithouse." From his window he could recognize all manner of foreigners by their distinctive clothing and strange manners (cf. Rublack 2010: 126–75). At night he is bombarded by the sounds of the street—wretches passing up and down singing lewd songs—and the noises of next door—the scissors of a tailor, the incessant cough of a toothless crone, and the shouts and shits of his ailing neighbour, whose apartment rivals the stench of a corrupted grave. In the morning, he hears the barges and gondolas on the "fetid, vile canal, with people shouting and braying with coarse and disjointed voices" (Chambers *et al*. 1992: 181–2). For Doni, who moved in literary circles and had close ties to both leading artists and political figures, such accommodations would not have been his natural surroundings, so he was free to turn squalor into humor. However, his text vividly portrays the unwanted sensorial intimacy that weak architectural barriers could not properly regulate. Spatial design was at the root of sensorial health.

In contrast, the ideal world to which Doni's readers aspired was supposed to be divided into distinct zones for the health and beauty of the city. For example, the noise of industry was not considered healthy for nobles, according to Giacomo Lanteri, who encouraged them in his treatise of family management (*Dell'economica*, 1560) to seek spaces of quiet and tranquility outside the city. Because nobles pursued a tranquil lifestyle, their dwellings should not be located along busy main thoroughfares and urban piazzas. Instead, they should find solace outside the city walls. It was acceptable, however, for merchants and artisans to live with the noise of commerce and industry precisely because they engaged directly with it (Dennis 2008b: 9). Noise, therefore, was a hierarchical phenomenon whose negative effects were only damaging to the delicate sensory apparatus of the upper classes. However, even though Lanteri himself was a nobleman, mercantile trade and manufacturing were still assumed to be an important part of the urban matrix. One of Lanteri's interlocutors notes that in Milan, where merchants and their workshops line the main streets, it actually makes the city more beautiful and delightful in the eyes of those who behold it (Lanteri 1560: 26). Cities were, by nature, heterogeneous entities but Renaissance theorists were increasingly concerned primarily with the rational spatial organization of the disparate elements of which they were made, which appealed primarily to the eye (cf. Atkinson 2012).

Lanteri advised that the most healthy and pleasant part of the home should be reserved for the master and that women's quarters should be as isolated as possible so that they could not be seen by outsiders, even in their gardens. Servants should be ensconced, naturally, in the most wretched part of the house. They could be summoned to receive orders by a system of handbells that highlighted the household's acoustic hierarchy and reduced the need for unseemly shouting, now considered inappropriate for the cultured classes (Romano 1996: 17–18; on the use of handbells, see Dennis 2008a).

According to Leon Battista Alberti (1404–72), the organization of a household had to mediate between degrees of encounter and separation, relative visibility and audibility based on gender, status, and familial relations in spaces of work, sociability, and intimacy. Grandmothers needed nearly complete solitude while men were to be protected from the noisy hordes of children and housemaids. However, servants had to be close enough to their stations to be able to readily hear commands (Alberti 1988: 120, 149; Dennis 2008b: 10–11). Noisy kitchens should not be so far from the guests that the hot food arrives cold to the table: "those dining need only be out of earshot of the irksome din of scullery maids, plates and pans" (Alberti 1988: 148). Palaces had to be designed to hide certain sights, sounds, and smells in order to create zones of sensory and social order that reflected the competence and status of the master (Romano 1996: 17–18).

If sound was a crucial component in the design of the domestic sphere, rooms were increasingly linked visually to the activities performed in them and the behavior expected of those inhabiting them. Both Alberti and the architect Filarete (1400–69) called for schemes of wall decoration that were relevant to the activities they housed (Filarete 1965: 129 [f. 74v–75r]; Rosenberg 1982: 531–3). Such a design ethic was concerned with compelling and reinforcing certain codes of behavior. Therefore, the visual and acoustic organization of domestic space appealed to the two senses humanists believed to be the most equipped to perceive beauty.

DISCIPLINING AND AESTHETICIZING THE SENSES

The design evolution of Renaissance palace rooms coincided with the emergent literature on manners and behavior that grew up around Baldassare Castiglione's treatise on the ideal courtier (*Il cortegiano*, 1528; on its European fame: Burke 1995). Such texts served the purpose of aestheticizing visual and aural perception as a means of elevating and disciplining the lower-order senses, since they could not, in practice, ever be avoided. All of this assumed that what people saw and heard would affect how they acted with others—eating, dancing, playing, and conversing. Not only was beauty thought to induce good behavior, it signified moral virtue and could not be present without it. For the social life of the senses this is crucial, since it was precisely the display of those materially bound senses that could make the meal so unappetizing to those who had to watch and listen.

One of the most widely read and translated texts on the subject was Erasmus' treatise on manners for young boys (*De civilitate morum puerilium*, 1530), which played a central role, according to Norbert Elias, in the emergence of modern civility (Elias 1994: 47–182, esp. 47–52, 60–9). It outlined a basic system of manners, while Castiglione's text described a more refined behavior proper to a more erudite intellectual world, enclosed within the Renaissance palace. Erasmus' text circulated in a more prosaic world of practical guides that would have found a receptive audience throughout Europe. In it, Erasmus locates the major sites in which proper behavior is required—on the street, in the church, at banquets, and in the bedroom, the most important spaces of Renaissance social life.

Erasmus makes all kinds of pronouncements about the natural but less than exquisite sights and sounds produced by the body. Prescriptions for meeting people on the street demanded a sensitivity to the way in which one's face and body betrayed respect, attention, distraction, or disdain. Not only should one look at the person directly, but one should also be aware of how *one's act of sensing*—looking, listening, touching—was perceived by others. Erasmus is highly sensitive to how unseemly it was to be "constantly changing your expression so that at one moment you wrinkle your nose, at another scowl, at another raise an eyebrow, at another twist your lips" (Erasmus 1978: 286–7). In other words, he calls attention to how the face, as the primary center of sense perception, conveys meaning in social interaction. Touching yourself was also part of this economy of sensual sensitivity. It affronts others to "scratch your head, pick your ears, to wipe your nose, to stroke your face as if wiping away your shame, to rub the back of your head." One should converse vocally, with the tongue, and not reel about wildly (Erasmus 1978: 287).

However, the author spends much more time discussing proper behavior at banquets, events at which all the potentially ghastly gestures of bodies were intimately on display. Bodily proximity required that arms and legs did not touch things and people in the wrong way. Hands should not be clasped, on the plate, or in one's lap. Elbows should be off the table and not be poking adjacent diners. Feet should refrain from kicking those across the table. Tasting the wine before eating sends a bad message. Lips should be wiped by a napkin before drinking, during which eyes should not look askance at someone. Although this was a time in which knives and forks were distancing hands from the food, which was still served in self-serve communal dishes, Erasmus detests the common practice of plunging one's "hands into sauced dishes" or "every part of the dish," or fingers into the salt-cellar. One should, instead, learn to navigate the food with plates and spoons, all the while wiping one's fingers on a napkin rather than one's clothes, refraining from consuming whole pieces in one unsightly gulp, or licking a plate because something sweet happens to have stuck to it (Erasmus 1978: 282–4). Such voracious eating makes the face ugly and produces annoying sounds like pigs smacking or human strangulation. Forcing the mouth to speak and eat at the same time distorts the proper rhythm of enjoying food, namely, hearing stories at pauses in the meal rather than watching someone "scratch their head, pick their teeth, gesticulate with their hands . . . cough, or clear their throat, or spit" (Erasmus 1978: 284).

The banquet, however, was an event for engaging with others—speaking and listening, but not alienating them through unsightly behavior or inappropriate looking. "It is bad manners to let your eyes roam around observing each person and it is impolite to stare intently at a single guest. It is even worse to look shiftily out of the corner of your eye at those on the same side of the table; and it is the worst possible form to turn your head right round to see what is happening elsewhere" (Erasmus 1978: 284). Neither snorts, smacks, elbows, sidelong looks, nor even the foul smell of a snuffed out candle should get in the way of enjoying food, wine, and conversation (Erasmus 1978: 286).

According to Jacques Revel, Erasmus' text was complemented by another approach to the same problem that emerged not from late medieval courtesy books, but from Italian court literature. Castiglione's *The Courtier* was also widely read, translated, altered, and plagiarized. As "'a basic grammar of court society' [it] offered its readers a very different model from that of Erasmus" (Revel 1989: 190). It takes the form of an elite improvised dialogue on the ideal courtier. Whereas Erasmus based his work on an internal piety linked to the authenticity of Christ's acts and words, Castiglione's courtier sought validation by winning the esteem from others through a wholly exterior display of grace, or "*sprezzatura*" (Revel 1989: 191). This quality manifested itself in the ability of the courtier to do everything with a seeming effortlessness and poise that turned even the most trivial acts into moments of beauty. Any indication of the effort involved in perfecting the performance of the body on display ruined the effect. If Erasmus had sought to make the sensual expressions of children less unsightly, Castiglione transformed the adult body into a moving, feeling, dissimulating work of art. Instead of Erasmus' goal of social transparency, Castiglione created a situation where outward form masked inward content, where the eye was deceived by the dazzle of carefully scripted bodies.

Although there were great differences in the motivations, techniques, audiences, and goals in these texts, both represent a more general trend in which Renaissance elites began to separate themselves from the more rough and tumble sensorium that would be considered characteristic of the lower classes. The more intimate, self-conscious sensibility imagined by Castiglione, as well as Erasmus' revulsion at the body's excesses, fostered a sensorial break in the idea of class. This emphasis on good manners played a part in the displacement of servants from the bedrooms and intimate spaces of their masters to dedicated quarters in Renaissance palaces, where spatial design minimized the contact between them (Classen 2012: 154).

At first glance, the courtier's obsession with looking and being looked at as a form of validation seems to reflect the more general historiographic assumption of the cognitive shift from the ear to the eye in Renaissance culture. The emergence of print culture led scholars such as Marshall McLuhan and Walter Ong to see media as the determinative factor in our understanding of the world. But the visual regime that the Renaissance was supposed to have unleashed at the threshold of modernity was really confined to certain experimental and intellectual sectors of the period. Subsequent scholars have shown how sight and sound were always integrated within a dynamic tension and that shifts in the way they structured knowledge were more like a cyclical dialectic than a momentous cultural shift. D. R. Woolf has shown how aural and visual culture were never mutually exclusive, pointing out how, even within the Ramist educational techniques that Ong relied on for his argument, the aural dimension persisted and complemented visual educational techniques in the post-Gutenberg world (Woolf 1986: 161ff.).

However, sight did take on new importance in certain practices beyond the visual mediation of print. In one sense, this was wholly practical, since the increasing use of lenses to correct impaired vision and technical improvements in mirrors aided sight in a way not available to the other senses, making the self both an internal subject and an external object of perception and interrogation. The rise of portraiture among non-noble classes as well as the development of painted panoramic landscapes are testaments to these developments (Braunstein 1988: 610–11; Classen 2012: 123, 153–4). With new technologies of vision such as linear perspective in painting, refinements in the telescope, and advances in geographic representations of the Earth's surface, sight was increasingly separated from the other senses but only in such specific areas of intellectual and representational specialization.

THE COURTIER UNMASKED: THE REVENGE OF THE SENSES

These arguments about the shift from the age of the ear to the age of the eye in the Renaissance have tended to assume that the fascination with new modes of vision and sensory discipline in the Renaissance, a fascination vividly brought to life by Erasmus and Castiglione, represented an eclipse of the role, not only of hearing, but of all the senses as valid means of expression. *The Courtier* was a Ciceronian dialogue of social elites offering different opinions for debate. Although it spawned a whole genre of less nuanced manners books, its dialogic form was endemic to Renaissance rhetorical culture, which meant that it was by no means the final word on the subject. Renaissance society was too conscious of the body's desires to ignore its more sensual appetites for food, wine, and love. *The Courtier* had to share space with texts that extolled the body's capacity to exceed itself through the senses, to physically interact with the material world around it and celebrate its abundance and excess, however ironic, complicated, or morally suspect those activities might be.

François Rabelais' satiric works about the lives of Gargantua and his son Pantagruel are the most salient examples of the celebration of the profuse consumption, evacuation, and reproduction of the body (Rabelais 2006). They make a mockery of the moralizing attempts of Erasmus and Castiglione to discipline the body's excess. Expansive bodies engage in a productive two-way transaction with the material world that surrounds them through all their sensorial membranes. The banquet is a central feature of the narrative but recasts the proscribed improprieties of Erasmus' polite society as the social adhesive of popular festive rituals. The grotesque body has free rein in these scenes, which are also intimately "connected with speech, with wise conversation and gay truth" (Bakhtin 1984: 281). Such a body is characterized by its open, unfinished nature, its interaction with the world, traits most fully revealed in the acts of eating and drinking. "Here man tastes the world, introduces it into his body, makes it part of himself" (Bakhtin 1984: 281). It is a thoroughly social affair where excessive eating leads to the delirium of linguistic inventions, where violence is mitigated by the grotesque beauty of the banquet (Jeanneret 1991: 100). The text revels in burlesque themes and scatological humor— monks eating feces—as it constructs a sensually dense image of consuming and excreting bodies that would have horrified Castiglione's courtier. It upends the prohibitions on food and eating found in Genesis, recounting how the body transcends prohibitions through its appetites, grows large and healthy, its newly invigorated vital organs giving birth to a race of giants. "What in the Bible is a first step toward death initiates here the conquest of life" (Jeanneret 1991: 106). The banquet becomes a sign of the individual and the social body's triumph over the world or moral constraints, over death, and sadness.

Mikhail Bakhtin saw the liberating potential of the grotesque body that exceeded its boundaries and connected with the world, even though such depictions of the lower classes could also be the object of upper class comic derision. In either case, however, such exuberant representations underline how the body's natural desires constantly threatened to undermine the new regime of manners imposed upon it. This regime disciplined sensorial relations so that they were experienced individually rather than collectively, defining the difference between a more visually and spatially stratified society. Rabelais' world marks the communal intimacy of eating that was lost by the abandonment of shared plates, cups, dishes, napkins, utensils, and seating, that Constance Classen connects to the increasing use of gloves which, depending on one's point of view, liberated or exiled the body almost completely from its intimate engagement with others (Classen 2012: 155).

If Rabelais constructs a world of puerile education in which Erasmus' young charge stares at his alter ego, Pietro Aretino's life and works lambasted the would-be courtier as a sycophantic, fawning, guileless fool who sought only fame and sex. His comedy, *Cortegiana*, pits servants against their hapless lords and allows us a glimpse of the sensorial life of the underclasses in Renaissance society. In one scene, two servants contrast the pleasure of eating to the misplaced obsession of their lord with carnal gratification. The tavern provides the locus of the critique, providing an alternative site for the construction of a more inclusive conviviality than the dining halls of the Renaissance palace. Rosso declares that "If you've never been to a tavern, you don't know what paradise is! What a friendly place!" It is a place where children learn how to act and where the senses are stimulated by the "lovely music the spits make when they're crammed with thrushes, or sausages, or capons ... the aroma of suckling calf, stuffed with succulent spices!" (Aretino 2008: 135). So delicious is the food, and so seductive the smells, that if the tavern were "next door to a perfume shop, people would be turned off civet" (Aretino 2008: 136). The appeal to taste and smell here is contrasted with the misplaced desire, on the part of the would-be courtier, for power and glory: "You know Caesar," Rosso continues, "who the boss admires so much? Now if he'd just had himself a good time in a tavern ... he'd have got fed up with his triumphal arches" (Aretino 2008: 136). And vision's status is undermined by Rosso's preference for the sight of a well-stocked table over the scenic view from the Vatican's Belvedere (Aretino 2008: 136). The tavern represented the persistence of Rabelais' world, even if it is hyperbolized in the comic nostalgia and outright hunger of Aretino's characters. There, it was the stomach rather than the eye, taste and satiation rather than elegant artifice that governed social interaction.

All the while, Rosso is holding two stolen lampreys intended for his lord's table but which he means to eat himself. As Stephen Biow has noted, hunger amongst the lower classes was a chronic problem in the Renaissance but it was also a literary commonplace. Aretino combined the real and the imaginary in his copious writings where he and his characters are constantly hungry and cravings for food are everywhere described and often satiated (Biow 2010: 64–5). But if manners were motivating the spatial segregation of the classes, taverns were places where people of disparate means mixed together, even though authorities were anxious about some of the violent and passionate activities such social relations fostered. Aretino himself was an inveterate feaster who also hosted very lavish banquets in his own home, which he imagined both as the setting for refined eating and a carnivalesque tavern "where it is always a delight to feed others, those who are friends and those in need" (Biow 2010: 88–9).

THE RENAISSANCE BANQUET: REFINING THE ELITE SENSORIUM

Between Rabelais and Castiglione, the tavern and the banquet hall, one can discern a cultural dialogue about the relative merits of the new regime of the senses that was emerging in Renaissance culture in defining difference and status. The issue of class, therefore, became an important one for the issue of taste, which, even as one of the lower senses, contained a hierarchy all its own. Baldassare Pisanelli's sixteenth-century treatise on food outlines which items were thought to be suitable to different classes. For example, fowl and fish were considered suitable for the upper classes. In general, the higher the animal lived, the more refined its taste. The same was true for the vertical difference that separated root vegetables from food that grew on trees. Such a system generally echoed the belief that proximity to the heavens and liberation from the earth allowed the senses to transcend the body, so that even when elites partook of a meal, it supposedly linked them to a more celestial experience than the earthbound food of their social inferiors (McTighe 2004: 307ff.). This is why Rosso's theft of the lampreys is so significant. It represents a violation of the social food code.

This divide is wonderfully illustrated by Guardabasso, a character in Aretino's *Lo ipocrito*, who blames his hunger on his employer, arguing that it is "necessary that sometimes there be meatballs, and at times little livers, and often tripe with some cheese to plug up the belly" (quoted in Biow 2010: 63). Capon was a mainstay of Renaissance banquets, while the products of four-legged earthbound animals—meatballs, liver, tripe, and cheese—were considered better for the poor, in however little quantities they were actually able to eat them. It was not that chickens tasted better than cows but that the taste of each suited particular classes, in the way urban noises suited merchants, but not nobles. Taste not only had a history but was also a marker of social status. This code is visually reinforced in Renaissance paintings that depict peasants eating next to abundant amounts of food (see Figure 1.1). As Sheila

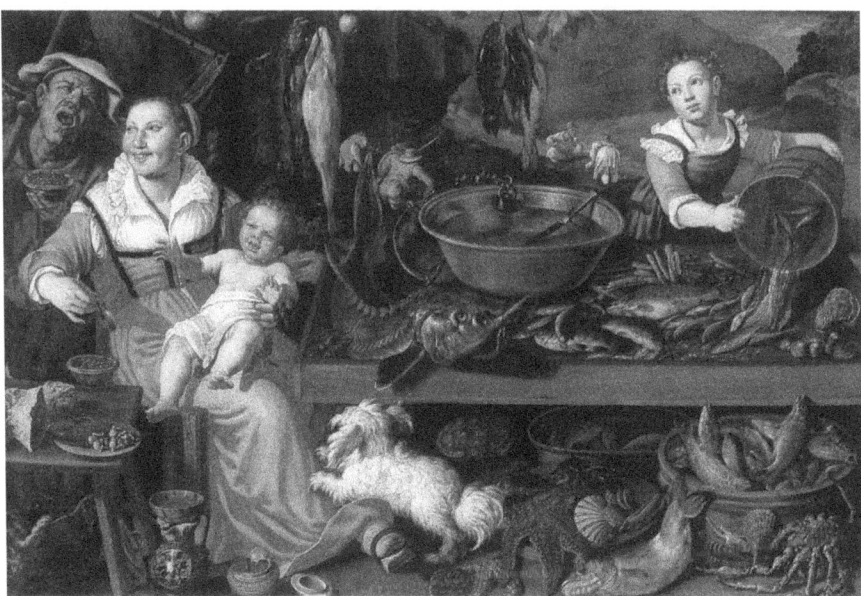

FIGURE 1.1: Vincenzo Campi, *Fish Vendors*, 1580s. Private collection.

McTighe points out, the rustics represented are never eating the food on display, but consume beans and cheese and other appropriate foods (McTighe 2004: 305). There is a clear visual separation between who consumes, sells, prepares, and supposedly enjoys or merits different kinds of food.

If such Italian images defined and reinforced class differences through the medium of food and distinctions of taste, northern painters could deploy the representation of food for different kinds of social messages. Consider Pieter Aertsen's *Market Stallholder* or *Christ in the House of Mary and Martha* (Figures 1.2 and 1.3). Both depict an enticing display of alimentary abundance in the foreground but contain backgrounds that induce conflicting modes of

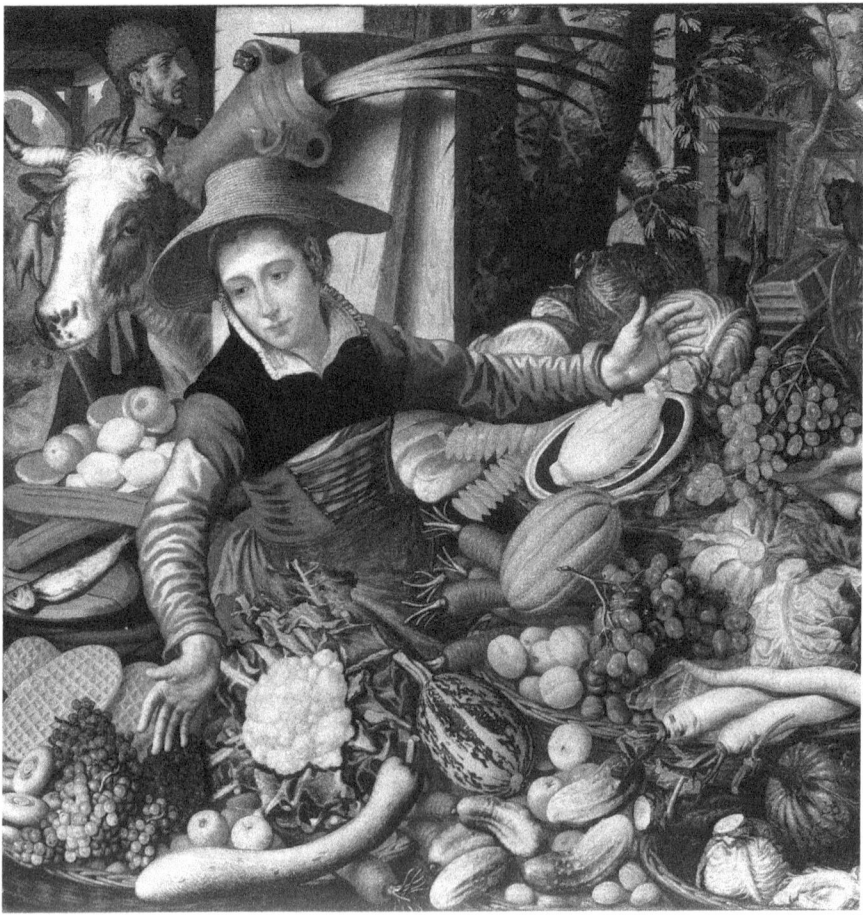

FIGURE 1.2: Pieter Aertsen, *Market Stallholder*, 1567. Berlin-Dahlem, Staatliche Museen Preussischer Kulturbesitz, Gemäldegalerie.

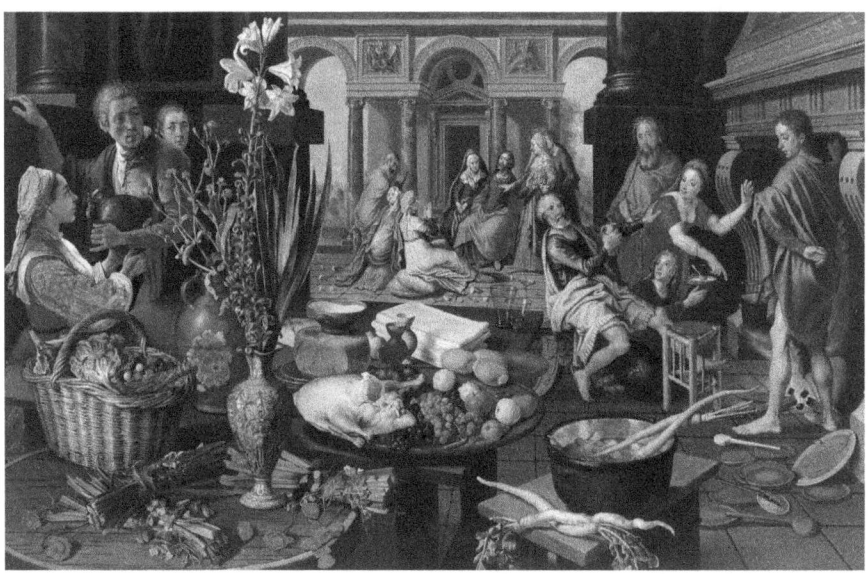

FIGURE 1.3: Pieter Aertsen, *Christ in the House of Mary and Martha*, 1553. Rotterdam, Boymans-van Beuningen Museum.

seeing. In the former, lovers embrace in the upper right corner, almost unseen amid the profusion of food. In the latter, an elegant domestic interior displays both the ingredients of a lavish banquet and its drunken effects, while the scene of Christ's visit to Mary and Martha opens up in the background like a misplaced theatrical performance. Günter Irmscher points out that market vendors, fishmongers, butchers, cooks, poulterers, fishermen, and vegetable sellers, along with pastry cooks and perfume sellers, were condemned in contemporary translations of Cicero's *De officiis*—a text Erasmus recommended memorizing— as practitioners of the most dishonorable trades (Irmscher 1986: 220). As purveyors of products that catered to the sensual pleasures of taste, smell, and touch, images of them and their wares were clearly understood as warnings against the pleasures of the lower senses through an appeal to lustful eyes, which would have been dazzled by the dangerous beauty of food and women (Irmscher 1986: 222). Hanging in the dining rooms of middle-class merchants—who as wholesalers were considered more honest traders—such images of alimentary abundance would have been meant to prevent the excesses of the lower senses by sublimating them within the realm of vision. The scene of Christ's meal with Mary and Martha dramatized the proper mode of looking, since it was Mary's consumption of Christ with her desiring gaze that was contrasted with Martha's misplaced desire to cook the meal (Irmscher 1986: 228).

This middle-class moralism contrasts sharply with the decoration of the most celebrated dining halls of the Renaissance. One of the most famous cycles was that begun in 1517 by Raphael for the wealthy Sienese banker Agostino Chigi's Villa Farnesina in Rome (see Figure 1.4). In the story of Cupid and Psyche, Cupid, the god of love, is enraptured with Psyche. At first fleeing from him but also plagued by his jealous mother Venus, they are finally united in marriage under the auspices of Jupiter, who makes her immortal (cf. Vertova 1979). Although understood as a Christian allegory of the immortalization of the soul in its union with divine love, Chigi's dining loggia was decorated as a grand bacchanal of beautiful naked bodies, surrounded by garlands and sexually suggestive foods, void of any moralizing scenes to temper any guest's lustful looking. Unsurprisingly, the dinners staged in this villa were nothing short of spectacular. Aretino was a regular guest here as a young courtier on the make and the experience would have offered him a glimpse of the profound decadence of Roman courtly society. In a letter of 1537, he describes how, a decade earlier, he himself had imbued the accoutrements and meals with such pomp that even Pope Leo X was overwhelmed (Larivaille 1997: 44). On February 27, 1518, as Leo's cortege approached the villa, firecrackers exploded. The house was decorated in precious silverware and an underground hydraulic system created water games in the garden. Other sources attest that the finest wines, and the most exotic foods from as far away as Spain and the Bosphorus were served on gold and silver plates, which were then, on one occasion, casually thrown into the Tiber river (but retrieved later from pre-placed nets in the river) (Larivaille 1997: 64; Pastor 1977: 117). Accompanying the meal were firecrackers, water games, theatrical performances, music, and triumphal arches, all of which would have intensified the visual decoration of love, beauty, and food (Frommel 2003: 63–4; Pastor 1977: 118).

Such epic design projects have left their traces in the accounts of master chefs (*scalchi, trincianti*), who coordinated the visual, olfactory, and aural delights that enhanced the taste of the meal and facilitated its digestion. Papal chef Bartolomeo Scappi records the extraordinary complex logistics of preparing and delivering individual meals to the cardinals and their staff during the conclave after the death of Paul III (Figure 1.5). Quiviger has pointed to the complex execution of such banquets that demanded the coordination of more than 100 dishes and where menus specify the "author, style, instruments, number of soloists, and sometimes their clothes" (Quiviger 2010: 157). Dining spaces were set up with tables, chairs, and the "credenza," a large sideboard exhibiting prepared dishes in a display meant to stimulate both awe and

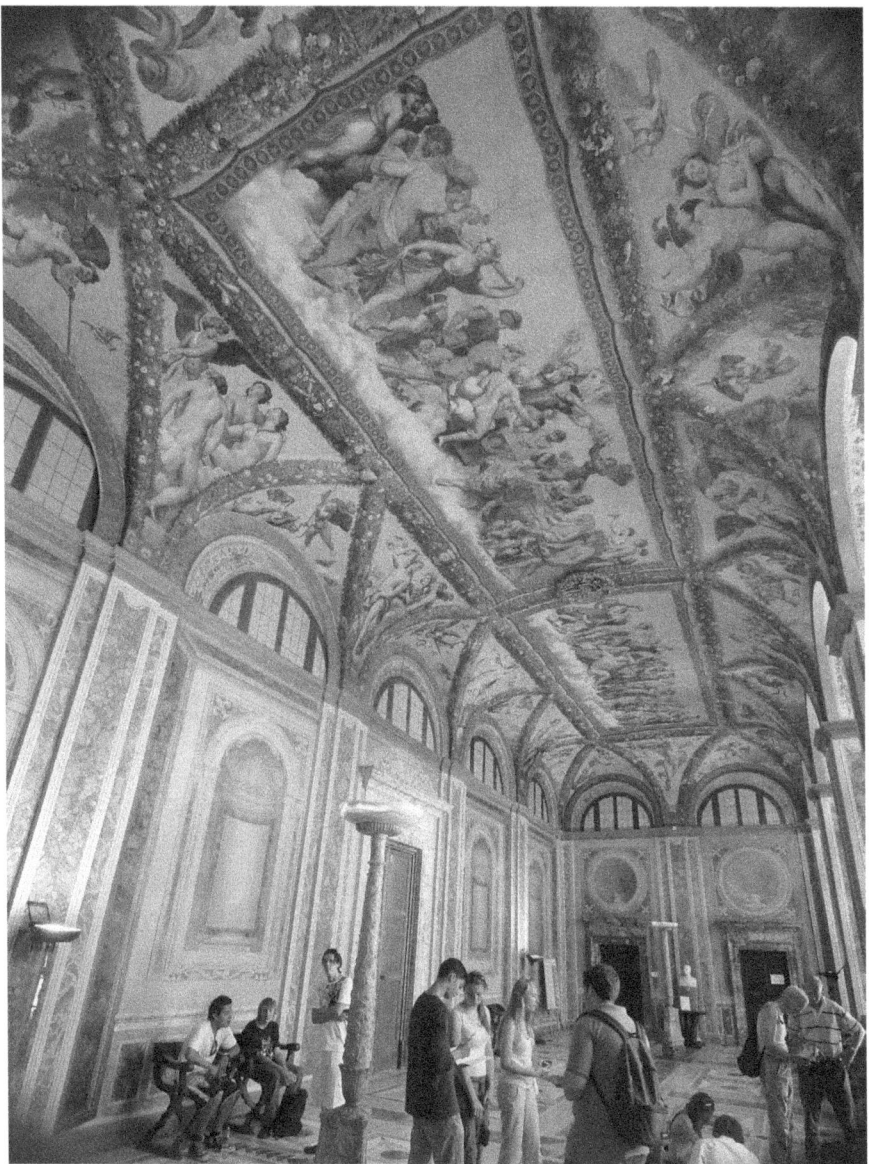

FIGURE 1.4: Dining *loggia* of the Villa Farnese with fresco cycle of Cupid and Psyche by Raphael and his workshop, 1517–19. Photo by Robert Baldwin.

appetite. They often included ephemeral sculptures made from sugar that unified meals around a certain theme, such as the twelve labors of Hercules that accompanied the twelve courses honoring Duke Ercole d'Este. Such sculptures, which sat amidst the finely decorated ewers and basins that held the

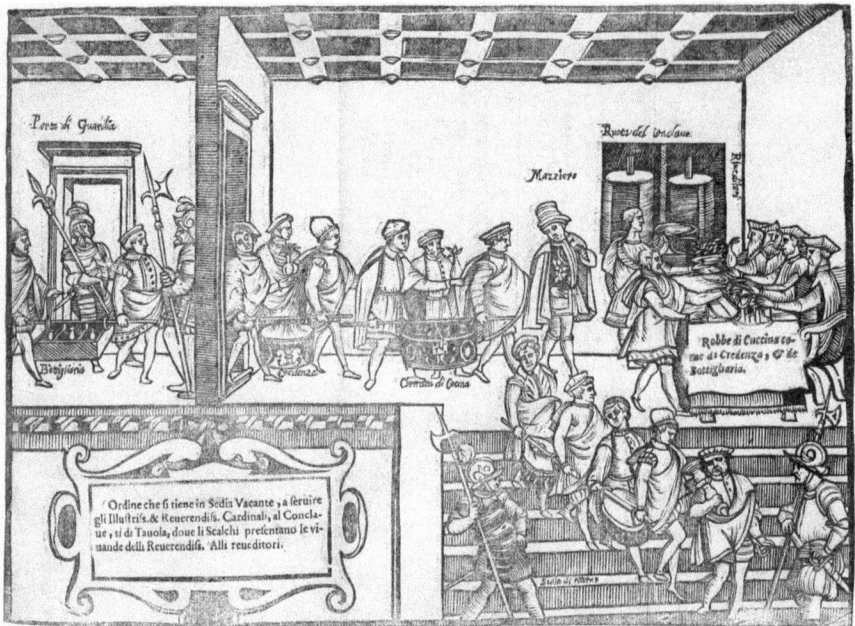

FIGURE 1.5: Illustration of the provisioning of the papal conclave, from Bartolomeo Scappi, *Opera*, 1596. University of Chicago Library. Special Collection Research Center.

various culinary creations, blurred the line between visual and culinary art, binding hungry eyes to stimulated taste buds (Quiviger 2010: 159–65).

Washing hands with perfumed water marked the beginning and the end of the meal. Such sensorial caesuras were complemented by nearly continual musical accompaniment, which was arranged "to give the guests the greatest possible contrast and variety of sound from course to course" so that music enhanced mouths that ate and talked (Brown 1975: 220). Ultimately, the dining halls were cleared for dancing before the guests finally went home. Scappi was conscious of how each dish within a meal contributed to the overall effect and underlined the importance of coordinating dishes prepared in the kitchen with those on the sideboards. The banquet was conceived, therefore, as a vast integrated work of art organized to dissolve the boundaries between the senses and bind them harmoniously through the careful manipulation of carefully timed and orchestrated stimuli. It was this meticulous orchestration that provided the setting for the courtier's most spectacular bodily display of elegance, refinement, and reserve.

Such banquets did not merely transform the less attractive aspects of eating, they overwhelmed the expression of the lower senses so that they receded into the background, lost in the visual and aural extravagance. The sounds, smells, and direct tactile experience of the meal were minimized by music, perfumes, and utensils. Aretino would grow to despise this kind of social ritual and wrote unapologetically about his love of and desire for food (Biow 2010). He was a fierce critic of the way the delectation of courtly culture masked an apparatus of moral turpitude, where courtiers become sycophantic lechers (Beecher in Aretino 2008: 107 n.8).

Conviviality and friendship were important themes of Renaissance social life. In a letter written in 1540, the humanist scholar Francesco Priscianese recalled dining at the house of the Venetian painter Titian. What is striking is the way that the meal itself, almost disappearing from view, is only one component of an integrated ritual of actively engaged perception. The delightful garden is both the setting and the subject of discussions of beauty and the house becomes the gallery that facilitates the viewing of Titian's remarkable paintings. The city outside fuses with the private interior, as Priscianese describes the sun setting on its canals teeming with gondolas and beautiful women, and resounding "with the varied harmony of voice and musical instruments which accompanied our delightful supper until midnight" (Chambers et al. 1992: 180). Although we learn nothing about the meal itself, it is clear that the sights and sounds that accompanied it were not an orchestrated assault on the senses. Instead, a private meal between friends harmonized with the natural rhythms of the city and the wider social phenomena it contained. Such an open and inclusive sensorial experience contrasts sharply with the exclusive extravagance of the highly staged banquets of popes and bankers.

ANALYZING THE SENSIBLE SELF

In contrast, Jacopo Pontormo (1494–1556), a well-established painter reaching the end of his life, meticulously recorded his daily, highly varied, diet. It consisted of boiled and dried meats, bread, eggs, cheeses, nuts, fruit, lettuce, and other vegetables, as well as a variety of Tuscan wines. He was constantly juxtaposing food, sickness, and pain and their mutual effects on each other. At times he felt healthy and in high spirits, at others his teeth hurt acutely, or he was hampered by a cold that forced him to moderate his consumption. All the while he records the body parts of the figures he was painting on church walls, so that heads, loins, sides, and stomachs of painted figures merge with the animal heads, loins, and other flesh he eats, not to mention his own aching stomach and bowels (Mayer 1979: g-167, esp. g-109). In Pontormo's self-analysis, paintings become unfixed from the ocular realm of the viewer and are mediated, in a profoundly tactile way, to the artist's feeling, hurting, and decaying body, conspiring with the food to sustain its health and exacerbate its ills.

We can see such experiments at work in a more comprehensive manner in the work of the French writer Michel Montaigne (1533–92), whose deeply personal self-analysis and concern for human happiness led him to reflect at length on the physical effects of food and the social function of eating. This meant that he was closely attuned to the workings of his senses, and even dedicated an entire essay to the subject of smells. He begins this short piece by noting that, in spite of extraordinary exceptions, bodily smells are not particularly pleasing. Even the sweetest and purest breath "has nothing more excellent about it than to be free of smell" and the "most perfect smell for a woman is to smell of nothing." He condemns the use of fragrance by women and this points to the particular condition in which his age found itself (Montaigne 1957: 228). Since soap was as foul-smelling as what it was meant to wash, all manner of scented liquids and cloths were meant to refresh the body's aroma, which was rarely thoroughly cleansed, by dispelling unpleasant smells. As a result, the sixteenth century produced a very dense landscape of competing smells, where "everything from letters to lapdogs was scented" (Classen *et al.* 1994: 71). No wonder, then, that Montaigne dreamed of a nearly scentless world. His home and his body would have been the site of the production and contestation of a whole range of competing odors. He hated the smoky and stuffy air that characterized many Renaissance homes—considered by some to be good for the walls and possibly for health as well (Classen *et al.* 1994: 63; Montaigne 1957: 4). But he took it as a matter of course that the scent of his gloves and handkerchiefs lingered in his thick moustache. In fact, he marveled at the skin's capacity to absorb and retain sensual memories, such as the "close kisses of youth, savory, greedy, and sticky," that stayed above his mouth for hours.

Like many of his contemporaries, Montaigne held a deep conviction that the good life resulted from sensual pleasure and variety, while mental and physical extremes, such as fasting and other rigid habits, hardened and weakened the body (see, for example Montaigne 1957: 830, 832, 847). Although he viewed intemperance as the plague of sensual pleasure, temperance was not to be "its scourge but it is its seasoning" (Montaigne 1957: 853). Temperance should not discipline the body, but enhance its enjoyment. The culinary metaphor is perfectly placed here because Montaigne found in the ritual of eating a profound locus of productive interaction between the bodily senses and the mind.

Although he had little use for a spoon or fork (Montaigne 1957: 830), he preferred to drink out of his own glass, one of a particular shape and size, transparent and not metal, so that he could taste with his eyes with each draught. He complained about the practice of crowding a meal with dishes that prohibited him from enjoying the developing taste of each course. He even attacks the upper-class taste for the daintiest foods that leads to disgust of ordinary foods where, quoting Seneca, "luxury beguiles the tedium of wealth" (Montaigne 1957: 843).

For Montaigne, the body's sensual relations with the world could never be separated from the world of the spirit. He hated it when "people order us to keep our minds in the clouds while our bodies are at table. I would not have the mind nailed down to it nor wallowing in it, but attending to it; sitting at it, not lying down at it" (Montaigne 1957: 850). A memorable meal was one where "each of the guests himself brings the principal charm according to the good temper of body and soul in which he happens to be" (Montaigne 1957: 849). He enjoyed shouting and arguing before a meal, but loved to rest and listen to stories in contented silence after eating (Montaigne 1957: 844–5). The meal constituted, instead, the place where the mind and the body were fully present, united together, because he could think of "no preparation so sweet . . . no sauce so appetizing, as that which is derived from society." The meal, for him, was not a spectacle for the senses, but a medium through which he generated close social relationships (Montaigne 1957: 846).

CONCLUSION: CONSTRUCTING A SENSORIAL REGIME

The reconfiguration of the sensorial regime in the Renaissance helped to define the particular ways in which elites separated themselves from their social inferiors. Although such social distinctions were not new to the Renaissance, the increasing codification of those distinctions within the body's sensorial apparatus served to ground them precisely at the point of one's physical apprehension of the world. This would have led to the assumption that different classes of people sensed the world in fundamentally different ways. Not only, for example, would they merit different foods, spaces, and sounds, but they would actually appreciate them better. As a result, the design of palaces created parallel worlds in which cross-class encounters were minimized. Cities were organized so that the ears of nobles weren't aggravated by the sound of middle-class commerce, and the separate worlds of taste were normalized by the hierarchical organization of foods.

For writers on architecture, manners, and food, extreme sensual indulgence destabilized the proper balance between all the senses, which was necessary for a meaningful social life. They knew that such excesses as greedily eating and drinking led to the disgust of others and even the injury of the self. Indeed, even though Montaigne believed it healthier to eat less more slowly, he often bit his tongue and fingers in his greedy haste (Montaigne 1957: 846, 848). However, for reformers like the Franciscan Saint Bernardino, indulging in this form of sensual excess could only lead to moral perversion in others. He excoriated his contemporaries for eating, drinking, and socializing in taverns, which could only lead to the reprehensible engagement in sodomy (Vitullo 2010: 107). Alberti saw a similar connection between food and sin, where people drinking at dinner "get overly excited because of their overindulgence, stupid conversations, inept smiles, immoderate gestures," which leads them to "go out again drunk with wine and certainly with anger that burns in them to do something foolish and wicked . . . displeasing and injuring everyone they can" (Vitullo 2010: 111). As Juliann Vitullo shows, the stakes were higher for Alberti, since such excess led to violence against the community itself. In contrast, Alberti wanted the banquet to be "the demonstration of joy in conversation and the pleasure of friendly company. This ornament and happiness of the table should be venerated and we can almost say that the table is the sacred altar of humanity" (Vitullo 2010: 113). By linking the banquet with the Christian Eucharistic communion, he shows how it could redeem the banquet's conflation of Adam and Eve's sin with sexual desire. However, Aretino's satire argues for a more honest and raw sensuality that concentrates on the positive link between food and sex. In his dialogues, he describes in detail a meal shared by two women in excited anticipation of an erotic evening, rounded out with quince jelly to settle their stomachs and candies to sweeten their breath (Aretino 2005: 63). Aretino defended such writings by comparing the gushing pleasure and life produced by the sex organs with shameful hands, which "gamble away money, swear false testament, make usurious loans, make obscene gestures, rip things up, pull, beat, wound, and kill" (Talvacchia 1999: 86). Making the distinction between economies of touch that give either pleasure or pain, he makes an ironic critique of his culture's tolerance of violence and anxiety about pleasure.

Despite the hyperbole and rhetorical posturing, Aretino was not alone in his defense of touch. The humanist and courtier at the court of Isabella d'Este and Federico II Gonzaga in Mantua, Mario Equicola (1470–1525), extolled touch in his compendium on love (*De natura d'amore*). He states that all the other senses merely ornament our experience but touch is absolutely necessary for our being. This claim derives from Aristotle's *De Anima*, which describes touch as the necessary condition for the existence of all the other senses (Aristotle 1907: 435b, Bk. 3, Ch. 12). It is the only sense that operates without mediation. Unlike the other senses, Aristotle states, where an excessive intensity of the phenomena they register merely damages their perceptual capacity—loud noises, bright lights, noxious smells, highly spiced foods—excessive heat, cold or hardness not only destroys the sense of touch, it brings death. As Ian Frederick Moulton states, Equicola used this argument to place touch and sexuality beyond the limits of moral evaluation (Moulton 2010: 120). His advocacy for regular but not excessive sexual activity (Moulton 2010: 125–6) echoes the arguments made by the papal librarian, Bartolomeo Platina (1421–81) in his work *On Right Pleasure and Good Health*. As a guide to good living, this text integrates eating into a comprehensive lifestyle that governs waking, exercise, reading, playing, going to bed, and having sex. Platina understood that certain foods were agreeable and flavorful to some and not others. Rather than moralizing or aestheticizing social behavior, he is more concerned with calibrating the senses so that the mind and the body functioned together harmoniously (Platina 1998: 105ff.).

It is this kind of moderation and sobriety that characterized most discussions about how to create, perceive, and consume beauty in the Renaissance. Castiglione's text criticized the excessively elaborate and scanty sartorial fashions of foreigners, preferring a more subdued ethic of blacks and dark colors for everyday dress, where foppish, trimmed, showy, or dashing clothing was not appropriate (Castiglione 1959: 121–2). Alberti shared Castiglione's aesthetic and applied it to architecture. "Extravagance, I detest!" he declared (Alberti 1988: 298).[1] For him, architectural ornament should conform to Castiglione's sensible taste in fashion. In a similar manner to the way in which temperance, for Montaigne, functioned as a spice rather than a purge of pleasure, ornament could only enhance an already beautiful building; it could not create one. Such sensory sobriety was a hallmark of an emerging sense of our modern idea of aesthetic taste. It navigated between extravagance and baseness, where true beauty lay. And although such beauty's worth was often predicated on its distinction between elite and vulgar society, Aretino, who had dined with Priscianese on that memorable Venetian evening, found pleasure in both and imagined, along with his contemporaries, a world in which *all* the senses could participate in constructing a beautiful social world.

CHAPTER TWO

Urban Sensations: Attractive and Repulsive

PETER BURKE

One of the ways in which the so-called "cultural turn" has affected urban history is in encouraging scholars to give more attention to the experience of living in towns, alongside relatively objective data such as the size of cities and the number of townspeople to be found in different occupations, from tailor to servant. The so-called "sensory revolution" forms part of this wider movement. In this vein, what follows is an attempt to imagine the impact of cities on the senses of both inhabitants and visitors in the course of the 200 years allocated to this volume, whether that impact was pleasant or unpleasant, what provoked cries of pleasure or admiration or, on the contrary, "What made eyes water, ears ache, noses wrinkle, fingers withdraw and mouths close" (Cockayne 2007: 21). A first step, for us who live over 350 years later than the end of the period discussed here, is to imagine cities without the sights, sounds, or smells to which we have become accustomed; the tall buildings made of glass, the streams of cars, trams and buses in the streets, the smell of petrol fumes, the rumble of lorries, the hooting of drivers, the ear-splitting sounds of electric drills, the sirens of police cars and fire engines, and so on. Taking all those sensations away, what should we imagine in their place?

The obvious question to ask at the start of such an investigation concerns the sources for such a reconstruction. The richest of those sources are descriptions of cities by travelers of the period in print or in manuscript:

"travelogues," as we may call them. Precisely because they are away from home and confronted with unfamiliar sensations, travelers are unusually aware of what they see or hear. Some sensitive observers might be described as connoisseurs of sensations. One of them, the Englishman Thomas Coryat ([1611] 1905: 306), declared that the church of San Marco in Venice "did ravish my senses." In other words, he was conscious of synaesthesia.

It is tempting and all too easy to produce a chapter that is essentially a mosaic of quotations from sources of this kind. We need to remember, however, that millions of people experienced cities in this period, whether as inhabitants or visitors, while we have access only to hundreds of travelogues. What is more, the authors form a biased sample of travelers, since they were predominantly upper class, male, and northern European.

It is obviously necessary to supplement these rich but biased sources with others, preferably presenting cities from inside and from below. Municipal regulations, for instance, offer a view from within the city, documenting attempts to control dirt, noise, stench, and so on. It cannot be assumed that these regulations were effective, but at least they testify to the ideals of the city's rulers. Paintings and engravings offer valuable testimony to the ways in which cities were viewed. The artists sometimes improved the appearance of particular buildings and streets, but these improvements, like regulations, offer valuable evidence of contemporary ideals. Private diaries and published plays, poems, stories, and biographies all add precious details. As for the experiences of ordinary people, these can be reconstructed, if at all, only in fragments, preserved in popular songs or letters, or in interrogations that survive in judicial archives.

THE SMELL AND TASTE OF THE CITY

The idea that smells have a history is a relatively new one that owes a good deal to a pioneering study by the French historian Alain Corbin, concerned with both "the foul" and "the fragrant" (Corbin 1982). To take the good smells first, they included spices such as cinnamon and cloves, a variety of perfumes such as civet and musk, and herbs such as lavender and rosemary. Many of these were displayed for sale in the open air, on Piazza San Marco in Venice, for instance, during the Ascension Fair, the *Sensa*. More common was the smell of baking bread, or the frying of other kinds of food, prepared and sold from stalls in the street. In Cairo, a fifteenth-century Spanish visitor remarked on cooks walking the streets "carrying braziers, and fire, and dishes of stew for sale" (Tafur 1926: 100). Other smells were more or less neutral.

Simon Schama has reconstructed the smell of Amsterdam, especially the part of the city closest to the river IJ, in the following terms: "A briny aroma of salt, rotting wood, bilgewater and the tide-rinsed remains of countless gristly little creatures housed within the shells of periwinkles and barnacles" (Schama 1999: 311).

As for bad smells (such as urine, excrement, rotting fruit and fish, and decaying corpses, especially in times of plague), Corbin argues that around the year 1750, the upper classes ceased to tolerate stenches that their ancestors had learned to live with, thus provoking a wave of sanitary reforms in Paris, London, and elsewhere. He is right about the sanitary reforms, of course, but the frequent complaints to be found in earlier sources suggest that the verb "tolerate" may be too strong. Montaigne, for instance, remarked that his appreciation of both Venice and Paris was diminished by the "sharp smell" (*aigre senteur*) of the lagoons in the first case and of the mud in the second (Montaigne [1580–8] 1962: Book 1, Ch. 55). Paris was singled out for its stink in the seventeenth century, especially by British visitors. The writer James Howell claimed that the city "may be smelt many miles off" (Lough 1985: 53). The virtuoso John Evelyn, who was interested in science, was more specific, writing that the city smelled "as if sulphure were mingled in the mudd" (1955, 1: 94).

The complaints were extended to other cities. In the early seventeenth century, William Brereton, a Cheshire gentleman who was familiar with both London and Amsterdam, described the smell of Edinburgh as strong and "noisome." "I never came to my own lodging in Edinburgh, or went out, but I was constrained to hold my nose, or to use wormwood or some such scented plant" (Brereton 1844: 105). In 1654, an English gentleman who lived in Cambridgeshire, Dudley North, complained of London's "sooty air," while in 1661 Evelyn published a pamphlet offering advice about ways to reduce the amount of smoke in the capital, an increasingly severe problem as wood supplies ran out and people turned to coal for their fires and furnaces (Jenner 1995). Outside Europe, the situation was no better. The Italian missionary Matteo Ricci, for instance, remarked on the foul smell of Beijing. The remark might be dismissed as the prejudice of a "foreign devil," but it is corroborated by the Ming dynasty official Xie Zhaozhe (who came from a small town in the south) in his *Fivefold Miscellany* (1608), noting "a lot of excrement and muck in the markets" (Elvin 2004: 404). At this point one appreciates all the more the claim—whether it was correct or not—made about Florence by the humanist Leonardo Bruni, that the city "is unique and singular in all the world" because "you will find here nothing that is . . . offensive to the nose (*nichil tetrum naribus*)," since whatever mess was produced during the night would be taken away in the morning (Bruni 2000: 5).

The complaints were all the more serious because it was commonly believed that bad air spread disease. What was to be done? One measure, offered by Evelyn among others, and sometimes enforced, was to confine trades such as butchers, dyers, tanners, and tallow-chandlers to the edge of the city so that the inhabitants of the center, especially the upper classes, would be free from these "horrid stinks." Smell management, including the removal of meat and cheese stalls from Piazza San Marco, was one of the duties of the health commissioners of Venice, for instance, the *provveditori della sanità*.

Another solution to the problem of stench was of course to clean the city. However, cleaning the streets of rotting vegetables was often left to pigs, who roamed the streets and brought their own odors with them. Serious cleaning was often an emergency measure. In 1580 the Lord Mayor of London ordered street cleaning for "the Avoydinge of the infection of the plague and the loathsome Stinckes and savours that are in the severall streetes of this Cyttie" (Jenner 2000: 131). In Italy, at times of plague, perfume was used as a means of disinfection. The use of perfume in order to fight one smell with another was even more common at an individual level. The upper classes wore perfumed gloves or carried perfumed balls known as "pomanders" in their hands, or relied like Brereton on using wormwood or holding their noses. In some northern cities, however, municipal hygiene was coming to be taken more seriously than before. The English gentleman Fynes Moryson, in Lübeck in 1591, noted that "the citizens are curious to avoid ill smells" (Moryson [1617] 1907, 1: 7). In the seventeenth century, the same point would often be made about Dutch cities, often as praise but sometimes as criticism, the cleanliness being described as "rigid" or "superstitious."

There is less to say about taste because explicit comment on the taste of food and drink is relatively rare in the sources; an exception is the English merchant Peter Mundy, taking his first cup of coffee in Istanbul, and comparing its taste as well as its appearance to soot. However, a few residents and travelers do at least record what they ate, giving an impression of the quantity and variety of food obtainable in cities (as the Milanese Pietro Casola noted in the case of Jerusalem), as well as references to local specialities such as the "excellent Sauciges" of Bologna (according to the English gentleman Francis Mortoft). In Macao, Peter Mundy discovered lychees, "the prettiest and pleasauntest fruit that ever I tasted," and also tea ("a certaine Drinke called Chaa") about which he was less enthusiastic (1907–19, Vol. 3: 162). The street cries of Paris, London, and elsewhere often refer to food and drink: to eel pies, for instance, to herring, to cherries, to peaches, to waffles ("Tartelettes friandes à la belle gauffre") and so on.

For a well-documented case-study one might take Samuel Pepys, a man for whom sensuous as well as sensual experiences were particularly important, who often records what he ate and drank. In the first month of his diary, January 1660, he refers to drinking ale, wine, and sack (including a "posset" in which wine was mixed with milk and spices), and eating turkey, "brawn" (boar's meat), venison, rabbit, beef, veal, mutton, goose, "pullets" (young chickens), larks, marrow-bones, ling (a kind of fish), prawns, anchovies, cabbage, and bread and cheese. The high proportion of meat and the low proportion of vegetables scored by Pepys were about par for the period, at least for his upper-middle social class (Pepys 1970–83, 1: 3–35).

As for cooking, in one now notorious trial, in Rome in 1603, the judicial archives inform us about different possible styles. The painter Caravaggio assaulted a waiter in an inn after being served with eight artichokes, four cooked in butter and four in oil. When Caravaggio asked which ones were which, the waiter replied "Smell them." Caravaggio's response was to break a plate over the man's head (Friedlaender 1955: 280).

THE TACTILE CITY

What were the most important tactile experiences in Renaissance cities? They were not necessarily pleasant. Crowded streets, for instance, meant jostling, elbowing, squeezing, and other forms of the invasion of personal space. A German visitor to London in 1602 found the Exchange "so filled with people that only by force are you able to make your way" (Gershow [1608] 1892: 11). Evelyn complained that Paris needed "a redresse of the multitude of Coaches, Laquays and throngs of Mankind" (1955, 2: 107). Mundy noted that in Agra, "in the Bazare ordinarilye there is such a throng that men can hardly pass without much trouble" (1907–19, 3: 207). Violence was common in cities, as indeed it was in the countryside, despite attempts to regulate it. The Englishman William Wey was not the only pilgrim to Jerusalem to record the fact that "as we entered, boys threw stones at us," doubtless because they looked foreign and might be Christians. On entering Florence in 1546, a German visitor discovered he was required to hand over his sword, while an Englishman had to hand over his pistols at the gate of Genoa in 1658 (Lough 1985: 41; Sastrow 1902: 172). What was more specific to cities was collective violence on a large scale, the violence of what would later be called the "mob," whether composed of apprentices trashing brothels (a common practice in seventeenth-century London), of crowds sacking the houses of the rich (as in Lyon in 1529), lynching unpopular officials (as in Naples in 1585), and so on.

At a more superficial level, itching may not have been a specifically urban experience, but it was probably worse in urban environments as a result of polluted air and the prevalence of fleas and lice in zones of high density of population. On the other hand, bath-houses were an urban institution, though a declining one after the 1520s, because they were increasingly seen in both Catholic and Protestant countries as a threat to morals, a step away from brothels, if indeed they were not brothels under another name. The *hamam* survived in the Islamic world (Boyat and Fleet 2010: 249–70), while bath-houses were commonplace in Japan, but public baths would not return to Western Europe until the eighteenth century. No wonder then that Western visitors to Istanbul, such as George Sandys and Jean de Thévenot, both in the seventeenth century, found the *hamam* so fascinating. Meanwhile, commercialized "sex in the city" continued to flourish, from the upmarket courtesans of sixteenth-century Venice down to the poorest streetwalker.

The tactile experience that the travelers noted most regularly, though, was that of movement around cities, especially on foot, leading them to comment on the quality of street surfaces. The Spaniard Pero Tafur was impressed by Venice in this respect, writing that "The city is as clean for walking as in a gracious chamber, so well paved and bricked it is, without the usual mud and dust" (Tafur 1926: 167). Ricci by contrast complained that in Beijing "Very few of the streets . . . are paved with brick or stone and it is difficult to say which season of the year is more objectionable for walking," the summer with its dust or the winter with its mud (Ricci 1953: 310). In similar fashion, the Englishman George Sandys noted that in Cairo, "the streets are unpaved and extremely dirty after a shower," while in Naples, to his relief, "the streets are broad and paved with brick" (Sandys 1615: 119, 259). Evelyn noted with pleasure the paving in Paris, which "renders it more easy to walk on then our pibbles of London," though his approval was not shared by another English traveler, Peter Heylyn, who claimed that a little rain made the streets "very slippery and troublesome" (Evelyn 1955, 2: 94; Lough 1985: 53). Bologna received special praise for its arcades, "so that one may walke here without feeling the heate of the sun or be in danger to be troubled by the raine" (Mortoft [1658] 1925: 176).

THE SOUNDS OF THE CITY

The sources allow much more to be said about the sounds of the city, so various and often so localized that it may not have been difficult for blind persons to navigate the streets by ear. Even for sighted people, it has been suggested, sounds were "significant in shaping people's sense of urban space" (Garrioch 2003: 14). Although "we have to contend with much louder sounds," as Bruce Smith reminds us, the soundscape of early modern London, for instance, was "acoustically dense" (1999: 49, 53). In the background Londoners could hear "the constant sounds of running water," from fountains, for instance. In Amsterdam, it was "the slap of canal water against the bridges" (B. Smith 1999: 57; see also Schama 1999: 312).

However, these sounds, to which it was easy to become so accustomed as to fail to notice them, were often drowned by inanimate noises such as clanging, clattering, clinking, creaking, grinding, hammering, rapping, rattling, ringing, roaring, rumbling, sawing, scraping, thundering, ticking, and tolling. To all these sounds one needs to add animate noises such as dogs barking, birds chirping, cocks crowing, pigs squealing, horses clopping and neighing, cats caterwauling, rats and mice squeaking, and humans speaking, shouting, or singing. A city was the scene of what the English satirist Edward Guilpin described in 1598 as a "hotch-potch of so many noyses" (Korhonen 2008: 338). Even in our own age of much greater noise pollution it remains easy to sympathize with the Florentine artist Piero di Cosimo, who could not abide the sounds of "children crying, men coughing, bells ringing or friars chanting" (Vasari [1550] 1966–76, 4: 69), or even with the character "Morose" in Ben Jonson's play *Epicoene* (1609), set in London, a man who is hypersensitive to what he calls "the discord of sounds," who "hath chosen a street to live in so narrow at both ends that it will receive no coaches nor carts nor any of these common noises."

Like smelly trades, noisy trades were supposed to be exiled to the edges of cities, but the rule was not always enforced (how could it be, as cities continually expanded?). In any case, this common regulation displaced the problem rather than solving it. Dante, who died in 1321, was already complaining of the noise coming from the Arsenal in Venice, where ships were under construction. In Bologna in the fifteenth century, Tafur noted the existence of a hundred watermills grinding wheat, sawing wood, and so on, and in Milan he visited a street where armorers were at work (Tafur 1926: 31). It was not desirable to live next to the workshop of an armorer, as some Londoners complained in 1378—to no avail (Cockayne 2007: 115). Morose, on the other hand, is represented as powerful enough to prevent an armorer from setting up shop in his parish. Like the sixteenth century antiquary John Stow, he hated the "loathsome noise" of metal-working in the city, the sounds evoked by the writer Thomas Dekker (a Londoner himself): "hammers are beating in one place, Tubs hooping in another, Pots clinking in a third" (B. Smith 1999: 54).

The chains of prisoners made a similar sound to the pots: not for nothing was a medieval prison on London's South Bank known as "The Clink." The noise of traffic must not be forgotten, especially the sound of horses' hooves and wooden wheels on cobblestones. Visiting Venice in the early 1640s, Evelyn was struck, as tourists still are today, by the quiet. They notice the absence of cars, while he found the city "almost as silent as a field," without the usual "rattling of coaches" and "trampling of horses."

To the noises of work in Christian Europe it is necessary to add the sound of chiming clocks and of church bells, marking the passage of time or drawing attention to major events, such as a papal election or the canonization of a saint, when cannons might be fired and bells ring all night. Bells rang, pealed, or tolled, distinctions in early modern English that reveal contemporary sensitivity to the different messages that bells could transmit. The tocsin, for instance, was a special bell that sounded the alarm, while the muffled sound of a bell that tolled denoted a death. Tafur described the Campanile in Venice and its different bells with different meanings, "one for Mass, one for Vespers, one to summon the Council ... and one when they arm the fleet," omitting the famous *marangone*, the great bell that told listeners when to begin work and when to stop (Tafur 1926: 164–5). The Dutch historian Johan Huizinga noted that in late medieval France and Flanders, individual bells were given names such as "Fat Jacqueline" or "Bell Roelant" and that "everyone knew their individual tones and instantly recognized their meaning" (Huizinga [1919] 1996: 2). Clocks on town halls, increasingly common from the fourteenth century onwards, could usually be heard as well as seen. The Prague clock, for instance, which is still active, was installed in 1410. In China, bells were also in use but urban time was often marked by drums, located in the drum towers of Beijing, Nanjing, and elsewhere.

Competing with these inanimate sounds and the cries of animals and birds was a babble of human voices. In the Islamic world, the call to prayer five times a day from the minaret of every mosque replaced the bell as a means of telling the time. In some places, main squares for instance, or the exchanges of London or Amsterdam, one might hear the buzz of many conversations. The English writer John Earle, obviously a connoisseur of sound, noted that in "Paul's Walk" (the central aisle of St. Paul's cathedral in London, still the old St. Paul's in this period) the dominant sound was the "humming or buze, mixt of walking, tongues and feet ... a still roar or loud whisper" (B. Smith 1999: 61). Elsewhere one might hear the shouting of children playing or neighbors quarrelling. Added to the mix were the "street cries" of many different trades, which the locals were able to distinguish and decode: the signature tunes of tinkers, knife-grinders, men and women selling fruit and vegetables, coopers making barrels ("Have you any work for cooper?"), and so on. In the early sixteenth century the cries of Paris inspired the composer Clément Jeannequin to turn them into a song for four voices.

Cities, especially large cities, produced a babel of voices in the literal sense of a mixture of languages, dialects, and accents. In Venice, for instance, one might hear not only Venetian, but also German, Spanish, Greek and Turkish, as well as the dialect of nearby Bergamo. In Amsterdam, besides Dutch (or the Flemish of immigrants from the south) one might hear French, German, English, and the Scandinavian languages. In Central Europe, even small towns might be multilingual. Sárospatak in Hungary, for instance, was described in the 1650s by the Czech scholar Comenius (Jan Komenský) as a place in which five modern languages could be heard (presumably Hungarian, Czech, Slovak, German, and Ukrainian) so that "one person understands another no more than in the Tower of Babel" unless Latin was used as a lingua franca (Bérenger 1969: 5). What linguists call "the urbanization of language" should not be forgotten. Foreigners apart, to a visitor from the countryside the accents of townspeople would have sounded strange or even unintelligible (Wright 2007).

The city was among other things a stage where a variety of performances could be heard. Drums rolled when soldiers marched into or out of the city, and also at public executions. Announcements were made by town criers, often accompanied by trumpeters or drummers in order to draw attention to their message in a noisy environment. In Florence, the main square and seat of government, Piazza della Signoria, included a platform called the *ringhiera* from which announcements and speeches ("harangues") could be made. Public squares such as Piazza San Marco in Venice served as stages for charlatans, who drew crowds by acting out their cures, and for singers of tales, *cantimbanchi* ("singers on benches"). In the late Middle Ages, religious plays were performed in churches or in the open air on the occasion of major festivals such as Easter or Corpus Christi, while purpose-built playhouses were constructed in major cities from the sixteenth century onwards. Sermons were another form of performance, dominated by the friars in the fourteenth and fifteenth centuries and by the Protestants in the sixteenth and seventeenth. A new form of church, the *Hallenkirche*, was constructed in the late Middle Ages to allow the congregation to see and hear preachers better. However, churches were not large enough to accommodate the most popular preachers, such as the Franciscans San Bernardino of Siena and Olivier Maillard, who performed in the open air, with some of their listeners perched on roofs or in trees. In the Protestant world, the Dutch pastor Jacobus Borstius was famous for the sermons he preached at Dordrecht and elsewhere. The crowd was sometimes so dense that babies fainted in their mothers' arms (Francken 1942: 210–11).

Late medieval or Renaissance cities were also the sites of many musical performances, as recent studies in urban musicology remind us, noting what one scholar calls "the sonic expressions of urban identity" (Kendrick 2002: 3; cf. Fenlon 2007; Getz 2005; Strohm 1990). Many cities employed musicians to play on special occasions, while individual pipers and fiddlers performed every day in the streets and in taverns. Ballads were sung rather than recited, by professionals and amateurs alike. Some London taverns had the texts of ballads pasted on the walls to encourage drinkers to join in performances, the sixteenth-century equivalent of today's *karaoke*. However, in this period, which ends with the rise of opera houses and concert halls, the best music, especially singing, was usually to be heard in churches. Visitors to cities often commented on the quality of the performances. The Dutch barber-surgeon Arendt Willemsz, for instance, who visited Venice in 1525, noted that "The canons of St. Mark's perform beautiful song, year in, year out," "intoning the psalms very pleasantly and magnificently" (quoted in Fenlon 2007: 75; Howard and Moretti 2010). One English gentleman in Rome remarked that "the best voices I ever heard are in the Pope's chappell," while another, visiting the church of San Apollinare, found the music "so rare and sweet that it would have Inchanted any man's Eares that heard it" (Mortoft [1658] 1925: 118; Somerset 1993: 233). The Protestant patrician Bartholomäus Sastrow, visiting the Catholic city of Trent at Easter 1546, confessed to hearing "most delicious singing" in the churches (Sastrow 1902: 143). The English merchant Robert Bargrave, an adventurous traveler, entered a church in Iasi, in Moldavia, and found the "anthems," as he called them to be "rather like the Turkish", while in L'viv, in the Ukraine, he found the church music to be "much sweeter and more regular" (Bargrave 1999: 136, 145).

Not all music was perceived as sweet or smooth, however. Judicial records contain complaints about street music as well as about hammering and shouting. "Rough music" (*Katzenmusik*), in other words a serenade played on pots and pans, was a not uncommon event in cities in this period in many parts of Europe, especially when an old man married a young woman, and the event usually took place at night (Cockayne 2002). Readers who think of preindustrial cities as sonic utopias because they are free from sirens, horns, and drills may be well advised to think again.

VIEWING THE TOWNSCAPE

The rise of the painted or engraved townscape in Italy, the Netherlands, and elsewhere took place for the most part after 1650, although Vittore Carpaccio, for instance, portrayed the streets of Venice in some detail around the year 1500 in paintings ostensibly devoted to religious subjects. However, in our period, literary sources reveal an increasing interest in the appearance of cities on the part of insiders and outsiders alike, especially a concern with uniformity and symmetry. Needless to say, both insiders and outsiders looked at other people as well as at the urban fabric, even if travel diaries say little about this. The age of the *flâneur* may not have dawned, depending as it did on the rise of the arcades and boulevards of nineteenth-century Paris and elsewhere, but to see and be seen were already strong motives for both men and women to walk or ride through the streets of the city. In London and elsewhere, "beauty," both of the body and its clothing, "was an essential ingredient of street culture," while Paul's Walk has been described as "the early modern catwalk" of fashionable London (Korhonen 2008: 336, 339). Male visitors from other countries remarked on the freedom of women in England. As Platter noted, "they often stroll out or drive by coach in very gorgeous clothes" (quoted in Korhonen 2008: 345). The Italian priest Pietro Casola, on pilgrimage to Jerusalem, complained about the use of veils there, so that "I was never able to see a beautiful woman" (Casola 1494: 257). Rich, colorful and shiny materials impressed some visitors. Visiting the Corpus Christi procession at Venice, Casola declared himself to have been dazzled by the brocades and jewels of the priest's vestments. At the Uffizi in Florence, what most impressed Mortoft was the furniture, especially tables made of jasper and decorated with jewels.

An interest in the "sights" of the city goes back a long way—witness the discussions in classical antiquity of the Seven Wonders of the World, all of them urban. Following this model, a mid sixteenth-century painting attributed to Pieter Claessens represented the "Seven Wonders of Bruges" (*Septem Admirationes Civitatis Brugensis*). Guidebooks to cities, notably Rome, to countries, notably Italy, and also to travel in general, already existed in this period. They told readers what to see and even, on occasion, how to see it. Some travel diaries of the period, although written by eyewitnesses (Evelyn, for example), reproduce passages from these books, suggesting that literature shaped perceptions. For example, one account after another of visits to Milan draws attention to the cathedral, the Castello Sforzesco, and the hospital.

In certain cities, such as Florence and Genoa, visitors were impressed by the height of the buildings, a reminder that in this period most people lived in houses of one or two storys. "Do not look up at the heights like a man from the country," the thirteenth-century Florentine Brunetto Latini warned his readers. Tafur probably did so all the same, for his description of Genoa noted that "all the houses are like towers of four or five storeys or more." Visitors also paid attention to the material from which cities were constructed. Tafur once again makes an eloquent witness, commenting on the "beautiful white stones" of the Temple of Solomon in Jerusalem, and the marble, porphyry and jasper to be seen in Santa Sofia in Constantinople. Again, Somerset called Genoa "one of the stateliest built townes of Italie," thanks to its use of marble (Tafur 1926: 27, 61, 139; see also Somerset 1993: 177–8). A number of travelers were concerned with cleanliness and dirt: one might contrast the Portuguese Jesuit João Rodrigues on Kyōtō, "extremely clean," "the streets are swept and sprinkled with water twice a day," with Somerset on Paris: "the streetes are at all times almost of the year verie durtie and mirie" (Rodrigues 2001: 168; Somerset 1993: 87).

Travelers not infrequently commented on the beauty of town squares. Like tourists today, they were impressed by Piazza San Marco. Again, Moryson found what he called the "market place" in Leipzig to be "large and stately," Brereton admired what he called the "fairest" and "most spacious" marketplaces of Delft and Haarlem, while Bargrave described the main square of the new town of Zamość in Poland as "very handsome and uniforme" (Bargrave 1999: 147; Brereton 1844: 19, 50; Moryson [1617] 1907: 9). The breadth of the streets in certain cities also impressed some visitors, indicating what they were accustomed to at home. Thomas Platter the Younger, for instance, who came from Basel, found the streets of Perpignan to be "extremely beautiful and wide" (*mechtig schön unndt breit*: Platter 1968: 323). Bridges were often considered to be worthy of note. Platter remarked, as people still do, on the "beautiful bridge" at Avignon, and Evelyn on its "very fair bridge," as well as the Pont Neuf of Paris, "a stately bridge." The Englishman Thomas Coryat also noted the "faire bridges" of Paris, while the Rialto at Venice was the "fairest bridge" that he ever saw. "Fair bridges" were one of the attractions of Rotterdam for Brereton (Brereton 1844: 7; Coryat [1611] 1905, Vol. 1: 170, 306; Evelyn 1955, 2: 161, 92; Platter 1968: 114).

Houses too attracted attention. As might have been expected, some travelers enthused over what Coryat called the "sumptuous and magnificent palaces" on the Grand Canal. Moryson was impressed by the "beautie and uniformitie of the houses" in Lübeck. Samuel Pepys, on a brief visit to The Hague, found "the houses so neat in all places and things as is possible", though Bargrave found those of Amsterdam "so superstitiously neat, as is fitter for sight than use" (Bargrave 1999: 167; Coryat [1611] 1905, 1: 306; Moryson [1617] 1907: 7; Pepys 1970–83, 1: 138). Brereton even praised the gallows at Leiden, "the daintiest curious gallows that ever I saw" (Brereton 1844: 38, also 49, on Haarlem).

The references to uniformity by both Moryson and Bargrave deserve comment. They are not alone. Robert Dallington ([1604] 1936: C4b) described the buildings of Paris as "fayre, high and uniforme," while Evelyn found some streets "incomparably fair and uniform" (Evelyn 1955, 2: 108). Somerset admired Antwerp because it was "one of the first townes built for uniformitie, that a man shall lightly see in Christendome; it hath marvellous fayre streets, and all the houses built answerable one to the other" (Somerset 1993: 283). Brereton admired Dutch cities for the same reason. In Dordrecht he noted "uniform and complete building," while the Keizersgracht in Amsterdam impressed him because it was "most uniforme . . . built alike on both sides" (1844: 13, 68).

By this time, towards the end of our period, the concern with regularity and symmetry was widespread. At the beginning of the period, though, this concern can already be found among the patricians of Florence, as some of the urban regulations of the time testify. In 1330, for instance, it was declared that Piazza della Signoria "ought to be more elegant and regular than anywhere else" (*magis deberat esse decora et equa, quam aliqua alia*), while in 1363 shacks (*domunculae*) were to be removed from Piazza San Giovanni (Piazza Duomo) because they "spoil the appearance and the beauty of the whole square" (*deturpant faciem et pulchritudinem totius plate*: Braunfels 1959: 104, 253). Later regulations required the facades of houses to be harmonious. No wonder then that Leonardo Bruni praised Florence as unique not only for its lack of bad smells but also for having "nothing that is disgusting to the eye" (*nichil fedum oculis*: Bruni 2000: 5). One might have expected this concern in the age of Bruni, Filippo Brunelleschi, and Leon Battista Alberti; what may be more surprising is to find it in urban regulations in the fourteenth century, when the Gothic style was still dominant.

The concern with symmetry went with an increasing interest in views or "prospects." Late in our period, travelers often described climbing towers in order to see a city as a whole. Moryson wrote of Lübeck as providing "a faire prospect," while he regularly noted cities "of a round forme," as if he had viewed them from above or had been looking at engraved plans. In Dordrecht, Brereton entered a turret that "gives you a full view of the whole town," while in Edinburgh he went up to the castle, where "you may take a full view of the situation of the whole city." In Milan, Coryat viewed the city from the roof and found it to be "a most beautiful and delectable shew." In Danzig (now Gdańsk), Bargrave found that "From the Topp of the Steeple is a fair Prospect of the City" (Bargrave 1999: 151; Brereton 1844: 13, 102; Coryat [1611] 1905: 244; Moryson [1617] 1907: 6, 9, etc.). The Dutch poet Constantijn Huygens climbed the tower of Strasbourg cathedral and wrote about the experience, though his verses say more about the danger of the climb than about the beauty of the view (Huygens 2003: 180).

Alternatively, the city could be viewed from afar or from the sea. Visiting Siena, Evelyn noted that "The Citty at a little distance presents the Traveller with an incomparable Prospect", including the many brick towers. In Genoa, he appreciated "the streetes and buildings so ranged one above the other, as our seats are in Playhouses." In similar fashion a little later, Richard Lassels described Genoa as "like an amphitheatre to those who behold it from the sea" (Evelyn 1955, 2: 201, 172; Somerset 1993: 178n).

In short, the city was becoming "a visually appreciated entity" (Strohmeyer 2007: 75, 80). The taste for wide views encouraged urban planning, and in its turn the results of planning reinforced the taste for views.

CONCLUSIONS

Reading these different accounts of cities gives the impression that visitors at least, especially visitors who did not live in cities themselves, suffered from as well as enjoyed the hyper-stimulation of the senses in an urban environment. One wonders whether visitors and citizens alike needed some kind of retreat and where they found it. Green spaces were common in cities at this time but they usually took the form of private gardens. Churches were a possible safe haven, at least outside the times of services, though as Dutch paintings of church interiors remind us, barking dogs as well as beggars might disturb the peace of anyone who wished to escape from the sounds of the city.

In any case, as I remarked at the beginning of this chapter, urban experiences were not the same for everyone. Men and women, old and young, rich and poor, immigrants from the countryside and upper-class foreign travelers are unlikely to have experienced cities in the same ways. For example, the sense of insecurity is likely to have been greater for women, the elderly, and visitors than it was for men, for the young, and for locals. Cities that were small by the standards of the twenty-first century were bewildering for visitors who came from villages. As a Russian traveler remarked in 1349, "Entering Constantinople is like a great forest" (Majeska 1984: 44).

It is also necessary to distinguish the experiences of night and day, summer and winter, working days and holidays. In this period the streets of cities were still dark at night, so that the stars were visible, while walkers and riders needed individual torches or lanterns. Given this norm, it is not difficult to imagine the effect on spectators of masses of lighted candles in theaters or in churches for the Forty Hours devotion, or the fireworks that celebrated happy events such as victories or the birth of a son to the local ruler. As for the sounds of the city, the night was not necessarily quiet. For example, "Shouting, yelling and screaming" (*jauchzen, jählen und schreien*) in alleys and houses at night was condemned in a Strasbourg ordinance of 1651 (Koslofsky 2011: 160, 337).

For a major event such as the feast of the patron saint (San Giovanni in Florence, for instance) or the entry of a ruler, the city would wear its best clothes, with triumphal arches erected in the streets and carpets hanging from balconies. Fireworks would light up the night sky and the soundscape would be transformed by music. When the emperor Charles V entered Milan in 1533, for instance, he was accompanied by singers and by musicians playing instruments. When Margaret of Austria entered the same city in 1598, she heard the trumpeters playing "antiphonally" at the Porta Romana, as well as the Te Deum sung by four choirs in the cathedral. When King Henri III of France visited Venice in 1574, he was accompanied everywhere by trumpets and drums, and frequently serenaded (Fenlon 2007: 193–216; Kendrick 2002: 4).

The Ascension Fair in Venice was "as much about viewing, touching, tasting and hearing as it was about making a profit" (Welch 2005: 183, 189). Carnival too was a feast for all the senses. It was a time of fancy dress. In Italy, for instance, people dressed as characters from the *commedia dell'arte*, such as Arlecchino, Dottore, or Pulcinella, while elsewhere people dressed as devils, wild men, or fools. There was much singing and dancing, in which the usual musical instruments were joined by special ones such as the Dutch *rommelpot*, made from a pig's bladder and squealing like a pig. Insults flew about like confetti on an occasion when many people felt that anything was permitted, while wearing masks gave them a sense of invisibility. Participants might throw eggs at one another, eggs filled with rose-water (or a liquid with a less pleasant odor), or they might throw oranges (in Provence), or flour, or stones. The streets were crowded and harassment (especially of women, of Jews, and of animals) was commonplace. Carnival was also a time of eating on a grand scale, especially meat, which Catholics were about to give up for Lent, as well as special carnival food such as pancakes and waffles. Those who could not afford to buy such items had to content themselves with the smell of roasting, baking, frying, and boiling. There was also heavy drinking, especially during the days leading up to Shrove Tuesday, with beer and wine first sharpening the perceptions of the drinkers and then dulling them (Burke 1978: 259–71). In similar fashion Peter Mundy, visiting Agra, noted that the Holi festival was "used in the same manner as Shrovetide is in France, by eating, drinckeing, feasteinge, playing, throweing sweete oyles and water with red powder," as well as what he called "affrontive Gambolls to those that passé by" (Mundy 1907–19, 3: 219).

Different kinds of visitor with different purposes came to the city with different horizons of expectations, and hence they viewed it in different ways. Pilgrims, for instance, saw cities such as Jerusalem, Constantinople, or Rome as assemblages of churches, relics, and images that were if possible to be touched as well as to be seen. For the English pilgrim Richard Guylforde, the sights of Venice included a golden chalice and two golden candlesticks from the treasury of San Marco, though he was also a knight and was equally impressed by the artillery at the Arsenal (Guylforde [1506] 1851: 7). Young men like Pepys (and there were probably many such, if few who were quite so frank in writing about their experiences) moved through the city on the lookout for pretty women. Visitors from abroad were naturally impressed by the contrasts with the townscape at home. In a dialogue by the Englishman Thomas Starkey, in the reign of Henry VIII, one speaker remarks that "Methought when I first came into Flanders and France, that I was translated, as it had been, into another world, the cities and towns appeared so goodly, so well builded, and so clean kept" (Starkey 1871: 92). Friar Felix Fabri, who came from Zurich, recorded his amazement when he entered Cairo at night, impressed by the density of the crowds in the streets, the shouting, bright lights, and so on (Fabri [1483] 1975: 400–1).

As Constance Classen has suggested, one reason that the senses have a history is that they are informed by cultural values, which change over the long term. The art historian Michael Baxandall wrote about what he called the "period eye" in fifteenth-century Italy, though the practices he described were, as Herman Roodenburg suggests, examples of synaesthesia, including haptic visuality and kinaesthetic empathy (Baxandall 1972; Classen 2012: 12; Roodenburg 2012: 4). One might equally well speak about the period eye in other places and times as well as about the period ear or nose. We have already seen how travelers in this period increasingly noticed and praised the regularity of certain townscapes, another case of the "Renaissance eye" or the classical sensibility. One might add that this regularity was appreciated all the more because it was still rare. By the time that it had become common, in the eighteenth century, observers were taking more pleasure in irregularity and other features of what would later be christened the "romantic sensibility."

One major cultural event affecting the perception of cities was the Reformation, bringing with it, in the Protestant parts of Europe, the taming of carnival and the disappearance of many images from churches (often following bouts of iconoclasm). Among the most obvious and important changes taking place as this period gave way to the following one around the middle of the seventeenth century were more lighting in cities at night, more paved streets, more traffic (especially the rapid rise of coaches in the seventeenth century), and more pollution (a result of increasing reliance on coal for heating). The rise of coffee-houses brought with it a new taste and a new aroma. Using London judicial records, one scholar has detected "a rise in the perceived levels of noise nuisance" after the year 1600, including increasingly negative reactions to street music (Cockayne 2007: 129). The soundscape of churches changed as Protestant ministers encouraged their congregation to sing hymns rather than to listen to them. Opera houses, beginning in Venice in the 1630s, spread through Europe in the course of the following century or so.

Turning to the history of the eye, the seventeenth and eighteenth centuries were the age of the rise of townscapes, especially Dutch and Venetian, by artists such as Berckheyde and Canaletto, both expressing and encouraging an interest in the appearance of streets and squares, an aesthetic or "picturesque" gaze. The style of travel writing changed, with later travelers paying more attention to the manners and customs of the inhabitants of the places they visited. A vivid example of the new style is the travelogue written by a young Englishman, Philip Skippon, who visited the Netherlands, Germany, Italy, and France in the 1660s. In Italy, for instance, Skippon (1732) made vivid observations on the local food ("they strew scraped cheese on most of their dishes"), clothes (with a sketch of a doge's cap), flagellants, funerals, blasphemies, silk production, a guillotine used in Milan, the voting system in Venice (complete with a diagram of a ballot-box), and even the ways in which three gentlemen walked together (with a diagram) or the manner in which the washing was hung out to dry on iron bars across the streets. For all these reasons, the years around 1650 make a convenient—if approximate—ending for this chapter.

CHAPTER THREE

The Senses in the Marketplace: Sensory Knowledge in a Material World

EVELYN WELCH

In September 1592, Robert Cecil, 1st Earl of Salisbury and Secretary of State to Queen Elizabeth I, was sent by his father, Lord Burghley, to track down goods that had been brought into dock in Plymouth in south-west England. These were exotic items from a Spanish ship, the *Madre de Dios* which had been captured by privateers off the Azores and returned as booty to England. In theory, these belonged to the queen. But long before any Londoner could reach the coast, local men and women had already begun to strip the boat. By the time he arrived, Cecil claimed that, "Every one he met within seven miles of Exeter, that either had anything in a cloak, bag, or malle which did but smell of the prizes, either at Dartmouth or Plymouth (for he could well smell them almost, such has been the spoils of amber and musk amongst them)" (*Calendar* 1867: 266–7; Claxton 2013: 55). Some of these goods—silks, porcelain and other items with the odors of spices, musk, and ambergris still clinging to them—were returned to the metropolis. But many disappeared, carrying their lingering scents into Devon homes that have often been regarded as being on the periphery of metropolitan culture and sophistication.

The arrival of a privateer's plunder at the end of the sixteenth century was only one example of the many changes that enabled the penetration of new commodities and sensory experiences into Europe's marketplaces. Two decades later, in 1609, Cecil went on to establish an elite shopping center in London that specialized in the sale of such wares. To celebrate the opening of the New Exchange, he commissioned the playwright Ben Jonson's 1609 production of *The Entertainment at Britain's Burse*. This began with a shop-boy emerging to ask the audience,

> What do you lack? What is't you buy? Very fine China stuffs of all kinds and qualities? China chains, China bracelets, China scarves, China fans, China girdles, China knives, China boxes, China cabinets, caskets, umbrellas, sundials, hourglasses, looking-glasses, buring glasses, concave glasses, triangular glasses, convex glasses, crystal globes, waxen pictures, ostrich eggs, birds of paradise, musk-cast, Indian rats, China dogs and China cats, Flowers of silk, mosaic fishes? Waxen fruit and porcelain dishes? Best fine cages for birds, billiard balls, purses, pipes, rattles, basins, ewers, cups, can voiders, toothpicks, targets, falchions, beards of all ages, vizards, spectacles? See, what you lack?
>
> Jonson [1609] 2002: 6–9; see also Baker 2005;
Levy Peck 2005; Scott 2006

The notion that the early seventeenth-century audience might "lack" these goods, in the sense that they were now essentials required for everyday use, was part of Jonson's overall conceit. But it also hints at the fact that by 1600 sensory excitements that might once have been regarded as rare or unobtainable had increased in both desirability and availability. Although still expensive, spices and perfumes, sugar, cotton fabrics, furs and felts, dyes such as cochineal, and medicinal products such as sarsaparilla, guaiacum, or holy wood (all of which were thought to cure syphilis), joined porcelain, colorful feathers, coffee, tobacco, and tea in the marketplace, sitting alongside new fashions such as fans, wax pictures, and billiard balls. While some of these goods, such as coffee and tea, would take more time to embed themselves, others—such as new perfumes, medicines, tobacco, and beaver felt hats—became part of the elite urban landscape with remarkable speed. While Jonson attributed the Exchange's novelties to "China," these new commodities came from across the globe. Their initial origins could become confused by the time they arrived in Europe. Claude-Louis Berthaud's 1608 poem praising Paris, *La ville du Paris en vers burlesque*, invited buyers into the *Galerie du Palais*, an elegant new shopping space in the Courts of Justice that can be seen in a print from the 1630s by Abraham Bosse (see Figure 3.1). Viewers were invited to admire:

Knives *ala Polonaise*
Leather Collars *ala Anglais*
A beaver from remote Japan
Come see a felt hat, oh so grand
That it repels the rain with ease
Just like those they wear in Turkey

Quoted in Newman 2007: 97

While the beaver fur that provided the raw material for the fashionable felt hats came from North America, Berthaud preferred to associate the headware

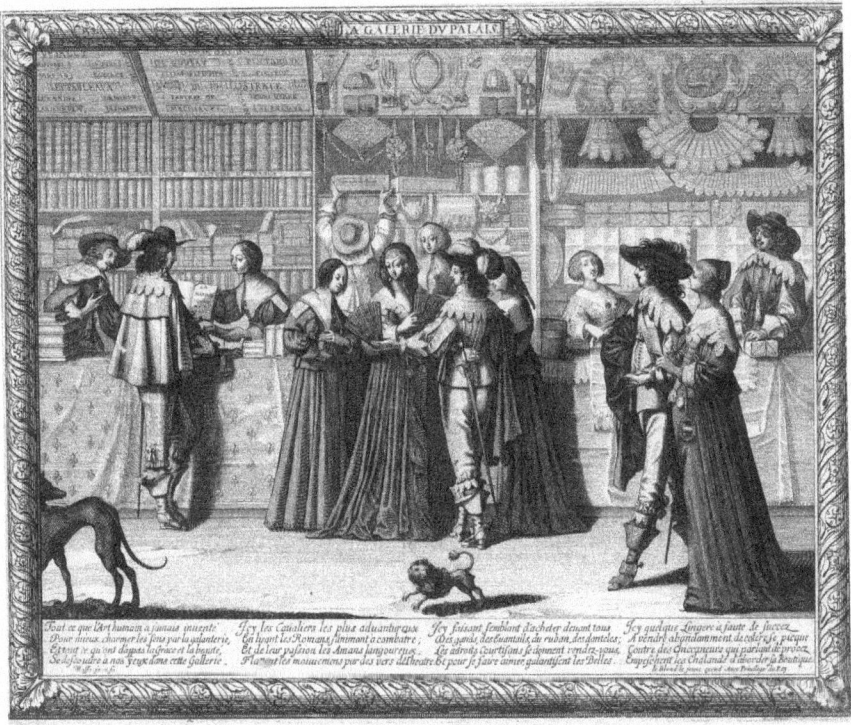

FIGURE 3.1: Abraham Bosse, *La Galerie du Palais*, etching, *c.* 1637–40. British Museum, London.

with Japan and relate it to the fez from Istanbul. For the poet, exoticism was more important than accuracy.

New connections brought conflict as well as prosperity. At the same time as the importation of global goods increased between 1500 and 1650, the period also saw famine, waves of disease, almost constant warfare, increasingly bitter religious divides, and political revolutions that disrupted ordinary commerce and daily survival. Whether they were elite aristocrats or struggling artisans, buyers might have access to Ceylonese fans or to New World tobacco, but they could not guarantee the price of bread or the availability of even the most basic goods.

In this environment of increasing global trade, European customers needed new knowledge about the unfamiliar commodities and continued reassurance over long-standing anxieties about fraud. The market was also a place to test all types of beliefs, from those in the truth of medical cures to the rising number of debates over the true faith. If bodily experiences could be fooled or distorted by fraudulent merchants and adulterated goods, how far could your senses help you differentiate between true and false gods?

This meant that, at its heart, the market was a place to undertake pragmatic testing of truths about the material nature of things. Wholesalers and speculators, hoping to introduce New World goods into European shops and stalls, needed to know that there would be a demand for their wares; retailers had to understand and promote the qualities of these items; artisans needed to manage the new properties of the materials to which they had increasing access; finally, customers needed to recognize what was worth purchasing. This wasn't only an issue for the well-off consumer. New products such as tobacco and sugar could be wrapped in paper and sold in very small amounts, making them affordable luxuries for the working poor, if not for the truly indigent (Zahediah 2010).

CHALK FOR CHEESE

In determining the qualities of their goods, Renaissance buyers and sellers shared the traditional Aristotelian notion of passive sensory perception based on the three internal (the *sensus communis*, memory and imagination) and five external senses (Milner 2011: 179). The merchant relied almost exclusively on the latter. In his 1634 *Merchant's Mapp of Commerce*, the English writer Lewes Roberts dedicated the entirety of his Chapter 9 to a discussion of how these five senses should be deployed to assess the goods encountered in an expanding world. In a lengthy passage, he explained,

[F]or I know it is practice and daily use that maketh a man skilled in this art, and many lets and impediments appear daily in many men, that hinder the true attainment thereof: for it must needs be granted, that he that is imperfect in any one natural Sense, or wants those helps that Nature affords to perfect minds, must neither be a merchant nor yet addict himself to the knowledge: for any one Sense being either depraved or defective in part or in whole, will force him to commit (against his will and mind) many Errors, and constrain him to take the bad for the good, or (at lastwise) the bad as soon as the good and sometimes (as we say) Chalk for Cheese, or one thing for another: for Experience tells us that all commodities are not learned by one Sense alone, though otherwise never so perfect in nor yet by two, but sometimes by three, sometimes by four, and sometimes by all ... But in general it must be granted that the Eye above all the rest of the Senses, still claim an especial interest and prerogative herein, and must every be admitted as one of the chieftest that must still accompany the rest in this distinction, and therefore many things are oftentimes found saleable that are pleasing thereto ... I know that it is Some [merchants] are noted againe to require the sence of feeling to be assistfull to the eye, as where the hand is of necessity be imployed, as is seen in cloth and such commodities. Some require the scence of hearing, as where the hearer giveth a help to the eye as is seen in some mettalls, minerals and such like: and some againe require the scence of smelling, as where the nose helpeth the eye, as is seen in some drugges, perfumes and the like; and lastly, some requireth the sence of tasting, as where the palate giveth the helpe, as is seen in spices, wines, oyles and many such commodities.

Roberts 1638: 37

In this description, Roberts was following the conventional hierarchy of the senses with vision as the most superior of the five, closely followed by hearing. The others were all inferior forms of perception (Harvey 2002). Yet a merchant could be easily deceived if he only observed his goods visually, mistaking, for example, "chalk for cheese." Hearing could be helpful, particularly when dealing with metalwork, but the other three lower senses: touch, taste, and smell, were essential to his trade. As examples, pharmacists had to determine the properties of herbs by their taste and smell while the qualities of textiles could only be determined through touch.

Using these skills, however, caused real challenges to the prevailing concepts of social status and dignity where touch was linked to manual occupations.

While it might be acceptable for a Venetian nobleman to be involved in trade, early seventeenth-century civic authorities who determined eligibility for senatorial status carefully investigated whether or not an applicant's ancestors had actually touched the goods they had sold. Would-be senators were only accepted if they could demonstrate that relatives had merely indicated to servants what should be done rather than manipulating or packing the goods with their own hands (Cowan 2007: 53).

Yet merchants were well aware that it was difficult, if not impossible, to determine the qualities of a commercial product without actually touching the goods directly. Lewes' emphasis on the multiplicity of senses required to make commercial judgments and the expertise and practice involved were echoed in other manuals where precise information was provided about what features should be sought. In his 1587 *The Marchant's Avizo*, for example, John Browne advised that when purchasing a valuable product such as salt, the buyer had to use both his eyes and his sense of touch, "Note, that of salt the brightest and whitest colour is best . . . which if it be new, it is perceived by the moistness of it, and by the sticking of it to your fingers, after hard wringing of it in your hande" (Browne 1957: fol. 24). When dealing with wine, Browne went on to warn that it was again impossible to assess this product by sight alone:

> Of wines: it cannot be set downe by pen or words, the right knowledge of it, for it is perciuable only by the taste and flauor. But the best sorts of wines generally are, when they doe tast pleasant and strong withall and when they drinke cleane and quicke in the pallet of the mouth, and whē they are cleere & white hued if they be white Wines, or of faire orient red, if they be red wines. But if they drinke weake, rough, foule, flat, inclining to egernesse, or long: they are not good.
> Browne 1957: fol. 27

Although these manuals were addressed to professional international merchants, customers also needed to know how to identify the varying qualities of what was on offer through similarly careful, multisensory observation. The Florentine astronomer Galileo Galilei offered a warning about how easily the senses could fool the unpracticed eye into mistakenly identifying base metals as gold or silver, or glass as gems:

> Sometimes there occurs to our senses, imprisoned so to speak by the kind and number of accidentals, the same thing that happened to the simpleton who, having found a piece of gilded iron or copper, or other substance

which appeared to be gold or silver by its surface, hardness or weight or some coloured glass ... which to the sight represented it to the intellect as a precious gem, esteemed both valuable until the expert jeweller or goldsmith ... makes him see that it is iron, copper or glass which he held to be gold, silver or a precious gem ... for any one of the senses is fallacious.

Quoted in Korrick 2003: 203–4

More worryingly, not only were the senses potentially fallacious, they could be manipulated by fraudsters who might misrepresent products to unwary customers. In Galileo's parable, the protagonist was a simpleton who made a basic error in his visual interpretation. But even experienced consumers could be fooled. Buyers needed to beware of grocers who added sand or water to grain to bulk it out; weavers who used poor quality silk in their less visible wefts; false weights and measures. They themselves might carry coins which were debased, clipped, or sweated with mercury. In all these cases, a customer would have to do more than look or listen in order to discover the deception; they would have to probe, question, and use their experience to avoid buying false goods. For example, in one description of the second-hand market in Paris, a mid seventeenth-century Dutch traveler described how unwary buyers might be fooled by skilled salesmen who used a combination of skillful patter and attractive displays:

[T]he second-hand clothes market (*la friperie*) is near the Halles. There is a large gallery, held up by stone pillars under which all the sellers of old clothes have their stalls ... there is a public market twice a week ... and it is then that these dealers, amongst whom there are it seems, a number of Jews, spread out their goods. At any hour going past, one is assailed by their continual cries, "Here's a good country coat! Here's a fine jerkin!"; And by the patter about their merchandise with which they seek to draw people to their stalls ... One can hardly believe the prodigious quantity of furniture and clothes they have; one sees some fine things but it is dangerous to buy unless one knows the trade well, for they have marvellous skill in restoring and patching up what is old so that it appears new ... you think you have bought a black coat but when you take it into the daylight, it is green or purple or spotted like leopard skin.

Quoted in Braudel 1982: 36

As this indicates, it was possible to insist (as market regulations did), that goods were only sold during the daylight hours, but even this might not provide full protection. Even if customers didn't reach out and touch the items on offer, they might be touched in turn. In 1475, for example, the Cook's company in London warned its members that they were not to pluck the sleeves of passers-by with their dirty sleeves, "whereby many debates and strives often tymes happen ayenst the peas" (quoted in Carlin 2008: 211). Such sensory assaults came in many forms. While some of the scents in the market were pleasant and welcome, others, such as the fetid odors of waste, particularly from the rubbish that accumulated around butchers' and fishmongers' stalls, gave rise to fears of disease (Dugan 2008, 2011). Raucous sounds were equally difficult to avoid. The constant cries of vendors and the unwanted patter of importuning peddlers and shopkeepers could create confusion about what was really on offer. With brothels often just around the corner from the marketplace, street vendors might be selling every form of bodily satisfaction.

MARKET SIGHTS/MARKET TOUCH

As this suggests, shopping was a multisensory experience where sight, sound, touch, taste, and smell all competed for the buyer's attention. A sixteenth-century traveler such as the Englishman Fynes Moryson was alert to the many sensations he encountered in the wide variety of markets and fairs he visited in his travels through Ireland, Scotland, Germany, and on into Italy, Turkey, and Greece. From his perspective, Dutch marketplaces were dominated by female buyers and sellers while in Italy and Turkey it was rare to see women making any purchases in public at all. He was shocked by the fact that Venetian aristocratic men bought their groceries themselves in the Rialto marketplace, going as far as to bring them home themselves, "The very gentlemen of Venice . . . carry home what they buy to eat, either in the sleeves of their gown or in a clean handkerchief" (Moryson 1617, I: 112). But he also noted that, for the most part, wherever they were located, markets usually had overseers who checked on the quality and prices of the most essential products. As he traveled, he could always find someone who would change his coins, find him a bed for the night, and charge him for the provisions that they would transform into meals. While what he ate and drank might change, swapping beer and ale for wine as he moved south, the markets and inns in which he found himself were described in remarkably similar ways, as places where the urban community invested heavily in ensuring secure provisions and a space for public spectacle.

With sight as the premier sense, European communities, both large and small, recognized that it was important to present a visible sense of order to visitors such as Moryson. The scale and orientation of markets varied enormously, from the

Frankfurt fairs which brought booksellers together from across Europe, to the small village squares offering a few vegetables, chickens, and eggs. In some cases cities created purpose-built market halls; more commonly, a town square was only used as a marketplace at specific times of the day or on designated days of the week (Welch 2005: 116–17). Often, products were restricted to specific sites and careful attention was paid to hygiene and cleanliness. Decaying matter that might generate pathogenic odors, especially from fish and meat, was considered particularly problematic; butchers were often gathered together and placed on the market outskirts or near water, with regular demands that stallholders keep their areas clean (Wheeler 2007: 27).

Whatever their scale, markets had rules about where they should be held, who was allowed to sell what goods at what price, and when selling should start and stop; licenses were supposed to be issued and taxes levied under the watchful eyes of market officials. In Paris, for example, it was obligatory to sell provisions from Les Halles on Wednesdays, Fridays, and Saturdays; in Venice, meat could only be sold from the *beccarie* in the Rialto and Piazza San Marco (Calabi 2004). Stalls were supposed to be sited according to the types of goods on offer; shops themselves were regulated in terms of the distance that their trestle tables could intrude onto the street itself. Annual or bi-annual fairs, which were larger affairs, usually required even more space and could spread out from the city and into the countryside. Indeed, any space that could be appropriated might be studded with stalls offering goods for sale. In Moscow, for example, shops were set up on the ice of the River Moscova during the winter and the so-called Frost Fairs of the late seventeenth century were London's response to an unprecedented period of cold weather (Braudel 1982: 32). But these were not without forms of surveillance; the winter fairs, like their summer counterparts, were carefully regulated by market overseers.

Written prices and the public display of weights and measures, such as the statutory lengths that are still inscribed in the town hall in Arezzo, gave further visual reassurance that the civic authorities were providing protection. Guilds provided marks, stamps, seals, and certificates that authenticated the quality of the goods on offer. Thus a customer who was not expert in woollen or silk cloth could, in theory, trust the lead seals that were applied to the weave. In Venice, offending products that failed to meet civic standards were publicly burnt. For example, one of the city's key products—theriac, a cure-all medicine with over sixty ingredients including live vipers—was created in full view of the College of Physicians; any ingredients found to be faulty were taken to the Rialto and destroyed (Welch 2008: 144–5). The highly spectacular nature of theriac's preparation (its public manufacture was accompanied by the sound of drums and trumpets) ensured that customers simply had to watch the spectacle in order to be convinced of the qualities of a medicine which became generally known as "Venetian treacle."

One of the most important ways of creating a sense of commercial security was by building impressive spaces for sales. Increasingly, cities and entrepreneurs invested in the specialist buildings required for different forms of exchange, whether this was for shipping, insurance and trade, or for the sale of lace, books, and prints. Buildings put up in the sixteenth and early seventeenth centuries included the Pand in Bruges and the Bourse in Antwerp and Amsterdam, Venice's Rialto market and Paris's Grand Palais as well as the Royal Exchange and the New Exchange in London (Calabi 2004). Antwerp's 1531 Exchange had a ground floor where merchants and bankers dealt with financial matters and wholesale overseas trade; on the floor above, customers could browse through paintings, books, and other luxury goods that were for sale in the shops that lined the balcony (see Figure 3.2). When Venice's Rialto area was destroyed by fire in the 1570s, this provided an opportunity for

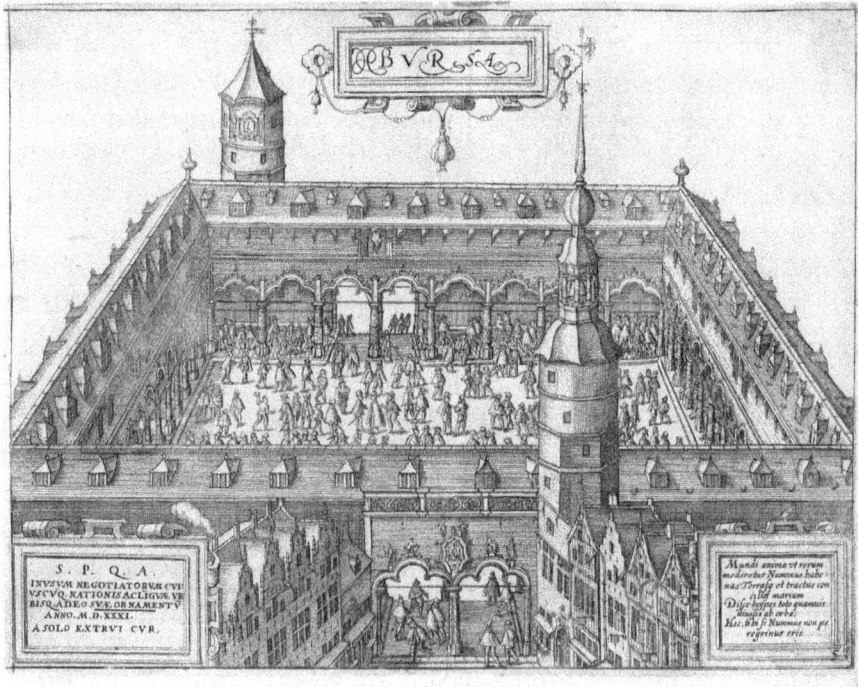

FIGURE 3.2: The Antwerp Exchange, engraved illustration in Ludovico Guicciardini's *Commentarii di Lodovico Guicciardini delle cose più memorabili* (Venice, 1565). British Museum, London.

redevelopment that included a heavy concentration of small shops on the main bridge and in the surrounding area which specialized in expensive products such as gold, jewelery, and silk. Around the same time in 1582 in Seville, city officials decided to move more elite sales off the street and into the so-called Casa Lonja while the New Exchange in London was deliberately restricted to sales by goldsmiths, mercers, stationers, picture-sellers, and perfumers.

These large semi-interior spaces were designed in stone to provide a contrast to the more common temporary wooden stalls and small shops. They provided a forum for wholesale exchange but they also allowed elite men and above all, women, to make their purchases in a safe environment where they would not be harassed or annoyed by peddlers, unwanted smells, or noises—these new spaces not only offered visual but also tactile, olfactory, and acoustic security. Transactions would still be visible, providing essential reassurance and oversight, but the interiors of these spaces were arranged for more comfortable inspection. This meant that women could arrive discretely by carriage to select from a wider range of goods than they could see at home. This was not, however, without its own challenges. Despite efforts to police the space, the committee responsible for managing the New Exchange in London received complaints about "diverse abuses daily committed in the Royal Exchange by idle boys, beggars, cheaters and other people of base quality" (Woodbridge 2006: 149). The Amsterdam Bourse, which opened in the late sixteenth century to provide a secure environment for trading stocks and shares, saw even the most elite of brokers reduced to highly physical and often unsettling interactions. Here, binding agreements were made by slapping and shaking hands twice; as the contemporary Jewish writer, Joseph de la Vega described, the last half hour of trading often disintegrated into scuffles, "Hands redden from the blows . . . handshakes are followed by shouting, insults, impudence, pushing and shoving" (Schama 1988: 349).

Even calm commercial environments could house dangers. In 1638, the engraver, Abraham Bosse, published *La Galerie du Palais*, a view of the shops in the newly built shopping spaces surrounding the Courts of Justice in Paris (see Figure 3.1). In this image, well-dressed young aristocratic men and women gather to examine the books, gloves, fans, and lace collars on display. The print seems to celebrate these new elegant forms of salesmanship, particularly since a box in the mercer's stall marked "eventails de Bosse" makes it clear that these were the paper fans that were produced by the engraver himself in that same year. At the same time, it offered a clear warning (Goldstein 2012: 126; Welch 2011: 236–7). Viewing and touching was laden with sensuous overtones: one man leafs through the romance play that the young saleswoman holds out to him while an aristocratic woman reaches out for the suggestive shape of the fan that her would-be lover presents. The flirtatious discussions over the "trifles" on sale are in stark contrast with the worthy classical tomes that they should be purchasing. It cannot be a coincidence that the item shown by the young bookseller to her customer is not one of the serious philosophical texts listed on the advertisements above her head, but a play entitled *Mariane: Trajédie*, which was first published in 1637, with a frontispiece by Bosse. Likewise the woman walking through the gallery wears both a watch and a mirror on her girdle, symbols of vanity and the passage of time as well as signs of fashionable status. Thus the print is not an unproblematic celebration of elegant acquisition in visually reassuring spaces. It is also a very traditional warning about the dangers of worldly goods where the appearance of new spaces did not necessarily signal the erasure of old anxieties.

MARKET SOUNDS

Bosse's print was probably connected to Corneille's play *La lingère*, which was produced in Paris in 1637 (Newman 2007). Also set in the Galerie du Palais, it centered on the concept that these spaces were sites where reputations as well as goods were made and broken. In this context what one heard in the market was as important as what one saw. For example, in a scene set in London's Royal Exchange in Thomas Nashe's *The Return of Pasquill* (1589) one character warned:

> Speake softly, Cavaliero, I perceiue two or three lay theyr heads at one side like a shyp vnder sayle, and begin to cast about you: I doubt they haue ouer-heard you. This Exchange is vaulted and hollow, and hath such an Eccho, as multiplies euery worde that is spoken, by Arithmaticke, it makes a thousand of one, & ympes so many feathers into euery tale, that it flyes with all speed into euery corner of the Realme.
>
> Quoted in Wilson 1995: 25

In this speech, Nashe is playing with the concept of mercantile knowledge. His lord or *cavaliero* is being overheard by men who are described as putting their heads to one side like ships under sail. The vaulted shape of the Exchange became a multiplier of information, distributing news across the country.

Market news came in a remarkable variety of auditory forms from bells and songs to shouts, whispers, and the sounds of horses' hooves or the clatter of stalls being opened. These sounds went well beyond the spatial confines of designated shops and stalls, filtering through the streets and penetrating into homes. An

Antwerp manuscript from around 1540 contains a poetic refrain where a drunkard continually complains that he cannot sleep because of the sound of street vendors: "How would any drunkard find peace?" His complaints continue as he hears the cries of "get your turnips, get your turnips," "herring, herring, tasty herring," "a fresh cod, a cod, a tasty thing," "tasty brandy," "all hot cakes, all hot" (Braekman 1999: 39). Around fifty years later, a song from the Amsterdam *Refereyn boeck* uses a similar conceit. This time a bed-ridden man ("How would a sick man find peace?") takes up the same complaints against the noises of the street of "Get whiting and haddock, they are cheap" or the shouts of those selling needles, spectacles, chestnuts, and rat-poison (Buijnsters-Smets 2012: 42–3).

The highly mobile sights and unseemly sounds of the market were made more respectable through their translation into print, paint, and song. For example, Dutch, Flemish, and Italian artists began producing oil paintings that depicted market vendors in careful detail such as the allegorical image of *Water* showing fishmongers by Joachim Beuckelaer (Honig 1998); artists and printmakers created collectible images of street-sellers (see Figures 3.3 and 3.4).

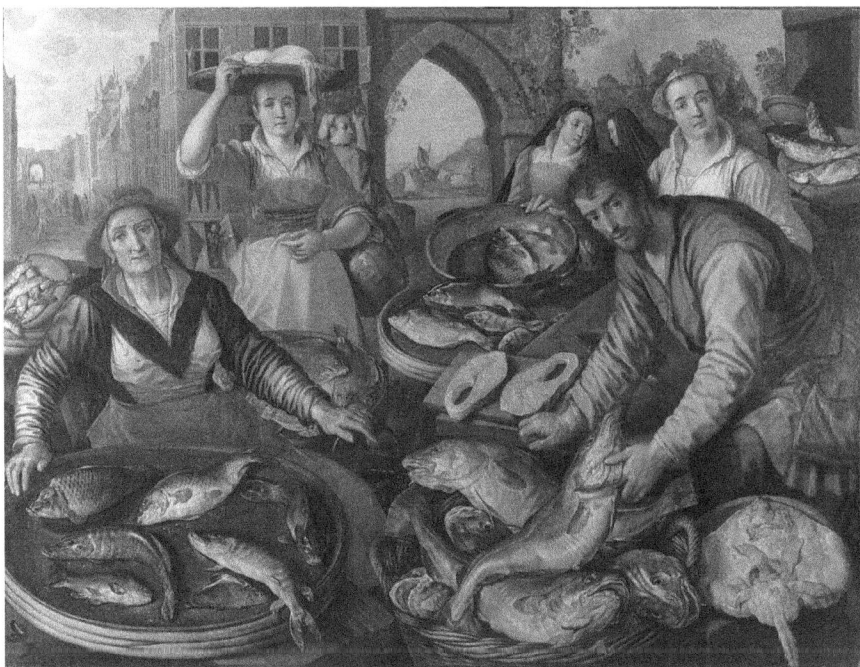

FIGURE 3.3: Joachim Beuckelaer, *The Four Elements: Water. A Fish Market with the Miraculous Draught of Fishes in the Background*, oil on canvas, 1569. National Gallery of Art, London.

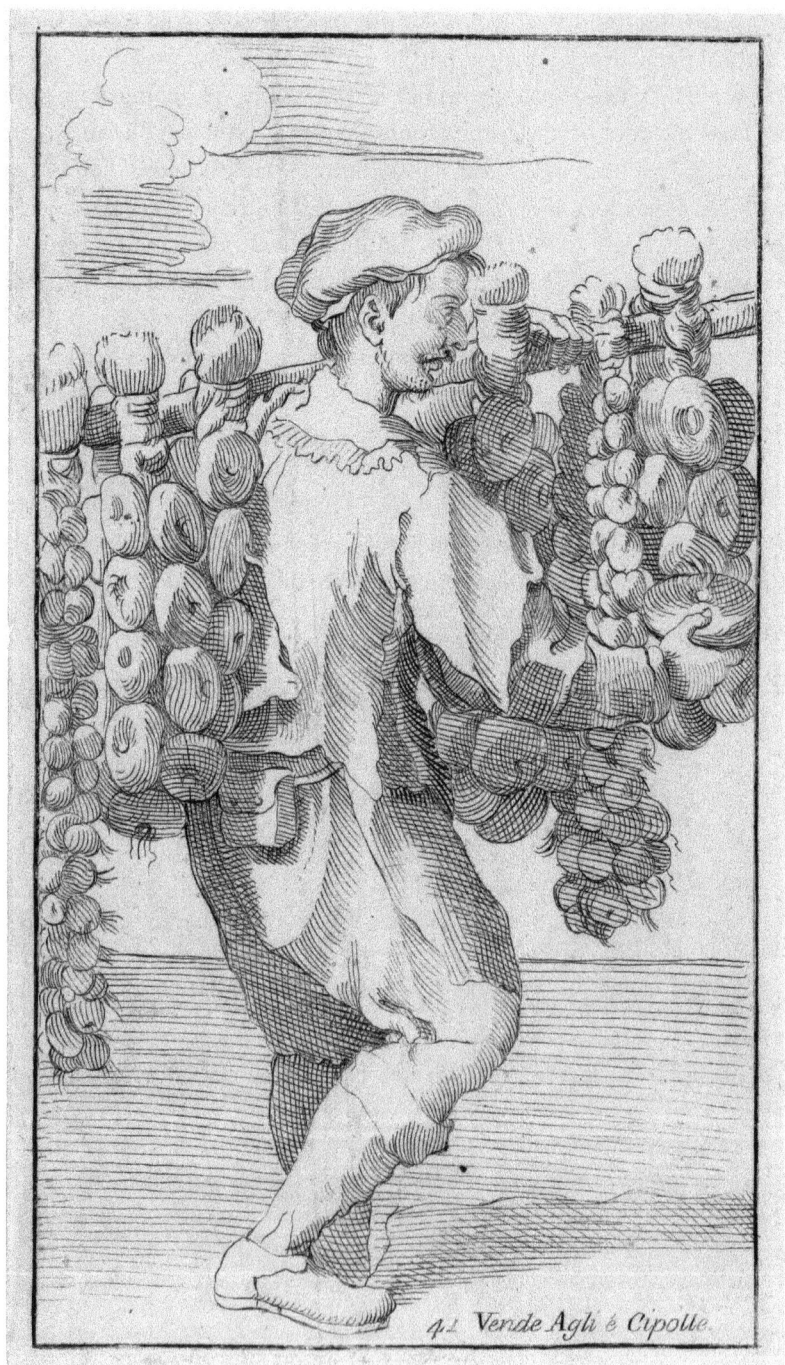

FIGURE 3.4: *Vende agli e cipolle*, after Annibale Carracci, engraving, 1646. British Museum, London.

At the same time the sixteenth-century French composers Claude de Sermisy and Clément Janequin created settings for songs such as "Voulez ouyr les cris de Paris?" Similarly Richard Dering's "Country Cries" and "Cries of London" (1599) and Orlando Gibbons' "The Cryes of London" (1614) shifted traditional English calls to buy oysters or have their knives sharpened into evocative polyphonic versions that could be sung by professional choirs (Korda 2008; Wilson 1995).

Sounds told the listener about more than just products and prices; throughout Europe new statutes or laws were publicly pronounced in the market squares. Transgressors were punished at the same sites. For example, in 1597, three women who had been accused of abandoning infants in the Royal Exchange in London were "tied unto a cart's tail and whipped . . . naked in Newgate Market, Cheapside, Leadenhall and in the Borough of Southwark having several proclamations openly made at every of the four said places declaring their several offences" (Gowing 2007: 141). The combination of the visible punishment and shaming, along with the shouts about the women's respective misdeeds, was meant to ensure the widest possible knowledge about the authorities' expectations of moral behavior.

The intersection between hearing and seeing was made even more prominent with the increased use of printing in the market. Instead of creating a silent environment for reading, it increased exchange as those who were literate informed those who were not. Amongst the shouts of Paris were those of "a boy who cries out 'new books: new farce, new prognostication'" (McIlvenna 2010: 84). Some cries could be highly political; the sixteenth-century French diarist Pierre de l'Estoile recorded the "defamatory libels against His Majesty coloured with all the most atrocious insults . . . printed in Paris and cried publicly in the streets" (McIlvenna 2010: 84–5).

The combination of the visible and the aural had a long history as shopkeepers, charlatans, and mountebanks had all traditionally used banners, seals, and certificates to testify to the efficacy of their wares. Now they used printed as well as verbal testimonials. For example, in a discussion about status in early seventeenth-century Venice, the merchant Santo Petrobonelli was described as one who "sat in a chair and discoursed on the quality of his goods to those who came to buy . . . he showed them his certificates from the Health Office so that they would believe that his goods were perfect, wholesome, unique and rare" (Cowan 2007: 54). With print, salesmen could provide detailed information about their wares and availability even when they were not present to offer a commentary. For example, a syphilitic patient asked a friend to read out a large handbill advertising medical cures that was posted by a pharmacy in the marketplace in Mantua (Gentilcore 2005: 57). Circulating printed or handwritten newsletters, known as *avvisi*, were similarly posted on walls and read aloud in the streets or shops. In 1596, a barber in Bologna subscribed to manuscript *avvisi*, and paid for a license to have them read in his shop (De Vivo 2007: 98). The Venetian apothecary and mountebank, Leonardo Fioravanti, described in 1564 how in barber shops

> one can hear all the news and the facts of private people, because sailors talk about their travels, the great fortunes they had, and the customs of the many lands they saw; soldiers narrate their battles and their victories; husbands recount how they married, and how they do with their wives; young lovers, how they fell in love, and how they follow their beloved ones; and one can hear a thousand jokes.
>
> De Vivo 2007: 98

It was not only barbers who offered such opportunities for news and conversation. An early seventeenth-century list of sites where professional informers should be stationed on behalf of the Venetian state included "bookshops, textile stores, taverns and the premises of mercers and shoemakers, as well as numerous barbers and apothecaries" (De Vivo 2007: 97). These were places where scurrilous songs, pamphlets, and prints spread quickly and often secretly, much to the concern of government regulators. In Rome's Piazza Navona, the site of the city's market for antiquities, a figure known as the Pasquino attracted commentaries on the papacy's flaws and cardinals' peccadillos, so-called *pasquinades* (San Juan 2001). In Paris, gossip about the sexual misdemeanours of the court was quickly translated into witty attacks that spread through both whispered gossip and illicit prints distributed in the corridors and stalls of the *Galerie du Palais* (McIlvenna 2010: 81).

With reputations at stake, the shouts and cries designed to attract a customer's attention could quickly disintegrate into arguments and disputes. In the early seventeenth century, a female vegetable seller in London came before magistrates complaining that another vendor had accused her of taking away his customers and had called her a "drunken whore" (Gowing 2007: 138). In 1590, women selling fruit at the city's Cornhill Gate were accused of "abusing themselves in cursing and swearing to the annoyance and grief of the inhabitants and passers bye" (Gowing 2007: 43).

The multi-sensory market experience had its fullest form in the charlatan salesman's performance (see Figure 3.5). In Venice the English traveler, Thomas Coryate was fascinated by troupes who used theatrical performances to gather

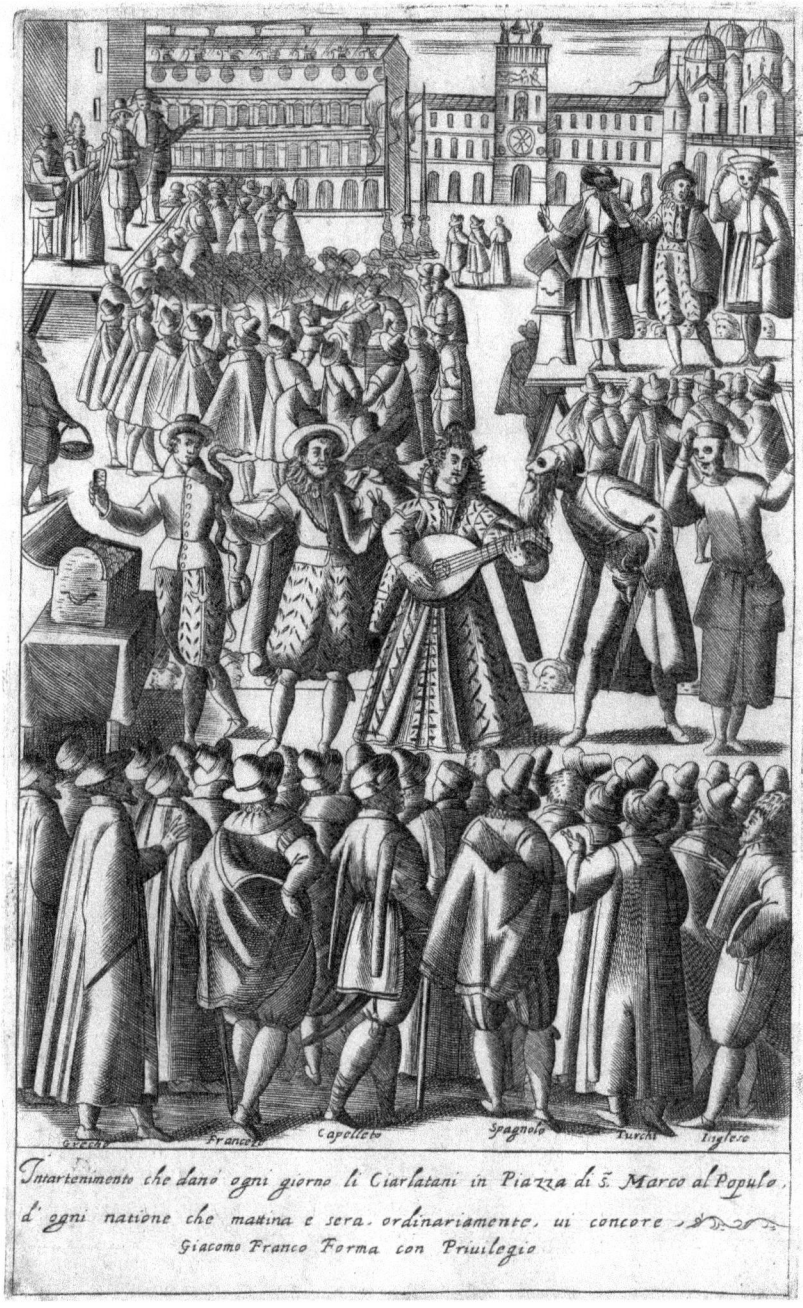

FIGURE 3.5: "Intartenimento che dano ogni giorno li Ciarlatani in Piazza di S. Marco al Populo d'ogni natione che mattina e sera ordinariamente ui concore," engraved illustration from Giacomo Franco, *Habiti d'huomini et donne Venetiane* (Venice, 1610). British Museum, London.

an audience which might go on to buy ointments and charms against venomous snakes: "These merry fellows do most commonly continue two good hours on the stage and at last when they have fedd the audience with such passing variety of sport, that they have even cloyed with the superfluity of their conceits, and have sold as much ware as they can, they remove their trinkets and stage until the next meeting" (Gambaccini 2003: 35).

While Venice was particularly famous for its charlatans and mountebanks, they could be found in many other Italian and other major European cities (Katrizky 2001). In 1627, for example, a Bolognese charlatan petitioned the Grand Duke of Tuscany to give him permission to "mount the stage with masked and unmasked personage, with music on workdays as well as holidays" in order "to sell oil for cold pains, compresses for the stomach, ointments to increase milk, rinses for the mouth and external things" (Gambaccini 2003: 41). The duke provided the requested permission but only on the condition that no female performers were included. This constraint would not have been welcome as women were a common part of a successful troupe. In 1616, one "Vettoria" was paid by a company of charlatans to work with them in Florence, "dressed like a boy, clean and neat." According to one description, she entertained the crowds in Florence with

> somersaults ... and divine dancing, with singing so soothing, and a glance so beautiful that in its sweetness [it] moves everyone to compassion, and being all put in a slumber they cry out, "oimee, oimee, my heart what is this?" Especially old men who look on her with their mouths open, because they would like to play games with her and give her a licking.
>
> Gambaccini 2003: 35

In Coryate's description, he uses the term "when they were fed" to describe the crowd's satiety at the end of the performance; likewise the lascivious description of the elderly men salivating over the cross-dressed Vettoria took bodily sensuality back to its most basic format. Here, just as the senses could inform, they could also dangerously arouse an audience, drawing on the basest of their senses.

MARKET TASTES/MARKET SMELLS

As the example of the mountebank indicates, bodily desires could quickly become bodily anxieties and governments were often keen to impose sensory discipline. A city with a full granary and streets that resounded with the cries of men and women selling fruit, vegetables, and cooked treats was a place of welcome abundance. But it was also a site that could, if not carefully controlled, become a place of sensory temptations. Rulers and magistrates had to ensure that vice in the form of lust, gluttony, avarice, and pride did not take hold in their towns and villages. At the same time, they had to make sure that the cities were fed. This often translated into both practical regulations designed to force farmers and peasants to supply the growing urban communities, and positive encouragement of inventors, through patents and other forms of protection, to develop new products to prevent imports from dominating the marketplace. Thus when printmakers copied foreign versions of city street cries, they were careful to adapt them to their own local conditions. For example, while prints made in England, Germany, and the Netherlands showing street vendors included women, their Italian variations such as the 1582 *Ritrato de quelli che vano vendendo et lavorando per Roma* did not (Welch 2005: 52–3) (see Figure 3.6). Although all the prints described "trifling

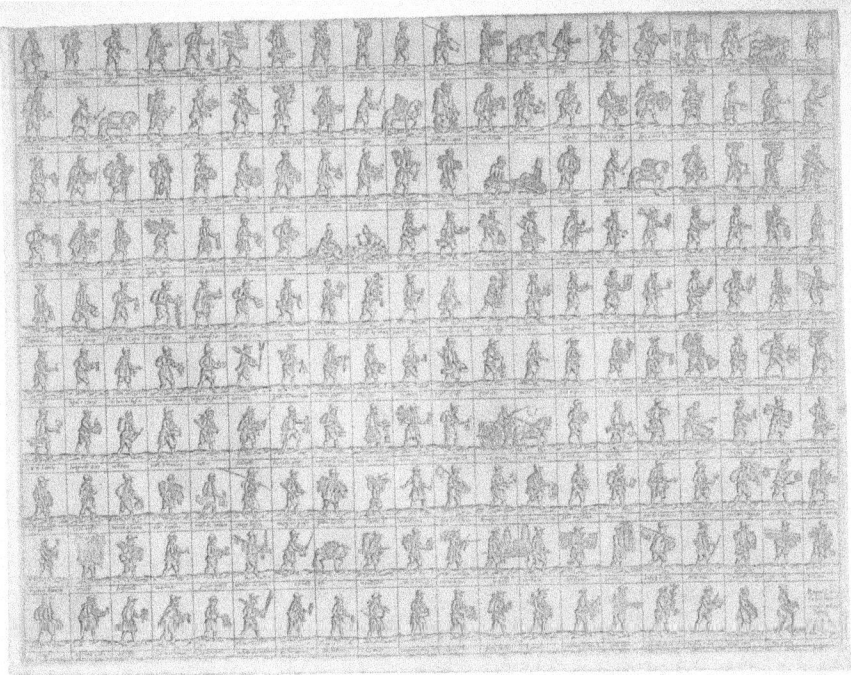

FIGURE 3.6: Ambrogio Brambilla, *Ritrato de quelli che vano vendendo et lavorando per Roma*, etching, 1582. British Museum, London.

goods" for sale such as tennis racquets and children's toys, they then concentrated on the foods that were on offer locally: oysters, pasta, garlic, and onions in Rome; strawberries, mussels, and hot pies in London. None of the variations, however, included the novel foodstuffs from the New World. The tomato and the potato remained obscure commodities until the eighteenth century (Gentilcore 2010). In contrast, sugar, already known as an expensive import from Madeira from the 1460s, was very much welcomed into a dietary regime that associated sweetness with health as well as with pleasure. Candies, sweetmeats, and conserves were often sold from pharmacies or made at home and then provided at the end of the meal to aid digestion. With the transfer of sugar-cane technology by the Portuguese from Madeira to Brazil and its development in the Caribbean, the trade was dominated by the Dutch, who had almost sixty sugar refineries in Amsterdam, whose heavy scent of cooking sugar and molasses would have hung over the docks in the mid-seventeenth century (Mintz 1986; Schwartz 2004). As the Dutch exported cones of refined white sugar and other countries began to develop their own industries, this once rare commodity became increasingly available across Europe in a multiplicity of forms from raw sugar to syrups to comfits. As sugar remained relatively expensive until the late seventeenth century, it was the more inexpensive savory goods that continued to dominate urban street smells. "London's Lickpenny," a fifteenth-century poem, provided a vivid image of the metropolis's offerings:

> Then I went forth by London stone
> Throughout all Candlewick street
> Drapers much cloth me offered anon
> Then comes one, cried, "Hot Sheep's Feet."
>
> Davis 2011: 1

While "hot sheep's feet" may not sound immediately attractive, with fuel in short supply it was not uncommon for urban communities to rely on communal ovens and bakeries for their hot foods. Customers would often bring their own uncooked breads and roasts and then wait as they emerged from the oven; hot pies, pancakes, sausages, and fish were offered by itinerant vendors and from inns or by women cooking on the street, ensuring that cities and villages were filled with the tantalizing smells. For example, an early seventeenth-century English series of prints on the Five Senses included a conventional image for "Smell": a woman holding a flower (see Figure 3.7). But the picture also included a bloodhound and the caption equated a man's ability to smell out

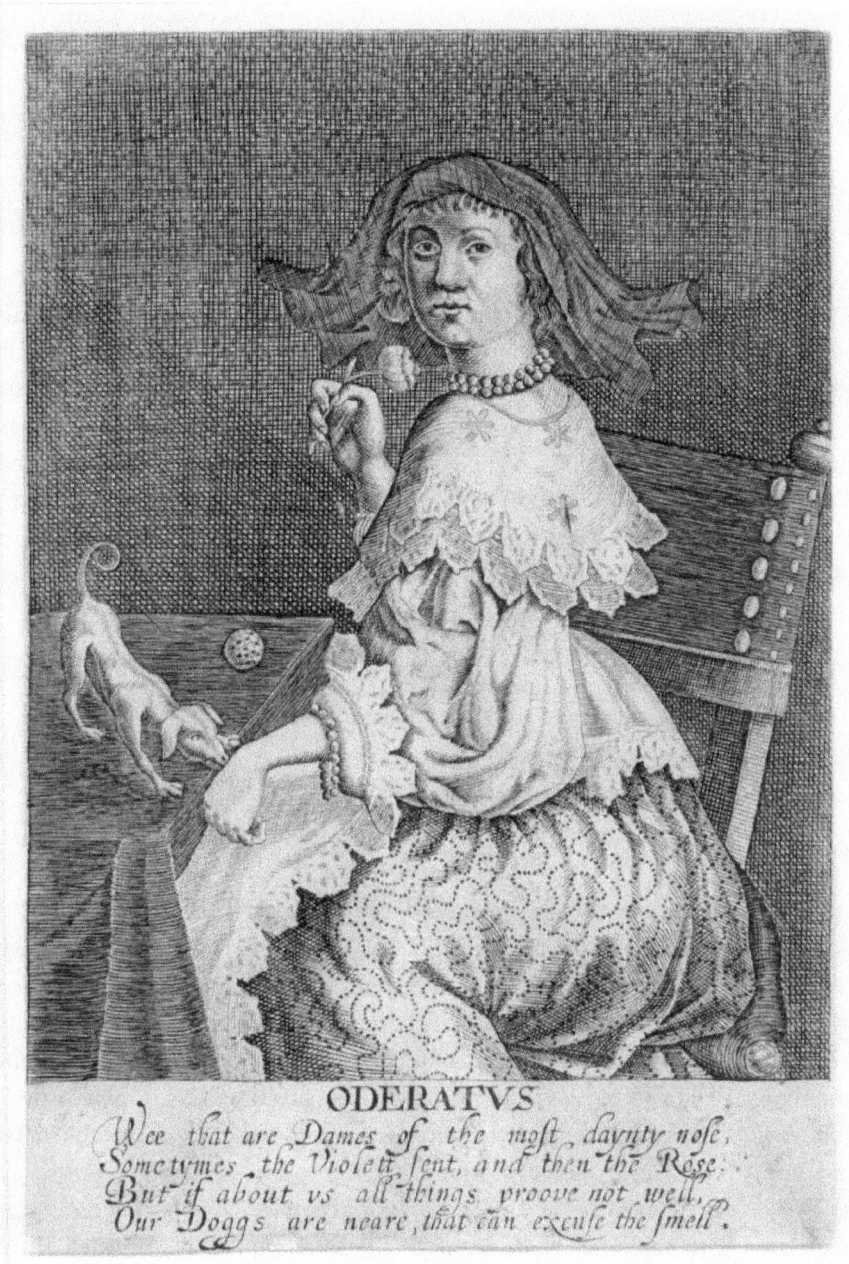

FIGURE 3.7: "Oderatus," engraving after George Glover, c. 1640. British Museum, London.

food in the stalls that surrounded St. Paul's Cathedral in London with that of a hunting dog:

> There are a crew of fellows I suppose
> That angle for their victuals with their nose
> As quick as Beagles in the smelling scence
> To smell a feast in Pauls 2 miles from thence.

In another set of contemporary early seventeenth-century prints on the senses, smell was more conventionally represented with floral imagery. But in this much imitated series, the iconography for "Gustus" or the sense of taste was radically different. Instead of the traditional iconography of women holding fruit or men sipping wine, "taste" was shown as a fashionably and somewhat immodestly dressed young woman smoking a pipe (see Figure 3.8). For knowledgeable viewers, the drying qualities of the tobacco, seen in a twist of paper at her side alongside a glass of wine, would have rendered her an overly masculine virago, a warning reinforced by the accompanying verse:

> Match me this Girle in London, nay the World
> For Feathered Beaver and her hayre well curld
> For none of our viragoes shee'l give place
> For healthing Sacke, and smoking with a Grace.
>
> Griffiths 1998: cat. 64

The appearance of tobacco under the category of taste rather than smell is understandable. In Aristotelian terms, the two senses were closely interlinked, using the same terminology of sweet and sour. Although tobacco was regarded as "stinky" because of its smell and its benefits were disputed, it moved from being an unusual medicinal product in the early sixteenth century to a ubiquitous commodity by 1600. With vendors selling coiled prepared leaves, pipes, snuff, snuff-boxes, and tinder flints, tobacco was undoubtedly one of the most important New World success stories in the European marketplace. Although by the end of the seventeenth century coffee and coffee houses would be closely associated with smoking, while tea and chocolate would take on their own, more feminized, rituals, using a pipe or taking snuff spread rapidly not only across Europe but also across the Indian Ocean and into China. This was not immediately welcomed. The English and Ottoman empires both attempted to ban it in the first decades of the seventeenth century; Sweden, Denmark, Russia, and some of the German estates followed suit shortly. But these sanctions failed

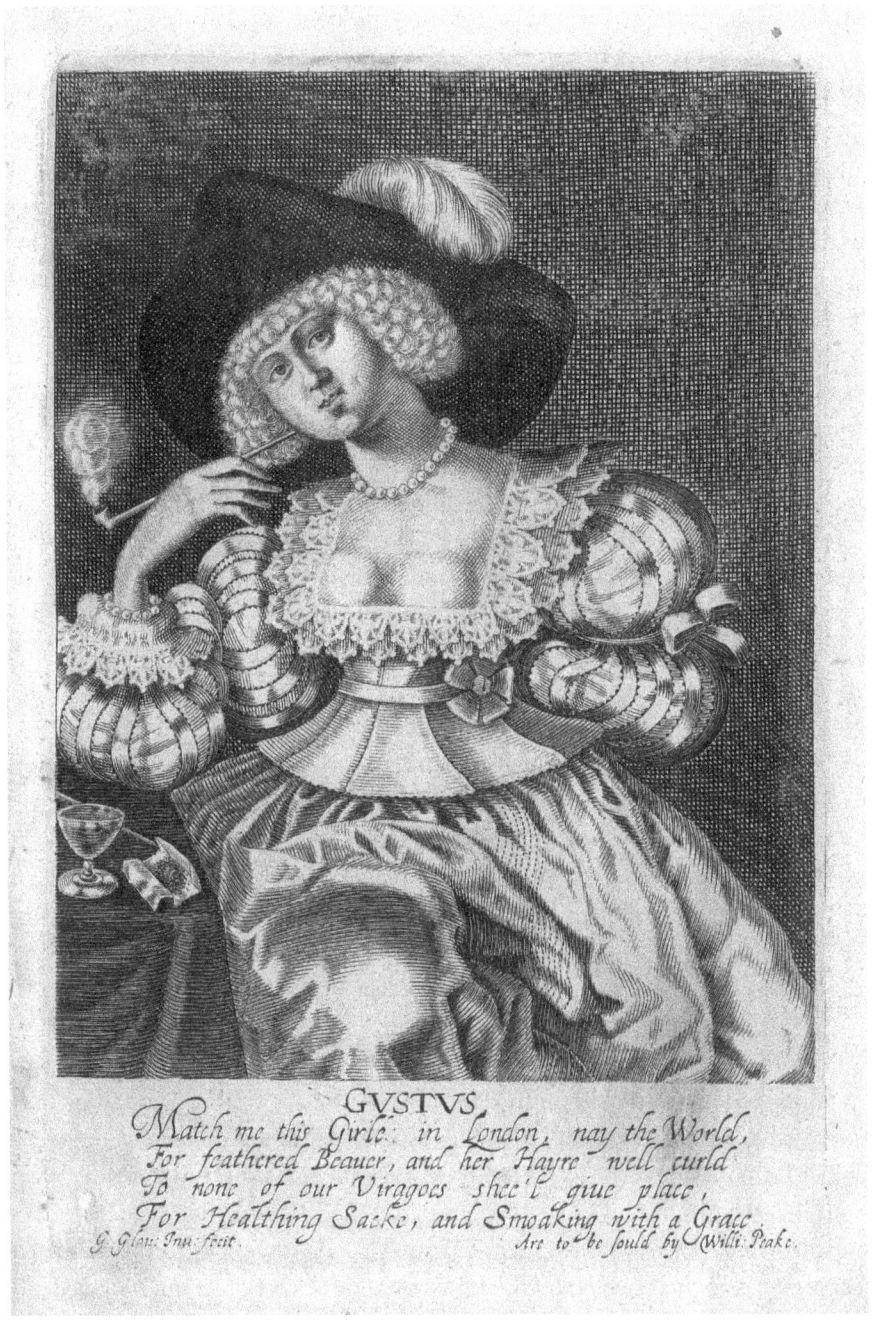

FIGURE 3.8: "Gustus," engraving after George Glover, c. 1640. British Museum, London.

and tobacco quickly became a common product for licensed grocers and tobacconists as well as street vendors who would cut off short sections for pipe tobacco; perfumers provided elaborately scented versions as snuff. Tobacco consumption in England alone rose from 100,000 pounds at the beginning of the seventeenth century to 12 million pounds by its close, changing the ways in which smells permeated public and private spaces and the very breath of men and women who used this new product (Zahediah 2010: 197–209).

From its initial arrival in Europe as Spanish cargo, tobacco was marketed as a cure for syphilis and the plague, joining a wide range of remedies that were recommended against these frightening diseases. Tobacco had its primary effects through its perceived heating, drying effects that might be appropriate for men but problematic for women with their supposedly moist, cold properties. Thus early medical advice prescribed smoking for migraines, toothache, and colds while proscribing it after meals in case its fumes damaged the brain and the liver (Dickson 1954; Goodman 1993). In his late sixteenth-century epigram, *On Tobacco*, Sir John Davis presented the New World product's virtues as if he were a mountebank offering cures:

> It is tobacco whose sweet substantial fume
> The hellish torment of the teeth dots ease
> By drawing down and drying up the rheum
> The mother and nurse of each disease . . .
> Oh were that I were one of these mountebanks
> Which praise their oils and powders which they sella
> My customers would give me a coin with thanks
> I for this ware so smooth a tale would tell.
>
> Loughlin *et al.* 2012: 1142

Davis' satirical praise of tobacco relied on his reader's knowledge of the mountebanks' trade; far from believing in the virtues of the new herb, they were expected to recognize tobacco as one of the many forms of "snake-oil" that were sold to gullible buyers. To truly know the qualities of a product, the wary consumer had to test all its sensible properties and its potential uses. Instead of trusting what they were told or even believing in what they could see, wise buyers had to develop their own expertise based on direct experience and knowledge.

CONCLUSION: SENSING AND KNOWING

This chapter has argued that being able to separate out the true from the false was a constant marketplace dilemma. In the fifteenth century, mathematical manuals and abacus schools trained young men in barrel gauging—teaching them how to use their eyes to quickly assess volume and weight rather than relying on what the vendor might claim (Baxandall 1971: 86–7). In the sixteenth century, numerous manuals provided advice on how to identify and use new products, exchange unfamiliar coins, and avoid the deceits and blandishments of mountebanks and peddlers. This sensory knowledge was as important outside as well as inside the marketplace. Alongside the entry of New World goods and knowledge, the period from 1450 to 1650 also witnessed dramatic changes in theology and challenges to the relationships between what men and women were able to witness and what they should believe. For some Protestants, true religion was not in "doctrines and precepts of touching, tasting and handling but (was) spiritual" (Milner 2011: 251). For others, the Catholic use of sensory appeals such as bells and incense at mass was as fraudulent as the spectacles put on by mountebanks. Here, in the debate between tangible witnessing and religious faith, the marketplace was often invoked as a model for either corrupting or honing the senses. Similarly, those trying to determine a new, more empirical way of understanding the world warned against unsubstantiated beliefs. In this environment, even words could not be trusted. It was no accident that in 1620 Francis Bacon could warn of "idols of the marketplace" in Aphorism 43 of his *New Organon*: "there are illusions which seem to arise by agreement and from men's association with each other which we call idols of the marketplace; we take the name from human exchange and community. Men associate through talk and words are chosen to suit the understanding of the common people. And thus a poor and unskilful code of words incredibly obstructs the understanding" (Bacon [1620] 2000: 42). For Bacon, his new "science takes its origin not only from the nature of the mind but from the nature of things" ([1620] 2000: xxii).

In this time of uncertainty, systems for testing veracity, whether of words or of things, were increasingly being developed from forms of torture designed to identify witches and heretics to more benign investigations into the nature of new products and processes (Bethencourt 2009; Mola 2013). Thus from the sixteenth century onwards, inventors seeking monopolies and patents had to present their ideas to commissioners who insisted on scrutinizing each idea before encouraging public support (Mola 2013). Increasingly, manuscript books of secrets belonging to late sixteenth-century apothecaries such as Stefano Rosselli (who supplied the Medici court in Florence) did not simply copy existing medicinal and cosmetic recipes—they tested them (Shaw and Welch 2011). Carefully noting the results of concoctions designed to temper steel or remove grey hair, they were clear that only results achieved under direct observation were believable. As princes such as Ferdinando de'Medici,

Grand Duke of Tuscany, and the Holy Roman Emperor Rudolph II turned to alchemical experimentations, a respect for empirical observations moved from the urban marketplace and shops and into the court and new scientific communities such as the Royal Society (P. Smith 1994, 2004). At the same time, physicians and naturalists recognized that the sensory skills required to evaluate the quality of spices, silks, and sugars from the New World were similar to those needed to discriminate between the different flora and fauna that they were cataloguing (Findlen 1994). Apothecaries were called upon to set up university botanical gardens; physicians needed to test the new products promising cures against new diseases; noblewomen and nuns created distilleries to provide medicines and scented waters; goldsmiths, alchemists, and princes joined together to test mercury's properties and to search for the elusive philosopher's stone (P. Smith 2004; Wallis 2008). For all its difficulties, or perhaps indeed because of its challenges, the sensory skills of visual observation and tangible testing, and the ability to distinguish between the valuable and the fraudulent, so long associated with commerce, now became part of elite understanding and scientific knowledge (Spolsky 2001). The marketplace was no longer only a place to buy necessities, it was also a place to demonstrate empirical knowledge and sensory governance.

CHAPTER FOUR

The Senses in Religion: Towards the Reformation of the Senses

MATTHEW MILNER

Renaissance Christianity was deeply shaped by contemporary sensory culture. In many ways its core preoccupations revolved around what religious sensing meant, and what place the senses had in true Christian beliefs and practices. The renowned sensuousness of Renaissance piety and artistry stand juxtaposed to asceticism and iconoclasm, and the Reformation as testament to the breadth of their possible variations. Religious life in the Renaissance drew heavily on the dominant Aristotelianism of late medieval sensory culture, but also eventually led to its transformation by exploring how religious expressions and experiences could or ought to be authenticated or have recourse to sensation. Central to this was an empirical attitude firmly built on traditional calls to use the senses to discern vice from virtue. Every sensation, to some degree, was framed by religious culture as the senses were the primary means by which believers encountered, explored, and experienced a religiously ordered and sacralized world. The religious upheavals of the Reformation dramatically recast how European Christians understood the relationship between religious life and sensing, and in no small way fostered the reconfiguration of the senses and sensory culture themselves.

The Renaissance and Reformation were defining moments for European Christianity; it is clear the senses lay at the heart of many of their conflicts. A key development is the emergence of religiously-configured aesthetic cultures in response to the need to integrate sensing with various religious doctrines. For scholars today these cultures are not the stereotypes of old. Gone are the accounts of overly intellectualized Protestant regimes struggling against overly sensual Catholics. Placing everyday practices alongside and in tension with sensory theories and religious doctrine yields some unexpected views of these religious cultures. No longer can we stereotype Reformation sensory changes as a switch from eyes to ears; visuality was important to Protestant piety, especially reading scripture, as hearing was to Catholic. Moreover, polemicists on all sides accused their opponents of sensuality. The tension over external piety was offset by intensely sensual inner spirituality, yet even the most ardent Protestants described their religious experiences with sensory language. Above all, however, is the sheer breadth of changes endured by European Christianity during this period, making its religious culture a crucible for the inevitable reformation of the senses.

RELIGIOUS LEARNING AND THE SENSES

The senses were an essential component of Renaissance religious instruction and learning. Lay spiritual and devotional teaching derived from guides which contained lists of the five corporeal senses amidst key prayers, the Ten Commandments, and the seven deadly sins. More complex discussions of the internal senses, like 'common sense', memory, or imagination, were rarer. Although Renaissance confessors' manuals tended to focus on particular sins, as did the *Defecerunt* of Antoninus of Florence, even these were bound with discussions of the senses (Casas Homs 1948: 125). Nevertheless, rarely, if ever, did preachers explicitly instruct churchgoers on the senses. Rather they mentioned them in expositions on Christian morality. At the other end of the cultural spectrum, scholarly works and commentaries continued to engage Aristotle's views of the senses as in his *Parva Naturalia* and *De Anima*. For non-academics, compendia like Georg Reisch's *Margerita Philosophica* (Frangenberg 1991: 78; Green 2011: 210; Woolgar 2007: 14, 19–22) provided summaries of Aristotelian sensory theories. Although Aristotelianism provided the vocabulary for scholarly discussions, Neoplatonism had a deep influence. The result is a wide range of themes and treatment of the senses in theological and philosophical works. In contrast to his *Defecerunt*, Antoninus of Florence's *Summa* took the senses in recounting the powers of the soul (Antoninus of

Florence 1582: 59–106). Marsilio Ficino's *Theologica Platonica* devoted considerable space to the senses and their function, as did Nicholas of Cusa's various works, like *De Docta Ignorantia* and *De Visione Dei* (Ficino 2001–6, 1: 199, 247; 2: 211–61, 353–63; 4: 31, 183–93, 215) (see also Cusa 1985, 1990). Charles de Bouvelles discussed the senses and forms of knowledge at length in his 1511 *Liber de Sensu*.

In all likelihood most men and women, prior to the Reformation, learned about the senses as a matter of practical morality. Devotional and humanist moral texts like Thomas à Kempis' widely translated fifteenth-century *Imitatio Christi* or Thomas Elyot's *Of the Knowledge* and his *Castel of Helth*, linked knowledge of how the senses functioned to the practices and habits of everyday life (Elyot 1539, 1549). These works taught readers that sensing instilled habits, affections, and passions that brought out virtuous or vicious living. Human beings shared sensory functions with animals. Sensing was passive, transforming and shaping the bodies of percipients. But unlike animals, human reason could override or permit sensory impulses which moved the body and will to certain kinds of actions. The avoidance of sensuality and vice was firmly rooted in the control of what was sensed and how one reacted to it. Only when subjected to and ruled by reason would the senses fulfill their God-given office of discernment. An awareness of sensory physiology was essential to the governance and control of the senses as a matter of godly Christian living. Erasmus's *De Civilitate Morum Puerilium* and Sebastian Brant's *Shippe of Fools* taught that such rational sensory control was what divided humans from beasts. We find the theme in numerous contexts; for instance, Jacques Lefevre d'Etaples urged readers in the preface of his French translation of the New Testament to avoid sensory curiosity (Brant 1517: K7r; Elyot 1549: 24v–26r, 32r–33v; Erasmus 1997: 601–4; Knox 1995).

Renaissance religious literature and imagery continued medieval examples of those who governed their senses appropriately, and those who did not. While Eve's taste brought about human fall from paradise, the disciple Thomas's insistence on seeing and touching the risen Christ went too far. Both failed to use their senses properly, either by allowing sensual desire to overcome reason, or by asserting sensory knowledge in matters of faith. Together Eve and Thomas were examples of worldly sensuality. The Virgin Mary and Christ offered models of good sensing. Mary's hearing at the Annunciation was the means of Christ's conception, a medieval theme which continued but was challenged by a growing interest in her sight as well during the Renaissance (Melion 2009; Steinberg 1987: 32). It was Christ's undamaged humanity that demonstrated the potential of human sentience unencumbered by sin. His suffering in the Passion was multi-sensory, his five wounds payment for the sins committed through the five senses. Christ's senses were the very locus of human redemption, his perfect sensing—both in terms of pain and his use of the senses—restored fallen humanity. Christians had to avoid the examples of Eve and Thomas, and aspire to those of Christ and Mary. The saints came closest to achieving a Christ-like governance of their senses, but most people failed because original sin prevented human will from perfect control over sensory desires and passions. The most spectacular failures were religious transgressors: the heretic and the idolater. Driven by their senses to delusion, heretics placed sensory opinion above the faith guarded by the Church, while idolaters misplaced their piety by worshiping sensible objects as divine (D'Alton 2005: 103–14; Dolan 1983: 345; Hogarde 1556: 28v, 71v).

The most fearful characters of Renaissance religious culture, the witch and the demoniac, misused their senses and harmed those of others. As an arch-heretic and arch-idolater, the witch was the most deluded in her senses and dangerous because she tried to manipulate the senses of godly men and women. Once captured she had to be gagged, blindfolded, and bound to protect her captors from her "suspect sensorium" (Classen 2005: 71–2). The evil eye was central to their maleficia, influencing the passions and actions of others, especially men (Clark 2007: 128; Classen 2005: 75–6). Joan of Arc, regarded by the English as a witch, had managed to blind the "wytes" of the entire "french nacion," such was the danger of her sensual prowess and deceit (Hall 1548: CXIIIv). The demoniac illustrated how susceptible the senses were to outside influence. Demons manipulated both matter and the senses themselves, creating apparitions and illusions that confounded those they possessed. They entered the body through the senses and rendered the possessed senseless by cutting off rational control of the body and the wits. Both the witch and the demonic had disordered senses, and employed or experienced illusions and sensory deception (Boaistuau 1598; Clark 1997: 19–21, 166–7, 265–6). Their work made sensing not only worldly, but deceitful and corrupting.

The upheavals of the Reformation found their genesis in this broad sensory religious culture, but also reconfigured it. For all of their attacks on the sensual idolatry of what Eamon Duffy called "traditional religion," Protestants tended to avoid discussing the senses in their catechisms, which focused on doctrine rather than moral conduct. Luther's catechisms and the Calvinist Heidelberg Catechism of 1616 only mention them obliquely in discussions of the sacraments. Protestant moral and devotional literature, however, did discuss the senses. Richard Albott's *Wits Theater* urged their keeping and offered some basic theory, while Richard Day's 1578 *A Booke of Prayers* contained images of the five senses (Albott 1599: 28v, 37r–40r; Day 1578: 40r). It appears that Catholic works were more likely to teach readers about the senses. The senses featured in explanations of Extreme Unction and other sacraments in the Tridentine catechism, which saw the heart as the seat of the senses and, unlike any Protestant catechisms, listed off the sense organs (Tridentine Catechism, 65, 100–2, 118, 209, 354). Guides like Luis de la Puente's *Meditaciones de los mysterios de nuestra santa fe* contained entire sections on the senses following the sins and the Decalogue, while Luis de Granada's *Guia de Peccadores* instructed readers to govern their senses and mortify their appetites as part of Christian devotion (de Granada 1594: 151, 231, 295; de la Puente 1609: 289–95).

The Reformation drew on traditional models of sensory use and misuse. For many, the fear of sensory deceit and illusion by devils and witches intensified: Reginald Scot wrote in his 1584 *Discoverie of Witchcraft* that the witch's evil was "alwaies accomplished and finished by the eie" (Scot 1584). But religious polemicists disagreed on what example the disciple Thomas offered the faithful, and whether the dead could indeed sense. Johannes Bugenhagen questioned whether Thomas had actually touched Christ. On the whole, Protestants tended to emphasize Christ's actions and words, rather than Thomas's. For Catholics, Thomas's story became an exemplar for Tridentine doctrine as seen best in Caravaggio's painting (Most 2005: 139–49). As for the saints and heretics, there was also disagreement. Canisius's work on Mary reaffirmed her holiness and proper use of her senses; Protestants brushed the saints aside in their focus on Christ. While Protestants quickly saw their opponents as devotees caught up in worldly idolatry, the opponents of reform were quick to see reformers as heretics deluded by their senses. Early critics of Luther wondered if he had suffered some kind of damage to his senses (Melion 2009: 223–42, 252; More [1523] 1969: 535–7, 569). Luther and Calvin distrusted the senses, highlighting how prone they were to deceit. But they tended not to question how they functioned. For Calvin deceit was a matter of intellectual or mental blindness rather than the workings of the eye. For both, those whose ears worked just fine and heard the gospel, but had no regard for it, were no better than dumb beasts (Behringer 2007: 408; Calvin 1561: Book 2, 11r–14v; Book 3, 131v, 169v; Eire 1986: 232; Wandel 2009: 148–50). Consequently, while reformers asserted that the senses had no role in salvation, and were problematic in the extreme in matters of faith, many embraced established sensory theories (de Boer 2012: 367–72; Donnelly 1976: 6–12, 194; Luther [1522] 1908–10: 676–7; MacCulloch 2010: 606).

Despite its diverse texts and practices, Renaissance Christian culture drew heavily on Aristotelian theories and terminology to explain why control of the senses was essential to Christian living. While the Reformation reordered the points of contact and questioned the trustworthiness of the senses themselves, the crux remained proper control and governance of the senses. Discerning when to surrender the senses to godly experiences, and how to avoid or shun sinful worldliness was what kept the believer on the right path. Failure led to sin and "dropsie of the mynde" (Ling 1598: 5v; Thomas 1549: Aiir, Biiir).

WORSHIP AND PIETY

Fifteenth-century European Christianity was aesthetically vibrant. Its variegated churches, practices, artwork, and music are renowned. From Norway to Spain to Hungary the mass, the saints, purgatory, devotion to the Virgin and the saints, shaped local and regional interpretations of core doctrine and worship, devotional expression, and artistry. Communal piety centered on the mass, believing the consecration mystically rendered the bread and wine the very body and blood of Christ, which lay beyond the limits of human senses. Around this aporia was a rich cultural realm of vestments, vessels, incense, clergy, and choirs, accompanied by the saints, martyrs, and angels painted or carved on church walls, and numerous images of everyday life that manifested and proclaimed the Church's witness. Masses could be extremely spartan or highly opulent. More often than not laymen and women did not take communion, but focused their visual attention on the elevation as a kind of ocular communion as the host was lifted by the celebrant. Surrounding the mass were other sacraments that refashioned believers through touch, and the aurality of the daily rota of devotional offices and preaching. A further penumbra of practices used all of the senses in various ways to celebrate devotion but also move Christians towards charity by healing them of bodily and spiritual illnesses (Rubin and Simons 2009). Sensory theories were anything but removed from pre-Reformation theology, which saw the touch of a priest's hands, or washing with holy water, as the means by which God worked to bring about changes in Christian believers. In the case of baptism such sensing left an indelible mark in the soul that was continually reinforced by encounters with the sensibly sacred (Reynolds 2005: 67–9, 73–9; Stanbury 2008: 172–90). This sensible piety undergirded all religious practices, making pre-Reformation Christianity's sacred sounds, sights, smells, touches, and tastes that means reforming of the individual towards godliness.

In many ways we can understand this sensual splendor as a demonstration of the belief that religious sensing led to the restoration of fallen humanity. Its transformative potential fueled the renowned works of Michelangelo and

Raphael, the sumptuous chapel frescoes of Domenico Ghirlandaio, or the masterful triptychs of Flemish artists. But this flowering was also musical: the fifteenth century saw choral polyphony come of age. The mass settings and devotional works of Franco-Flemish composers like Josquin des Prez and Jacob Obrecht stand as musical analogues to the visuality of painting and sculpture. Though we can remark on the works of individual artists and composers, the provision of this sensual abundance was a communal endeavor. It took rich cities, merchants, or rulers to see through grand projects like the doors of the Duomo's baptistery in Florence, or the churches of Venice, or the altarpiece of Toledo cathedral. Religious communities, whether parishes, confraternities, or religious houses, participated in this culture of provision within their means. Since this religious material culture aided the spiritual well-being of everyone, dead or alive, funding it was also a charitable work.

Renewed interest in Neoplatonic thought inspired the exploration of the religious potentials of human imagination and sensation through such religious artistry (Hankins 2006: 149). For Marsilio Ficino the senses were the means for mystic ascent; properly guided sensory desires could elevate and purify the mind (Kraye 1988: 312–13; Levi 2002: 124; Vinge 1975: 12). Artistry was a powerful tool in this enterprise, and the artist a kind of god whose imaginative creations mediated the sensible and insensible realms (Carman 2009: 181; Jurkowlaniec 2009: 211–23; Pugliese and Kavaler 2009: 19–29). Neoplatonic thought vindicated Renaissance artistic expression, transforming it into a route to the restoration of human righteousness. The German prelate, scholar, and mystic Nicholas of Cusa drew heavily on these themes in his mystical and devotional writings which abound with sensory theory, especially visuality and optics (Green 2011: 212, 222). Ficino and Cusa are prominent examples of the extremely complex interplay between the senses, affect, morality, mysticism, and artistic ingenuity in fifteenth-century Christianity. The largely northern European Devotio Moderna movement took up many of the same issues, but sought to apply them to practical piety. Inspired by the works of Geert Grote, and highly influenced by Augustine, the Devotio taught how highly sensory meditation on the life of Christ, rather than new artistic creations, reformed believers. Thomas à Kempis's *Imitatio Christi* urged careful discipline of the senses to bring about an inner moral conversion (à Kempis 1997: 5, 10, 27, 67; Levi 2002: 140–5; MacCulloch 2010: 565–7).

Many of these strands fed into humanist culture and scholarship, reinforcing belief that sensing led to actual and real moral reform of individuals. The *studia humanitatis* so central to the Renaissance was always *studia pietatis*, linking the moral concerns of sensing in classical works and contemporary piety (Caffero 2011: 187; Levi 2002: 92–3, 109–11). The late fifteenth century saw a shift in humanist works, however, towards Christian over classical virtues, which drew on patristic authors and in no small way was influenced by the Devotio. Best seen in the works of Erasmus, this *philosophia Christi* urged strict regulation of conduct and the senses as key to inner spiritual growth. Erasmus laid out his practical program for pious moral reform in his 1503 *Enchiridion Militis Christiani*. Its rules, which boil down to a simple quotation "to be holy, ignore the demands of your senses," placed control of the senses at the heart of the Christian quest for virtue and the conflict between flesh and the spirit. The Christian, Erasmus urged, was to "develop a fine sense of discernment" to combat the blindness caused by original sin, and to ensure that he or she maintained a life that imitated Christ's (Dolan 1983: 52–3, 60–4, 71–5; Eire 1986: 30–4; MacCulloch 2010: 594–601).

It is difficult to overestimate the importance of the sensory practices of discernment to Renaissance Christianity. Sensing brought with it immense risks because contemporary theories gave so much agency to things believers sensed. The most dangerous vices were those that had the veneer of virtue. The fear was that the sensory-fueled human artistry of the Renaissance counterfeited the divine. This apprehension played into growing anxiety over the devil and his deceits (Clark 2007: 39–49; Dolan 1983: 66–70; Levi 2002: 124). The unease surrounding the authenticity of religious sensing in the fifteenth century is evident in the founding of the Spanish Inquisition in 1478, the growth of witch-hunting and the publication of the *Malleus Maleficarum*, and unease over possession and spiritual visions. These were accompanied by increasingly complex lists of sins in confessors' manuals (Gentilcore 2008: 605). Each, in their own way, as Behringer has noted with the discretion of spirits, entailed "elaborate procedure[s] of evaluation" (Behringer 2007: 406; Clark 2007: 223–6; Levi 2002: 250; McGinn 2011: 200) where the senses were used to root out diabolic verisimilitude. Savonarola's burning of vanities in Florence in the 1490s illustrates what might occur when these strands and an ardent sense of Christian morality mingled with secular politics (Caffero 2011: 190; Clark 2007: 126; MacCulloch 2010: 591–3).

This growing culture of discernment meshed with the *philosophia Christi*, bringing about real concern that the sensual splendour and practices of Renaissance piety were inappropriate, or even ungodly. In his *Enchiridion* Erasmus asserted that outward actions, or "external ceremonies," had no efficacy or meaning on their own without spiritual engagement on the part of believers (Dolan 1983: 65–8). In his *Morae Encomium* Erasmus, like his compatriots Thomas More, Lefevre d'Etaples, John Colet, Juan Vives, and

Cisneros, mocked the sensory piety of his contemporaries. Not only was it void of spiritual meaning, it was dangerous. Calls for clerical purity and reform, from humanists and observant clerics like Colet and Giles of Viterbo, were fueled by the fear of the sensuality of fifteenth-century piety (Gregory 2007b: 590–1). Interest in reform preceded the sixteenth century because the moral concerns of sensory governance and right worship were treated in the same breath. In the end it is apparent that while Renaissance religious culture exploited the senses to reshape Christians, its experiences were completely contingent upon the authenticity of its practices and artistry. As Stuart Clark has put it, the Renaissance culture of discernment, coupled with anxiety and sensing that transformed individuals, created a paradox because the dangers and benefits of sensing constantly intensified the need to verify what was going into European senses (Bouwsma 1980: 225–30; Clark 2002: 227–32).

These anxieties about the authenticity and sensuality of Renaissance Christianity took on new dimensions when Luther questioned whether any good works had any role in salvation. This not only included sacraments, or giving to the poor, but piety, artwork, and devotion. For Protestants, Christians were saved because of a divine promise of redemption. Faith, which came from hearing the gospel, did not encompass the sensible practices of the institutional Church (Cameron 2012: 13–200; McGrath 2005: 214; Romans 10:17). This shift meant reformers could observe the traditional prohibition on using the senses to determine faith while opening up all religious practices to sensible scrutiny. The other cornerstone of their theology was the paramount authority of scripture (Luther [1522] 1908–10: 663; MacCulloch 2010: 580). Undermining the authority of the Church raised doubts about which religious experiences and practices were godly. The traditional call for Christians to discern all things, so important in pre-Reformation Christian morality, consequently obliged the use of the senses to compare scripture with the state of the Church. Reformers found it wanting and sensually dangerous.

The fear of sensuality, both as misgovernance and as deceit, made religious reform a vast exercise in discernment. If its impetus was traditional, what reformers sought to discern was not. Though Thomas's sensing warned about using the senses in matters of faith, reformers went about to identify false religion with their senses and replace it with godly piety. Regardless of doctrinal differences, all reformers embraced a sense-based compare and contrast approach to the status quo as the means for setting Christianity on the right course. Both sides called for proper use of the senses, to root out either heresy or idolatry, and highlighted their opponents' failures to do so. William Tyndale succinctly told his readers, because traditionalists had lied, true Christians ought to "judge them in all thinges" (Tyndale 1845: 90). Lutheran artwork exemplified this early on. Cranach's 1521 *Passional und Antichristi* contrasted the pope's Church against scriptural piety (Uppenkamp 2009: 251–3). The trope became a Protestant hallmark and was historicized in works like John Foxe's *Acts and Monuments* or *The Magdeburg Centuries*, which told the tale of Rome's culture of dissimulation and sensuality. Catholic polemicists weren't far behind: Konrad Schlüsselburg's *Haereticorum Catalogus* cast Protestants as just more in a long line of heretics who threatened the Church. For Protestants scripture was the template for reconstituting godly piety, while for their opponents it sat alongside the practices and hierarchy of the Church. Not surprisingly, actual reform entailed describing the sensible attributes of true Christianity in confessional, doctrinal, and regulatory documents (Clark 2007: 78–80, 128, 174; Wright 2005: 98).

Initially, reformers sought to put the "rein Evangelium," the pure gospel, into the eyes, ears, and hands of European Christians through new scriptural translations and vernacular preaching (Pettegree 2005: 19, 27–8; Taylor 2002). Access to scripture fueled reform, and Protestant attacks on traditional piety turned quickly to focus on abuse and idolatry. The first great conflict arose over images in 1522 when Luther's colleague, Andreas Bodenstein von Karlstadt, instigated their violent removal from Wittenberg's castle church and instituted a trimmed down vernacular mass. Luther returned in haste from the Wartburg where he was translating the New Testament into German and opposed Karlstadt on both counts (Eire 1990: 58–61). For Lutherans, images remained didactic tools for the illiterate. In contrast, Swiss and later Reformed Christianity claimed they were idols. The difference arose from the numbering of the Ten Commandments as Reformed churches adhered to the Jewish belief that the prohibition on images was its own specific commandment (Aston 1988: 183, 372–8, 435–7; Bucer 1535: B3r, B4r, C7v). And so Lutheran churches retained much of their medieval artwork, while Reformed churches were stripped bare. Sometimes iconoclasm proceeded peacefully under the direction of a magistrate, but it could also be the work of crowds or mobs, as in the summer of 1566 in the Low Countries. The destruction of statuary is particularly telling of the Reformed belief that finite artwork was no home for infinite divinity (Eire 1986: 197). The eyes of statues were gouged out, hands, ears, and noses knocked off, denying their senses any potency. In a gruesome twist, a papal "heretic" was even burned using the wood of an idolatrous statue in England (Clark 2007: 166–79; Marshall 1998: 351–74).

More broadly conceived iconoclastic fury also focused on tastes, sounds, and smells. Sacramentals like salts, creams, spittle, holy oils, and incense disappeared, though when and how varied. Incense remained an important fumigant, but all leading reformers urged its removal from worship (Baum 2013: 336–42; Karant-Nunn 2007: 376). Attacks on the mass captured the full extent of the dangers of traditional piety. Its liturgy was like the whore of Babylon, whose sensuality lured in unsuspecting believers. Even gestures were idolatrous; kneeling and the sign of the cross were done away with in many reformed jurisdictions, earliest in Zurich (Becon 1844: 354, 389; Eire 1986). Vestments were a thorny issue. Reformed Christians, on the whole, opted for academic dress for ministers, though England was an exception. Lutheran ministers continued to garb in surplices, and unlike the other Churches retained auricular confession. Paraliturgical practices like processions were curtailed or suppressed, carnival was attacked as sensual in Nuremberg and elsewhere, and the tradition of *Rauchnächte* cast aside too (Johnston 2000: 550; Karant-Nunn 2007: 374–5).

The stereotype of Protestantism as a religion of the ear comes from its focus on the Word and scripture in preaching and vernacular worship. Both made the gospel accessible to those who heard it. Along with the administration of the two remaining sacraments of baptism and the Eucharist, preaching was a sensible mark of the true Church. It was accompanied by communal prayer and often sung psalmody. Luther himself was a skilled musician, and Lutheran churches made quick and effective use of new hymns set to well-known tunes. England retained its cathedral choirs and love of polyphony, but by midcentury Reformed churches had embraced metrical translations of the psalms set to new tunes. Preaching, prayer, and psalmody made these churches auditoria (Coster and Spicer 2005; Mochizuki 2008). As Richard Hooker put it, prayer made others ear-witnesses to faith. We would be remiss, however, to think it was all ears. Authentic worship was visual since it required witnesses. Baptisms, or the laying on of hands, where it was retained, were only lawful if they were seen. The laity received the taste of communion more frequently, and the elements stayed bread and wine, rather than body and blood. Nevertheless, Protestants were anything but agreed on what constituted the sensuality of worship (Benedict 2002: 301–16; Calvin 1567: 20r; Eire 1986: 72, 201; Karant-Nunn 2007: 373, 378; MacCulloch 2010: 577–9; McGrath 2005: 45).

Those loyal to Rome, in contrast to the sensual fear of idolatry, sought to rein in the unbridled sensuality of heresy. Though there was agreement that certain practices were abused, and some sympathy for reformers' views on justification, until the opening of the Council of Trent in 1547, the opponents of reform focused on heresy, the excesses of traditional piety, and the prohibition on using the senses in matters of faith. When it met, the Council only turned to religious practices after clarifying doctrine. Much of traditional piety was reaffirmed, but stricter regulations were placed on local piety. The mass remained central alongside the other six sacraments, prayers for the dead, devotional images, clerical vestments, the cult of the saints, and the sacramentals. Preaching took on a renewed life. Between 1568 and 1614 a new set of liturgical texts appeared, binding the Church in external ritual forms. As François Quiviger's contribution illustrates, Trent also saw a renewal of religious artistry and its role in Catholic worship. Equally as important was the role of music and sacred theatricality, seen in Cavalieri's first oratorio in 1600, *Rappresentatione di Anime e di Corpo*, which stressed the need for sensory control and inspired the renewal of public religiosity (Karant-Nunn, 2007: 379–80; MacCulloch 2010: 681–3; Wright 2005: 198–208).

Mission in the New World mixed Tridentine aesthetic fervor with indigenous cultures. In the Americas Catholicism literally built upon the ruins of its predecessors; churches sat in temple grounds, or even, as at Santaria Nuestra Señora de los Remedios, on a pyramid. The "capilla real" at Cholula is a blend of cultures, based on a mosque-turned-church in Spain, which in turn was based on the al-Aqsa mosque in Jerusalem (MacCulloch 2010: 698–9). Myriad influences resulted in stunning interiors towards the end of the seventeenth century, as at Tonantzintla and Tepotzotlan. New materials like copal resin (whose name "Jesuits' Balsam" suggests its use in holy oils), native flora and fauna, became part of Christian worship. The maize papier-mâché crucifixes, *Cristos de Caña*, were more often than not made from old Aztec documents (Ryu 2011). Over the past decade musicologists have rediscovered the existence of lively musical cultures in Bolivian Jesuit missionaries. Nahuatl compositions of Mexico sit alongside Latin liturgical music as the earliest examples of choral music in the Americas. Scores and crucifixes made their way back to the Iberian peninsula, influencing European Christian piety in return.

Radicals went further in their reform efforts. They denied the authority of magistrates as well as bishops, and saw scripture as a literal template for worship, or only as inspiration. Anabaptism tends to be dated to the rebaptism of believers at Zurich in 1527. A ritual form, a *Form of the Supper of Christ*, appeared that year, but on the whole Anabaptist worship tended to follow principles rather than texts. It was simplistic, emphasized preaching, even by women, and congregational participation (Roth 2007: 370–3; Rothkegel 2007: 170–8). The Eucharist was a memorial. Generally singing was allowed, though instruments were prohibited; Conrad Grebel, the "father" of Anabaptists, forbade singing altogether. Worship was usually clandestine due to persecution.

Spiritualist radicals placed less need on external practices and piety. Followers of Caspar Schwenkfeld even stopped the Eucharist, and thought that baptism was not necessary because of inner baptism by the spirit.

Protestantism's early affinity with humanism collapsed, and took with it the links between piety, practice, and the senses which had formed over the previous century. Erasmus and Luther's mid-1520s clash over free will went to the heart of this divorce. Luther argued not only that the sovereignty of God and the sacrifice of Christ rendered human actions inconsequential, but that to assign any value to them, including sensing, was a grave transgression of divine work (Levi 2002: 300; Luther [1522] 1908–10: 614–16, 634–6). His rebuttal of Erasmus proclaimed the utter depravity of humanity and its enslaved, corrupted will. It was a dramatic reversal of the Renaissance lauding of human capabilities. Salvation by faith alone severed the links between sensing and salvation that lay at the heart of Catholic doctrine. No longer, for Protestants, would sensing save by transforming believers. However, the Catholic emphasis on good works meant religious sensing and experiences still had a role in salvation. This fundamental difference profoundly shaped how piety related to the senses. Protestant preaching shifted away from identifying with Christ's sensible pains to focus on the emotional horrors of human sin. Not only could Christians not imitate Christ, imagining his suffering was ineffective. Anxiety over sin was on much more stable theological ground as it drove believers towards repentance (Karant-Nunn 2010: 71–85, 97–122). In contrast, Catholic preaching continued to embrace sensory experiences as the means to moral betterment and salvation of believers. Focus on the humanity of Christ sensibly moved and affected believers to imitate and identify with him as the key to personal spiritual transformation (Karant-Nunn 2010: 30–64, 169).

Individual piety is difficult to analyze precisely because it is where sensory culture actually met sensing. Believers mediated external and internal spiritual senses, but also reconciled, disagreed, or took up religious practices and their aesthetics. Protestant scriptural religion emphasized the private taste and tactility of reading printed scripture. Despite their churches, Reformed Christians still had religious images in their homes and new translations of scripture (Pettegree 2000: 118). Nevertheless, Catholics simply had more devotional options. The Rosary stands out; it was more than a mnemonic device as its beads were ideally made of odoriferous woods or compacted rose petals. The smell of its prayers wafted as incense to divine nostrils, while the rose imagery invoked the Virgin herself. The forty-hour devotion to the host was extremely visual (Gentilcore 2008: 612; Wright 2005: 213). Catholic devotion to the sacred heart and the passion, in which believers like Ulrich Pinder engaged Christ's sufferings and pains in artwork and imaginative devotions, employed sensing as the vehicle for heartfelt transformation of believers (Karant-Nunn 2010: 219–21; Wright 2005: 217–18). Bernini's *Ecstasy of Saint Theresa* captures this heartfelt piety most succinctly.

The transformative potential of pious sensing continued to fuel Catholic devotional and ascetic practices. Francisco de Osuna's 1527 *Spiritual Alphabet*, and the spiritual exercises of Ximenez de Cisneros, developed the regimented approach evident in Erasmus's *Enchiridion*. Its pinnacle remains the *Spiritual Exercises* of Ignatius Loyola which lay at the heart of Jesuit pedagogy and devotional culture. These exercises drew heavily on the Bonaventurian tradition which asked users to envisage moments in the life of Christ, but also sought highly sensualized meditation on personal sins and the pains of hell. For Loyola, mortification of the flesh conquered worldly desires, while intense spiritual sensing formed the mind for the religious life (Loyola 1914: 136–8; J. Smith 2002: 29–39). The *Exercises* saw sensory regulation as the means to the truly devout Christian life; their spiritual devotional regimen, which emphasized control of worldly sensing, was critical in the Jesuit-led reconversion of lost areas of Europe. Both Canisius and François de Sales lauded its ability to save souls.

Catholic personal piety drew heavily on the fluidity between external and internal sensing where imagination collated sensory experiences and spiritual themes (McGinn 2011: 190–1). The rich sensory language of Teresa of Avila and the devotional poetry and works of John of the Cross epitomize this movement from inner sensory piety to the ineffable mystical moment. Teresa urged Christians to visualize each word of the Pater Noster as they prayed. John of the Cross warned, however, that even ascetic practices could be deceiving (Bensimon 1974: 248; Kavanaugh 1999: 105, 112). Only by avoiding the "contradictions of sensuality" could the believer approach the divine; the self-imposed purified darkness of blindness prevented sensory deception (Kavanaugh 1999: 37, 61, 65). Protestants also retained rich sensual spiritual devotion. Writers and poets like Pierre Viret, George Herbert, and William Perkins described their piety in intensely sensual ways, while such practices in many ways defined spiritualist radicals like David Joris (Clark 2007: 190–1; McLaughlin 2007: 122–40; Perkins 1600: 816; Schwartz 2008: 640–2; Wainwright 2011: 225–8, 238; Waite, 1990). The problem was whether faith itself was a kind of feeling. Thomas More ridiculed William Tyndale for this in the 1530s, but the theme persisted. While Luther (not surprisingly) contradicted himself on the matter, Calvin strongly argued against thinking that feeling was an indication of election (Karant-Nunn 2010: 83). Nevertheless, many Protestants sought to see spiritual sensations as proof of true faith. As Protestants stripped bare their external pieties, especially the Reformed, they made up for it by exploring the guts of Christian contrition and the possibilities of internal sensing.

The greatest consequence of the Reformation for European sensory culture was the Protestant view that while piety thrust the rhetoric of Christ's saving acts into the eyes and ears of churchgoers, sensing had no role in salvation (Davies 1979: 100–2; Tyndale 1848: 360–1): sensuality remained sinfully sensory. The sensible signs of true piety, like weeping or moaning, reminded others of their own sin and Christ's promise, but did not transform others. Even so, the senses remained the source of human woe and sin. But this presented a dilemma for Protestants as the old remedies for sinful sensuality had been godly sensing of sacred images, relics, and the sacraments. Reformers removed these idols and provided for scriptural religion, but it was difficult to prevent reorientation of this sensual piety onto scripture, preaching, or fasting. Claims that touching scripture, or merely hearing rather than listening to a preacher, did something beneficial went against Protestant doctrine. This was the precise reason Luther warned against iconoclasm: that it itself would be construed as a good work (Eire 1986: 69). Yet distinction between hearing the gospel as message and its aural or tactile experience of it as the last relic was difficult to make in practice (Clark 1997: 284–91; Hunt 2010; Wabuda 2002: 68–77; Walsham 2008: 510–16). Zachäus Faber of Chemnitz mocked the Catholic belief that the anointing of the senses at extreme unction had medicinal effects (Karant-Nunn 2010: 142–3; Jütte 2003: 104–5). The lack of good efficacious sensing was most acutely felt among Protestants when dealing with demonic possession. It is in the belief that religious experiences continued to have some kind of spiritual efficacy where the history of the senses meets the histories of magic and historical accounts of disenchantment or desacralization that are so important to the early modern period.

SENSING AND RELIGIOUS CONFLICT

These sensory concerns and dynamics extended well beyond doctrine and worship. The discernment necessary to carry out reform was politically, as well as morally, configured, as it hinged on whose senses were best suited to the task. Though baptism traditionally allowed an individual the ability to discern between good and evil, it did not grant the right to adjudicate for the entire community. The Church's great prelates, the bishops, were defined by this right: episcopacy was an ocular office. The magistrate or the king was the other model for the Christian governor, and had Christ as his prototype. Bishops and kings or magistrates obtained the abilities necessary for good governance with their office, and both, as censors, were tasked with keeping the senses of others. The Renaissance saw another round in their long contestation. In Protestant lands, magistrates won the day; even where bishops remained they derived their powers of oversight from princes. The independence of bishops, with their episcopal rights and gifts, was a tricky matter for the Council of Trent, which attempted to steer clear of the issue for fear of undermining papal authority. We need only to look at Philip II of Spain, though, to assuage any belief that Roman Catholic monarchs thought differently than their Protestant counterparts (Clark 1997: 619–32, 2007: 12; Hunt 2008: 29; Wright 2005: 162–3). At the same time many Renaissance scholars emphasized the effects of godly erudition and good learning on men who properly controlled their senses. Whether the capabilities needed for good Christian governance and the discernment of true religion were endowed by an office, or could be acquired, remained an important source of contention that shaped the politics of reform.

Consequently, accusations of sensuality were a crucial element in religious polemic, and were linked to social discipline. Bishops, monks, priests, and especially popes, appeared in early German woodcuts in the 1520s as anthropomorphized animals, making them out to be sensual beasts. These apes of antichrist were driven by their sensuality to lechery, gluttony, false religion, and idolatry; they danced their way into the jaws of hell with the incense, relics, and images of their deceitful religion (Marprelate 1580; Ryrie 2003: 43–4; Scribner 1994: 74). In contrast reformers cast themselves as men of discretion and good sensory governance. To their opponents, such claims were absurd. Like Thomas, heretics put their senses over faith. Canisius wondered whether Luther was blind (Melion 2009: 245). Charges of sensuality aimed to discredit opponents, even rulers, as delusional or mad. Luther called Henry VIII of England a vicious insensate wooden post, while debates over the rights of magistrates connected tyranny with misguided sensing (Iunius 1599: 79–80, 84–5, 130–1; Luther [1522] 1908–10: 192, 195, 206, 215; Maier 1980: 173–81; Pettegree 2005: 32). Not surprisingly, claims of sensory control often accompanied claims of authority. Seats on Protestant church councils and consistories that monitored moral comportment, as well as religious practices and finances, were filled by men of "discretion." Church governance was intimately linked to social discipline and regulation of speech, eating, sexuality, and the needs of everyday life. The oversight of Christian virtue and persecution of vice was fueled by the continued fear of diabolic and worldly sensuality

(Benedict 2002; de Boer 2001; Gentilcore 2008: 617; Gorski 2003; Parker 1998; Po-Chia Hsia 1992: 122–73; Spierenburg and Roodenburg 2004; Wright 2005: 227). Those who rebelled, or did not conform, were often seen as deviants who had failed to govern their senses. The lines between persecution, prosecution, and good sensing, though, were porous: the punishment of heretics or idolaters was demonstration of God's justice in the eyes of persecutors, while for their brethren, such suffering was an indication of true faith.

The sensuality of suffering and demonstrations of political and military power were crucial to early modern religious conflicts. Violence between religious groups was as much a religious experience as devotional imagery, as it was the cultural and social "psychomachia," or battle between vice and virtue, writ large. Whether iconoclastic fury or persecution, religious violence was a sensible expression of godly fury or the pain of a godly martyr. The gore of the Peasants' War of 1524–6 was followed by over a century of religious warfare that included, among others, the massacre of Anabaptists at Münster in 1534–5 following their failed utopia under Jan van Leyden. The subjugation and slaughter of religious rivals were sensible displays of rulers' godly power (Klötzer 2007: 217–56). Though conflicts emerged in the British Isles, Italy, the Low Countries, and the Empire, the St. Bartholomew's Day massacre in Paris in 1572 stands out for its sensible brutality. Pregnant Protestant women were cut open and thrown into the Seine by Catholics, their foetuses dangling out of lacerated wombs; blood coloring the water and pavement. Autos da Fe, the carrying of faggots in penance, beheadings, drownings, or burning at the stake were highly sensory. Burning flesh smelled, as did the release of bowels at death, smoke, and fires. The cutting touches of swords and halberds accompanied the sights and screams of slaughter, in the square or the battlefield. French street fighting saw Protestant psalm tunes used as battle songs. A heretic or martyr's death came with the jeering of crowds, the smell of incense, and the sight of vestments (Davis 1973; Gregory 2007a: 469–71). As Christianity spread to the Americas and Asia, missionaries brought this violence with them. Iconoclasm itself was central to conquest: in the Americas religious sites underwent the same kinds of destruction for fear of idolatrous sensuality, and in this case it was carried out by Catholics. But missionaries also were tortured and died for their faith in Brazil and Japan (Metcalf 2007; Whitehead 2009). Sensible pains of religious violence were experienced spiritually by those who underwent and witnessed them often allowing suffering to be transformed. In Europe, Anabaptists sung of the cathartic pains of martyrdom in their hymns, while histories like Foxe's *Acts and Monuments* recalled patristic and scriptural accounts of martyrdom that turned the smoke of fires into incense (Foxe 1563; Gregory 2007a: 475).

Despite their common cultural inheritance, how communities reconciled new doctrine positions with the everyday needs of worship and Christian living resulted in increasingly distinct sensory cultures that defined religious or confessional identities. An appreciation of the senses or religious aesthetics shifts the focus of confessionalization away from institutional social processes, to the more blurred and complex processes of cultural translation arising out of religious practices. As Susan Karant-Nunn has shown with emotions, confessionalized aesthetics grew as much from the culture shared by European Christians as the perspectives and practices created by doctrinal changes and rigidity (Karant-Nunn 2010: 245–55). The senses were instrumental in shaping what it was to be Lutheran, Anabaptist, Reformed, or Catholic. These confessional cultures leaked across borders and bureaucracies. The godly recognized each other by their pieties (Willen 1995: 20). Confessional identity was aesthetic: everyday shared gestures, sights, smells, and sounds bound communities together in ways that doctrine or language might not. Even national Churches could have different languages, as did the English Church with its Latin, French, and Welsh prayerbooks. Nevertheless its worship maintained the same gestures and aesthetic parameters. The prohibition on music in Zurich, the persistence of images in Hungary, and England's insistence on set liturgical text, choral music, and vestments were contentious precisely because they transgressed larger trans-national expectations more than doctrine per se. Equally the continuation of the Mozarabic and Ambrosian liturgies in Catholicism did little to disrupt the aesthetics of Tridentine Catholicism. Christians at home and abroad, like Sebald Welser, wrote of these distinctions in journals and diaries, describing both the beauty and profound dangers of the lands and peoples they encountered, including rival confessions, whether in Europe or abroad (Ozment 1996; Whitehead 2009: 86–95). Sensory discernment and regulation were essential to the grafting as much as the rejection of new and different sensations and experiences into what was becoming worldwide Christianity.

SENSES, RELIGION, AND EARLY MODERNITY

Perhaps the most important watershed for the history of the senses in the Renaissance was the belief that sensing might not be as transformative as medieval thought suggested. Religious co-existence forced practical consideration that bodily experiences of a rival religious expression might have no inherent danger on their own. Of course many argued against this, Calvin chief among them, asserting that merely attending the mass was detrimental. But as with proving election by feeling, the crux was sensible demonstration. Whether in the fatigue evident in Montaigne's skepticism, or Melanchthon's notion of *adiaphora* or indifference, we find a growing sense that religious sensing had no effect without intellectual and rational engagement. Persuasion was always a part of Reformation rivalry, but this suggests that believers had to consider whether religious experiences and their sensations moved or failed to move them, regardless of what authorities asserted was authentic or not. No longer were human sensibilities of a piece, in terms of religious experiences, with those of animals. Sensuality, and its religious and moral implications, were in the eye of the beholder (Gregory 2007b: 565, 597; Wandel 2009: 149–51).

At first more a hint than a sentiment, seventeenth-century natural philosophy and epistemology radically altered how the senses, choice, and the mind related to one another, reinforcing these trends. Cartesian philosophy grew out of the fraught sensory cultures of the Renaissance, drawing clearer demarcation between the mind and the body, and placed sensory deceit, rather than the mind, at the heart of epistemological problems. The collapse of Aristotelian philosophy brought about a re-evaluation of the senses, coinciding with the end of the Renaissance, and the emergence of an ardently confessionalized Christianity. When the dust settled in 1648, the Treaties of the Peace of Westphalia not only legalized Calvinism in the Empire, they gave men and women the freedom of conscience and right to emigrate for religious conviction. The ups and downs of religious conflict and upheaval had failed to assert any clear answer, while the new philosophy and medicine suggested new ways of thinking about the senses. Galileo remarked in correspondence on the similarities between the interests and methods of the new science and Protestant uses of the Bible (Feldhay 2008: 731, 746). The Renaissance, its religiosities, and sensation defined each other in critical ways. How religious upheavals catalyzed changes regarding the senses *in toto*, and how the history of the senses might recast the well-manicured landscapes of the Renaissance and Reformation, is only just beginning to be appreciated. With recent work we obtain a glimpse of the work that remains (de Boer and Goettler 2012).

CHAPTER FIVE

The Senses in Philosophy and Science: From the Nobility of Sight to the Materialism of Touch

DANIJELA KAMBASKOVIC AND CHARLES T. WOLFE

> One of the greatest difficulties in Physics lies in understanding the operations of the senses.
> Mersenne 1636, I.v.1, prop. LI: 79

> Someone should write a book on the epistemology of the sense of touch.
> Bennett 1971: 102

> The hands—despised for their materialism.
> Diderot 1975–, IV: 140

The choice of a particular sense in the construction of a metaphysical hierarchy, a rank-ordering of the world, is a classic motif, on display notably in the Platonic and Aristotelian privileging of sight as the noblest of senses. The meaning of *theoria* as contemplation takes center stage here, with the thinker being defined by her contemplative distance from the object experienced;

indeed, most Indo-European terms for mental activity apparently derive from words for vision or the visible (Biernoff 2002: 66). To privilege one sense is of course to downgrade others. If sight is privileged in the idealist philosophical tradition, as the contemplation at a distance of the objects of perception, touch, the contact sense, the dirty sense, is all the way at the other extreme. This is the case, whether in a libertine sense or in the way early modern "empiricks" or barber-surgeons get their "hands dirty," whereas learned professors of medicine do not (including by touching someone's beating heart, as William Harvey describes in his encounter with the nobleman Hugh Montgomery, whose heart was covered with a metal plate after a wound that healed, leaving an opening (Harvey 1653, Ex. 52; Salter and Wolfe 2009).

Touch is spread throughout the body and is the least abstract, and therefore basest. But, as shown by medieval and early modern theological debates regarding the pivotal role of touch in following the path of virtue or vice, not all is bad. Touch may be spread throughout the body, but it is also located in the hand, the focus of worthy and noble human activities. In *The Allegory of Touch* (1618; one of five paintings representing each of the senses, a collaboration between Rubens and Breughel the Elder), Elizabeth Harvey has called attention to the hand's crucial role as an organ of touch that bridges mind and body, showing how it oscillates in the image with a more diffuse somatic theme: the protective armor that shields the body from harm. She quotes John Bulwer asserting, in his *Chirologia; or, The Naturall Language of the Hand* (1644), that the hand is the "*Spokesman* of the Body," speaking a universal language that is understood by all (Bulwer 1644: 2–3, in Harvey 2011: 396). The hand defines the self, as it is impossible to touch without being touched. It takes on the role of a teacher of the mind, both through pleasure, and through the pain that it gives.

Other senses have other narratives and other valuative investments. Martin Luther constructed an entire metaphysics of hearing, for the Word is not something to be seen or touched, but heard (see the analysis of Luther and Kant in Schürmann 2003). Luther glosses Matthew 11:15 and Revelation 2:7 as:

> He that hath ears to hear, let him hear, and he that doth not, let him be left behind, earless, unhearing, deaf," and "a right faith goes right on *with its eyes closed*; it clings to God's Word; it follows that Word; it believes the Word even when all creatures are against it, even if it should seem to the flesh that nothing is less likely to happen than what the Word wants believed.
>
> *Lectures on Jonah* 1:1, in Luther 1974, 19: 8, emphasis added

The distantiation-function inherent in hearing—as I wait to hear The Word—is used by Luther as a counterpoint to both the idealism of the scholastic theologians and the naïve "touch" empiricism of the humanists. The theologian and natural philosopher Marin Mersenne also deemed hearing a better, more reliable sense than sight or touch, which often cannot distinguish between bodies, and sounding rather like Luther, added that "this may be why God wanted revealed truths to be received by the ear, which is less likely to be deceived than the eye" (Mersenne 1636, I.i, prop. XI: 20).

Taste and smell are subject to equally contrasting interpretations, but tend to be associated with our animal nature. It would appear that no sense is immune to the essential ethical ambiguity that characterizes human life. In this chapter we examine some key moments in the evaluative metaphysics of the senses—the role a given sense will play in the construction of a metaphysics but also a system of value—in the centuries prior to the emergence of a unified, experimental life science. We pay particular attention to sight (including optics), unsurprisingly, but also to touch, which has often been the "poor relative" of sight and hearing—an opposition which Bakhtin famously presented as that between high and low culture, in his project to exhume a history of the body and its urges: a Rabelaisian, explosive body with its socially destabilizing potential (Bakhtin 1984). Moments of the revalorization of touch discussed here—sometimes provocative, sometimes innocent—include medicine, theater, and metaphysics.

After all, no less a philosopher than the very ahistorical Jonathan Bennett recommended that "Someone should write a book on the epistemology of the sense of touch" (Bennett 1971: 102)—for it is not just Plato, Descartes, or the metaphysics of light: philosophy per se tends to privilege sight. But unlike Bakhtin or, today, *mentalité*-inspired historians like Alain Corbin (Corbin 1988), we will not try to reconstruct particular historical regimes of the senses. Our attempt, if fleshed out further, would be closer to what John Sutton calls "historical cognitive science," which "works between two projects": "the analysis of other and older theories of mind, how they relate to and differ from current approaches, and what forgotten or neglected explananda they bring into focus" but also, "relating to cognitive practices rather than theories": "the task of working out how such views about mind and self reflect or partly cause different historical forms of mental activity" (Sutton 2000: 117). One might hear echoes here of Benjamin's inquiries into the historicity of perception, in his celebrated 1936 essay "The Work of Art in the Age of Mechanical Reproduction" (Benjamin 1968) and throughout his writings (on Baudelaire, Paris, photography, etc.), which themselves may echo Marx's own intuitions regarding the historicity of the senses (Howes 2005b).

A papyrus purchased in Cairo in 1901 by Ludwig Borchardt, upon examination, contained two distinct texts (recto and verso), the second of which was the work of an author whose hitherto unknown or missing works had led him to be excluded from the front ranks of Stoicism: Hierocles, a major disciple of Chrysippus (Heller-Roazen 2007: 117ff.). In this verso text, Hierocles comes closer than perhaps any other author before the early modern materialists to expressing the knot which binds together the senses and the world of value: "Sensation [*aisthēsis*] contributes to the knowledge of the first thing that is one's own and familiar and it is precisely that discourse which we have said constitutes the best principle for the elements of ethics" (1.36, in Heller-Roazen 2007: 119). To the above-mentioned investigations into the historical, cognitive, affective sedimentation of particular sensory regimes (à la Febvre) we add the metaphysical, valuative dimension that Hierocles orthogonally points to: the senses as construction and valorization of a world.

THE NOBILITY OF SIGHT AND THE SOLAR EYE

The Platonic and Aristotelian sources of medieval and Renaissance thought (and beyond) privilege sight and depreciate touch. Plato spoke of "the eye of the soul" (*Republic* VII.527d), also equating the eye with the sun, and allocating this organ the highest ethical capacity. Aristotle famously interwove sight, contemplation, and philosophy itself at the beginning of the *Metaphysics*: "We prefer sight, generally speaking, to all other senses . . . [O]f all the senses, sight best helps us to know things, and reveals many distinctions" (*Met.* A. 980a25), and was hostile to natural philosophers such as Democritus who "represented all perception as being by touch" (*De sensu* 4.442a29; Kirk *et al.* 1983: 428), even if he elsewhere stressed that he was located in between the *phusiologoi* and the Lovers of the Forms. When writing in a biological mode, he privileged touch much more: "the organ of touch," "correlated to several distinct kinds of objects," is "the least simple of all the sense-organs" (*De part. anim.* II.1.647a15). But the predominant understanding passed on by these texts is that *sight is privileged because it is "eidetic": it is a grasping of essences*.[1] In Hans Jonas's terms, sight alone allows the distinction between the changing and the unchanging, whereas "all other senses operate by registering change and cannot make that distinction. Only sight therefore provides the sensual basis on which the mind may conceive of the idea of the eternal, that which never changes and is always present" (Jonas 1966: 145). The privileging of sight runs through various prestigious moments in Western metaphysics and science, including Aquinas' *Summa Theologica* (II.1. xxvii):

> Those senses are most concerned with beauty which are most concerned in apprehension, namely sight and hearing, which ministers to reason. For we speak of beautiful sights and sounds but do not give the name of beauty to the objects of other senses, such as tastes or smells ... what simply satisfies desire is called good, but that whose very apprehension pleases is called beautiful

Leonardo in a fragment of his *Libro di Pittura*, asserts the primacy of vision, and by extension of painting over any other kind of art or science:

> And if you call painting dumb poetry, the painter may call poetry blind painting. Now which is the worse defect? to be blind or dumb? Though the poet is as free as the painter in the invention of his fictions *they are not so satisfactory to men as paintings*; for, though poetry is able to describe forms, actions and places in words, the painter deals with the actual similitude of the forms, in order to represent them ... And if the poet gratifies the sense by means of the ear, the painter does so by *the eye—the worthier sense.*
>
> 16 a–b, in Leonardo da Vinci [1888] 1970, I, ix
(The Practice of Painting): §§ 653–4

Similar enthusiasm resonates through the major figures of the New Science: Kepler wrote to Galileo in 1610 that Bruno was more "godlike" than them; they were his followers because his insights were arrived at without even seeing the phenomena (Kepler 1610: 10 recto). Such appeals to the mind's eye resonate with the metaphysics of light, from Plotinus to Renaissance Neoplatonism. André Du Laurens, the physician to King Henri IV, described sight as the noblest object, "born from the heavens," "God's eldest daughter" (Du Laurens 1597: f. 24r). We can still hear this centuries later, in Goethe: "If the eye were not solar / How would we perceive light" (Goethe 1970: liii).[2]

Galileo, in *The Assayer* (1623), analysed the senses and secondary qualities in corpuscular-mechanistic terms, in order to reduce them to primary qualities; he discussed the microstructure of taste and touch but was careful to repeat that sight is the "most excellent and noble of the senses," related to light itself (Drake 1957: 277, translation modified). For the great neuroanatomist Thomas

Willis, "Seeing" was "the most noble Power, because this faculty apprehends things at a great distance, under a most subtil Figure, by a most clear perception, and with great delight," "next in virtue to the Eternal and Immaterial Soul," embracing bodies within "Heaven and Earth in a Moment," "far remote from our touch," although he then expresses gentle irony about the claim (Willis 1683, XV, "Of the sight": 75). Sight is the most noble sense, also due to its "great distance"; for Robert Hooke, too, of the "differing ways of Sensation," "the 1st and most Spiritual is plac'd in the Eye" (the fifth is "over the whole Body"; Hooke 1705: 12). Kepler, Galileo, Willis, and Boyle perform a metaphysical valorization of sight which occasionally resembles a mystical commitment, yet they are also giants of the New Science, in a fitting testimony to the hybridity of genres.

On this view, sight is the purest, most philosophical sense; it is closest to light (hence the equation between *theoria* and contemplation, sight and intellection). Attribution of ethical perfection to sight may also indirectly have affected the organization of societal codes of appearance. Failure to wear colors and fabrics prescribed for particular stations in society has been associated with social disarray and uncertainty, and brought on severe repercussions since ancient times. Jewish Holy Commandments, for instance, stipulate that "women must not wear male clothing nor men that of women" and command lepers to always appear "bareheaded with clothing in disarray so as to be easily distinguishable";[3] in late medieval Florence and Venice, laws were passed in both cities outlawing cross-dressing by prostitutes as males to attract customers (Ruggiero 1993: 25); and in sixteenth-century England, Parliament regulated color-coding enabling the viewer to determine rank of individuals on sight (Hager 1991: 4), with the association of status and rank with the specific fabric worn regulated personally by the monarch.[4]

As regards the hierarchy of the senses, this privileging of sight is clearly opposed to the Epicuro-Lucretian valorization of touch, from antiquity via Rabelais to Julien Offray de La Mettrie's materialism. For Lucretius, touch is primary, it is "the sense of the body" (*De rerum natura*, II. 434), which further implies that "the nature of the soul and of the mind is corporeal": touch requires materiality, hence there must be something in the mind/soul (*animus, anima*) which is material (III.161–6). This valorization of touch is present in Gassendi's invocation of bodily experience against Descartes in his Objections to the *Meditations*, and in the Epicurean physician Walter Charleton, for whom "All Sensation is a kind of Touching" (Charleton 1966, III, ix: 248, which implies, contrary to Rey 1995, that it was not in Le Cat's 1740 *Traité des sensations* that sight and hearing were first reduced to touch). It is a recurrent motif in a minority line of early modern thinkers (often physicians), running through Guillaume Lamy and La Mettrie. Prominent medical figures such as William Harvey and Franciscus de le Boë Sylvius also praise touch (see below), but without these radical Epicurean overtones or underpinnings.

Yet even if we do not "stoop" to the base materialism of touch, sight itself is not master in its own house: it is fickle, and it allows for a process of mechanization which demystifies—one might even say "secularizes"—the solar eye.

THE FICKLENESS OF SIGHT AND THE MECHANIZATION OF VISION

Renaissance treatises on painting point, also, to the moral fickleness of sight. Leon Battista Alberti described perspective as an exercise in representing an objective, but also a deeply subjective, reality. "The painter," Alberti wrote, "strives solely to fashion that which *is seen*; anything which exists on a surface so that it is visible"; "no one would deny that the painter has nothing to do with things that are not visible" (Alberti 1956, I: 42). Shakespeare throws light on this interplay between the mirage of "objective truth" arising from a deeply subjective viewpoint, which not only engages with treatises on perspective, but also foreshadows tenets of philosophical relativism. "The truth" emerging from what is seen, in Alberti's phrase, becomes redefined in Shakespeare's *Sonnets* as the question of refraction through a unique artistic consciousness. There, Shakespeare advocated awareness of "the painter's skill," rather than uncritical immersion; such critical awareness, he seemed to suggest, serves to enhance the exquisite, morally complex and formative experience of seeing through, and beyond, an individual artistic take on the "truth" and "value" of what is seen:

> Mine eye hath played the painter and hath steeled
> Thy beauty's form in table of my heart;
> My body is the frame wherein 'tis held,
> And perspective that is best painter's art.
> For through the painter must you see his skill
>
> Sonnet 24, 1–5

The fickleness of perspective can be translated to the dramatic space as well. Everyone can see Hamlet's father's ghost in the opening scene of the play; but later, in the bedroom scene with his mother, Hamlet is the only one who can see it (*Hamlet*, 3.4.107). In this scene, for Hamlet, the ghost's appearance is "reality"; but from Gertrude's perspective, Hamlet addressing empty space looks very much like his madness. Shakespeare is asking here whether something can ever be considered "real" or "true" if only one person can see it; in other words, he questions the limits of vision as the purveyor of truth, and proposes that visual phenomena require social confirmation before they can be accepted.

Indeed, to turn to a central figure of the New Science, even Descartes, who stated in his treatise on optics, the *Dioptrics* (1637), that "it is the soul that sees, not the eyes" and, right at the start of the treatise, that "The entire conduct of our life depends on our senses, amongst which that of sight is the most universal and noble,"[5] lays out a vast project for demystifying vision.

The science of optics grapples in its own way with this tension between a metaphysics of light and a demystification of the sense of sight—including Kepler's unique conceptualization of the eye as an optical instrument. An issue had been the transmission of information through vision, the "age-old problem of contact between the observer and the visible object" (Lindberg 1976: 39): was there a "flow of material substance," in which the medium is all-important, or rather chiefly an act of seeing by the organ of the eye? For Leonardo, to take an example, "sight is exercised by ... the mediation of light ... the senses which receive the image [*similitudini*] of things do not send forth from themselves any power" (da Vinci [1888] 1970, II: 99). Kepler, in *Ad Vitellionem Paralipomena* (1604), relying on the anatomical descriptions provided by his contemporaries, tried to account for the diffusion of light through the eye. To elucidate the way light rays propagate inside the eye, Kepler compared it to a camera obscura, with the pupil being like a window and the lens a screen (Kepler [1604] 1968, V: 2); he criticized Della Porta, who was the first to describe the eye as a camera obscura, but thought that the image formed on the lens rather than on the retina. Descartes, in *Dioptrics* I, says:

> I would have you consider the light in bodies we call "luminous" to be nothing other than a certain movement, or very rapid and lively action, which passes to our eyes through the medium of the air and other transparent bodies, just as the movement or resistance of the bodies encountered by a blind man passes to his hand by means of his stick.
> AT VI: 84 / CSM I: 153

Here, vision is analyzed on the model of touch; a mechanist account of vision requires that the visible be "set at a distance, in order to objectify it" (Bellis 2010, II: i.A.2). Bellis notes that the properly scientific objectification of vision in Descartes' *Dioptrics* is matched by its metaphysical distantiation in the *Meditations*: "I shall consider myself as having *no hands or eyes, or flesh, or blood or senses*, but as having falsely believed that I had all these things"; "I will now shut my eyes, block my ears, and divert all my senses. I will erase all images of corporeal things from my thoughts" (First Meditation, AT IX-1: 18 / CSM II: 15, emphasis added; Third Meditation, AT IX-1: 27 / CSM II: 24). The figure of the blind man here (differently from its later usage in Molyneux's Problem: if someone born blind is familiarized with the sphere and the cube, will [s]he spontaneously recognize them if his/her sight returns?)[6] is used as a thought experiment (so to speak), in which the phenomenal qualities of light can be eliminated, and indeed the visible as such. This is mechanization of vision as an ontological reconstruction of the world (Bellis 2010: Ch. II), what Hamou elegantly calls a "déprise du sensible" (Hamou 2002: 72f.), comparable in its boldness to the (symmetrically opposite) Epicurean reconstruction based on touch and materiality.

Such a reconstruction of vision on the model of touch (a form of reductionism) could be tantamount to materialism, perhaps most notoriously in Hobbes' reduction of all sensation, including touch, vision and all of cognition, to a type of motion. As he writes in his autobiography:

> I thought continually about the nature of things, whether I was traveling by boat or by coach, or on horseback. And it seemed to me that there was only one true thing in the whole world, though falsified in many ways ... the basis of all those phenomena which we wrongly say are something—the phenomena of sense-impressions, which are offsprings of our skull, with nothing external. And in those internal regions, there could be nothing but *motion*.
>
> Tuck 1988: 248; for the original translation, Hobbes 1994: lvi–lvii

The way Descartes' blind man "sees with his staff" is a kind of extended touch: "one might almost say that they see with their hands, or that their stick is the organ of some sixth sense given to them in place of sight."[7] Once sight becomes percussive, i.e., a form of touch, then touch becomes metaphysically primary; in the previous, typically Aristotelian context, what we grasped in sight are forms of qualities that move across matter—a qualitative change in matter, not a movement of matter itself—and thus transparency, not collision, is fundamental to understanding how sight works. We cannot improve on Catherine Wilson's diagnosis, in which rationalist philosophers move between a conception of vision that they construct as a phenomenon of embodiment, explained, conditioned, and sometimes degraded by its involvement with the material and the corporeally dense, and a conception of vision they construct as an intellective act, implicating geometrical principles, as a way of having while keeping one's distance, as a satisfaction—but of a thirst for light and knowledge. From this melange ... we can extract what prefigurations we like: community or terror; embodiment or transcendence; engagement or dissociation; the active gaze of Augustinian concupiscence; or the retreat into the shadows of philosophy and the colorless, formless world of midcentury ontology.

Wilson 1997: 135

However, it is possible to say that contact senses reduce to touch, without committing oneself to an Epicurean-type ontology in which *touch is the pre-eminent sense* (in the metaphysical and ethically laden or "valorized" sense).

This idea of "seeing through one's staff" also extends, in Descartes and beyond, into the theme of the instrumental or artificial enhancement of our cognitive powers (and by extension, Spinoza would add, our power of acting). At the end of the *Dioptrics* (AT VI: 226), Descartes speaks approvingly of the advantage we will gain from optical lenses such as the microscope—an optimism explicitly rejected by thinkers such as Locke, who we consider as paramount empiricists (Locke, the physician Sydenham, and others in their milieu were suspicious of the imprecision of these new techniques, but also, more philosophically, of the microworld as a space unsuited for human perception).

Sight is thus gradually demystified, no longer so noble or "solar," which *mutatis mutandis* makes it easier to imagine increasingly *embodied* discourses (Wolfe 2012). Yet there is no linear process of unfolding, from one historico-conceptual regime of the senses to the next. For, as has been noted by cultural historians (Bynum 1995), instead of a phobia of touch and a fascination with vision, earlier centuries seem characterized instead by a more "overflowing" presentation of the sensory world, as is fervidly manifest in a singular "incunabulum" of 1499, the anonymous *Hypnerotomachia Poliphili*. This work, which can be described with equal fairness as a utopian phantasmagoria, an aesthetic treatise, an erotic novel, and a masterpiece of visionary, speculative architecture, tells the story of Poliphilus (the "lover of many things" but also of Polia), who tosses and turns during a restless night after being rejected by his beloved Polia (or "many things"). In Poliphilus's dream-world, he journeys to the utopian location of Cythera, with long descriptions of the buildings encountered (and sumptuous woodcuts of these), in a kind of oceanic paean to beauty and the (virtual) promise of the senses. However much sight and touch are in tension (for all the hundreds of prominent statements praising sight, there are almost as many like Robert Burton's declaring that touch is "the most ignoble" of the senses; Burton [1621] 1989, I: vi, "Of the Sensible Soul"), a tension which is partly resolved by reducing the former to the latter, we need to pay attention, if not to the cornucopia of the *Hypnerotomachia*, at least to the other senses—hearing, taste, and smell.

OF STINK AND CONFETTI, OR, EMBODIMENT

In his commentary on Plato's *Symposium*, Ficino described sight and hearing as "spiritual senses," directly linked to the higher human capacity for ethical thought and higher reasoning; any need to involve other senses in the contemplation of the world is classified as appetite (Ficino [1544] 2000: Oration I). This is the reason why Thomas Kyd's sixteenth-century play *The Spanish Tragedy* describes the courtship of Bel-imperia and Horatio as one which starts virtuously—involving eyes and ears only—and then deteriorates morally though the gradual engagement of all the other senses (Kyd 1987: 2.4.40–55). Late in the sixteenth century, Shakespeare quietly opens the tradition to scrutiny in *Titus Andronicus*: when Lavinia is raped and her tongue and hands cut off by her violators, she becomes a grotesque embodiment of ideally virtuous feminine sensuality, a move with which Shakespeare questions the validity of such ideals.

In Renaissance England, music, and the sense which perceives it, hearing, were seen as instruments of order or disorder. Order, degree, and harmony in music thus emerge as categories related to harmony of the macrocosm, the universe and the body politic, as well as the microcosm, or the body natural, bound in a cycle of psychosomatic feedback. In *Troilus and Cressida*, Shakespeare famously used the metaphor of an instrument falling out of tune to illustrate the precariousness of social and universal order (1.3.85–110). The role of the senses, particularly sensory pleasance and hearing, began to be seen as an important source of mental and physical health, but also of disturbance. In his *Treatise of Melancholie*, a major statement of humoral theory influencing Shakespeare among others, Timothy Bright argued that music will cure "a disordered rage, and intemperate mirth" and brings order which should normally be imparted by reason, but is more easily done by music. As "musicke as it were a magicall charme bringeth to pass in the minds of men, which being forseene of wise lawgivers in the past, they have made choice of certaine kindes thereof, and have rejected the other, as hurtful to their common wealthes" (Bright 1586: 248).

If we agree with Luther that hearing can touch the deepest part of the heart, then there must also be dangers associated with being open to words. If the beloved opens her ears, for instance, hears the lover's pleas and is swayed by his praise, she may become amenable to sin. This is a grave danger, and, in this context, hearing also becomes perceived as another gateway for wickedness and excess (on love as danger, see Kambaskovic-Sawers 2012). Examples of this abound in literature. Boccacio's *Fiametta* writes a lament for all women to hear what happens to women who believe their lovers' sweet promises (Boccaccio 1562). One thinks also of Satan attacking Eve's morals in Milton's *Paradise Lost*, with his Petrarchan poetic praise.

Not unlike the conundrum of the base touch being situated in the noble hand, the speaking function of the tongue is also placed in the instrument for tasting. Both functions of the tongue are ethically ambiguous, and this ambiguity is well documented in the early modern period and modern-day critical discourse. Dichotomous metaphors involving noise and silence, life and death, succour and injury, are all used to indicate this ethical ambiguity. When "sins of the tongue" are mentioned, this usually refers either to ethics of speech on the one hand, or the soundness of rhetorical construction on the other, rather than gluttony. The mouth, the location of the tongue, is also a problematic place as it is, at once, the seat of life (food, breath) and the location of pleasurable sensations (smell, taste, sensation) leading to the danger of sin.

As the pleasure of eating was ethically questionable, so was its source, food, and by extension, the sense of taste, which of course has Epicurean overtones. On the one hand, wholesome and tasty food is necessary for survival, health, and flourishing of the human body. But on the other, pleasant-tasting food is a category to be treated with caution, as it can become a source of obsession leading to gluttony, one of the seven deadly sins, semantically connected to lust (Vitullo 2010: 106). Imagery of honey used in love poetry suggests purity, natural sweetness, and artistic merit. When taken in moderation, honey "not only cleanseth, altereth, and nourisheth, but also it long time preserveth that uncorrupted, which is put into it" (Elyot 1595: H4r–v). By contrast, the sweetness of sugar, a man-made sweetener, was associated with lies. The Latin *confictio* means "to fabricate, to cheat, to deceive, and to manipulate," and is the root of the English words *confectionary* and *fiction*, but also the Italian word *confetti*, the art of sugar-coating with the aim of improving the shape and taste of food (Palma 2004: 42). Then there is the solitary pleasure that Spenser's speaker in *Amoretti* takes in prolonged contemplation of the lady's body:

... her brest the table was so richly spredd
my thoughts the guests, which would thereon have fedd.

Spenser 1999: 77

The process of being tempted by delectable food is semantically linked to much of the sexual overtones of Renaissance love poetry and religious and medical treatises warning of the spiritual dangers of gluttony.

The sense of smell was associated with cognitive capacity in the form of intuition, engaging the function of what we know today to be the amygdala. Calvin referred to non-verbal, unconscious cognitive processes in his commentary on the Bible, and suggested that the Fear of God must precede the conscious judgment of "the sight of the eyes or the hearing of the ears," and be intuitive, as if smelled out. The Hebrew origin of the word is, in fact, "smell": the Fear of God is a shrewdness that should come intuitively, like awareness of a smell, rather than learned consciously: "The verb ריח, (riach) which is here put in the Hiphil conjugation ... is peculiarly applicable to the person of Christ ... Christ will be so shrewd that he will not need to learn from what he hears, or from what he sees; for by smelling alone he will perceive what would otherwise be unknown" (Calvin 1609, Ch. 11: 120–1).

Moral judgment is often implied in early modern literary metaphors involving a sense of smell, as in Hamlet's observation that "something is rotten in the state of Denmark" (*Hamlet*, 1.4.67). *The Garden of Eloquence*, a 1577 handbook on rhetoric (revised 1593), makes clear the ethical implications of Shakespeare's usage of such a symbol, explaining "that abominations of sinne do stink and are odious to God and all good men" (Peacham 1593: 5). Faecal matter can also serve as a symbol of moral purging. Sir Philip Sidney often refers to "rhubarb words" in *Astrophil and Stella*—they allow him to purify his soul of all the foul-smelling, putrefying love and hatred that Astrophil feels for Stella—and the smell of faecal matter is often invoked in political context (P. Smith 2012: 5).

THE EXQUISITE SENSE OF TACT AND THE DOCTOR'S TOUCH

If sight is both the paramount sense, the philosopher's sense, and also a crucial player-and-victim of the dismantling of hierarchies brought about by the Scientific Revolution, and other senses such as taste and smell are deeply embedded in (and saturated by) the cultural, religious, and affective fabric (scholars speak of a "permeability" of the senses in this period), we are still missing a crucial piece of the puzzle. We have alluded several times to the presence of a "hatred or phobia of touch" (e.g. Ficino in his commentary on the *Symposium* describing the lower senses such as touch as the source of "lust or madness"; Gilman 1993: 201)[8] or at least a depreciation of its value (as when Boyle calls it "the most dull of the five senses": *Effluviums*, Boyle 1772, III: 694). And conversely, we have mentioned the combination of praise and blame for organs like the hand, as in Bulwer. But we have left out the massive appeal to touch in the medical tradition.

If one recalls the old distinction, usually associated with Avicenna, between the *via medicorum* with Galen and the *via philosophorum* with Aristotle, it is striking that in the former touch is emphasized as important, especially the fingertips. Along with sight, touch was the most important diagnostic sense for Galen (Nutton 1993); for Fernel, touch was the best sense (Fernel 2003: 228, 230; Giglioni 2013). From this it is not a great step further to what Marie-Christine Pouchelle calls the medical "rehabilitation of the flesh," with medieval surgery promoting "the solely secular value of the body" (Pouchelle 1990: 204), but also, the anatomical revival and the emergence of medical humanism, which both nourish Renaissance medicine—for example, the Padua school (Klestinec 2011; Mandressi 2003; Sawday 1994). The new emphasis on medicine in the Renaissance, with its re-evaluation of touch, has broader implications for a culture of touch, but also the emergence of a new kind of "embodied" empiricism (Salter and Wolfe 2009). Our own interest here in the ranking and hierarchy of the senses—here, touch—will appear more clearly once we have set out the medical situation in more detail. Two prominent cases of the medical privileging of touch are Harvey and Sylvius.

Touch was the pre-eminent bodily sense for Harvey: it is privileged in his inquiries. Harvey drew on touch because, as he wrote in *A Second Essay to Jean Riolan*, it offers more possibilities and is more powerful (Harvey 1958: 60ff.; Salter 2010). He spoke of the "powerful authority" of sense and experience as the "rule of the Anatomists" (or "anatomical habit"), founded on "touch and sight" as opposed to demonstrative reasoning "by causes and probable principles" (Harvey 1958: 58). He also emphasized the experimental and diagnostic priority of the "testimony of sight and touch" as regards generation—here, the womb: "It resembles the softness of the brain itself, and when you touch it, did not your own eyes give evidence to that touch, you would not believe your fingers were upon it" (Harvey 1653, Ex. 68: 415).

Sylvius follows Harvey in speaking of "the testimony of sight and touch," and personifies sight and touch as witnesses for Harvey's model of the heart's action against Descartes' speculations: "I bring forward a pair of faithful

Witnesses of this Truth, which are enhanced with every qualification, Sight and Touch," these being the two paramount senses for anatomists (*De febribus* [1661], IX, 22, in Sylvius 1679). The two "faithful witnesses" testify that the arteries pulse and dilate whenever the ventricles of the heart contract, that the blood pours out from the heart with each contraction, and that a finger placed in the heart through a hole cut in the tip can feel the contraction. The testimony of touch, moreover, proves that the blood is poured out and a finger inserted in the dissected ventricles of the heart near the tip is sensibly compressed, whenever the aforesaid ventricles are contracted; and then at the same time the concurrent dilation of the arteries can be discerned by that same touch, through a hand brought up against them.[9] Sylvius described Harvey as teaching according to the testimony of the senses, unlike Descartes, who "trusted more in the laws of his own Mechanics, rather than in his external Senses," and thought that "the Ventricles of the Heart and the Arteries were Dilated and Contracted simultaneously" (this empiricist-like criticism of Descartes was common amongst physicians in the later seventeenth and early eighteenth centuries, notably Steno and Boerhaave). Sylvius clearly elevates touch to be the equal of sight as an epistemic witness.

In other period contexts, the sense of touch is associated—consonant with Harvey and Sylvius—with learning about the world and the forging of the soul through the sensations of the body, as in Sir John Davies' philosophical poem *Nosce Teipsum* (1599):

> By touch, the first pure qualities we learn,
> Which quicken all things, hot, cold, moist and dry;
> By touch, hard, soft, rough, smooth, we do discern;
> By touch, sweet pleasure and sharp pain we try
>
> Davies 1599, XVI: 45–6

It should not come as a surprise that touch, the basest of senses, can be praised. Touch is characterized by an essential ethical ambiguity: on the one hand, it was perceived as most common; on the other, as most necessary (Harvey 2011: 386–9).

Using the example of early modern prints depicting the human senses, Sharon Assaf argues vividly that the sense of touch perhaps most frequently evokes the erotic and seductive. Citing Badius' *Stultiferae naves*, an early printed book combining prose, verse, and woodcut illustrations, which she calls "the first text of the sixteenth century devoted to a moralizing appraisal of man's five senses" (Assaf 2005: 77), Assaf points out that Badius restated commonly-held notions about touch: that it is the last in the hierarchical ranking of the senses, that it is common to all living beings, and that it is spread throughout the body. Yet, at the center of the woodcut illustration is the hand. In each, the hand is perceived as the organ of touch, but in the former it is depicted as an offending appendage, whereas in the latter it is shown engaged in a worthy activity. In addition, the first print series devoted to the five senses by the Nuremberg *Kleinmeister* Georg Pencz presents the ambivalent meaning of the senses in the guise of nude female personifications, simultaneously seducing the viewer and presenting him with a moral lesson about each sense (Assaf 2005: 78).

Touching in its various guises—sexual, tender, exploratory, and, especially, creative and fashioning—appears in medieval and Renaissance poetry. Petrarch's word for Laura—*scolpito,* "sculpted or chiseled," also means "restored to wholeness," with a sexual connotation (Petrarch 1999: 543). In sonnets 32 and 51 of the *Amoretti* (Spenser 1999), Edmund Spenser the speaker compared his lady to iron "mollified with heate," then beaten, in order for her "stubberne wit" to be bent into shape he deemed appropriate. It is the fashioning of the lady not only through the poet's sexuality, but primarily through the power of his creativity, that is made to be the focus of the forging image. Early modern applications of the word in practical rhetoric seem to revolve around *learning* by being hurt, wounded, or tested by ordeal, giving touch a distinctly moral reading: "God hath touched me, that is, hath grievously smitten and wounded me. Another example, And they were pricked in their hearts (Act 2.) meaning, pearced with sorrow and repentance" (Peacham 1593: 7).

That poets, physicians, and other virtuosi can praise touch as an "exquisite sense," including in anthropocentric terms where it becomes a marker of our own superiority over the rest of the animal world, is noteworthy, not least given the initial privileging of sight we witnessed. "Of all the creatures, the sense of tact is most exquisite in man, because his body is most temperate," Alexander Ross declared in his 1651 *Arcana microcosmi*; Willis considered that "there should be many sensories in perfect animals," for the sake of self-preservation and "propagation of their kind"; at the other end of the spectrum, the more "imperfect" animals, such as oysters and limpets, are "gifted only with the sense of touch."[10]

Some recognize the importance of the "networked" character of touch, which is increasingly emphasized with the addition of musical (vibratory, harmonic) metaphors; Willis muses that even if touch seems "a faculty of a lower order," in some respects "it is more excellent by far than the rest," because it "receives and knows the impressions of many sensible things, and

... so obtains a most large and ... general Province."[11] That touch "knows many things" or interacts with different sensory modalities—nose and skin, but also inner and outer, self and other (witness the numerous medical discussions of ticklishness) makes it something of a "common sense" (*koinē aisthēsis*, *sensus communis*; Heller-Roazen 2007), or what we would call proprioception: "it is scarcely to be distinguished from the having of a body that can act in physical space" (O'Shaughnessy 2000: 658). This proprioceptive dimension was later highlighted by Condillac, for whom it was through this "fundamental feeling," touch, that we acquire a sense of ourselves, but also, that there is something existing outside of us (Condillac [1754] 1984, II.i.3: 158). Similarly, for D'Alembert, "touch undoubtedly teaches us to differentiate what is *ours* from that which surrounds us; it makes us circumscribe the universe to ourselves" (D'Alembert [1759] 1986, VI: 45). But this tactophilia is not a metaphysical-ethical valorization of this sense. For that, we need to turn finally to the materialism of touch.

"IL N'Y A POINT DE PLAISIR SENTI QUI SOIT CHIMÉRIQUE": THE MATERIALISM OF TOUCH

Let us distinguish two attitudes towards touch, not specific to either philosophy or "science": the reductionist and the holist. According to the former, the world is made of microparticles in motion. From heat to taste, from rain to sound, all the qualitative munificence on display in the *Hypnerotomachias* of this world is reduced to a quantitatively specifiable set of components and properties: "in those internal regions, there could be nothing but motion." But the holist attitude displays, as with the "common sense" theme, a fascination but also serious interest in the "network" or reticulated character of touch, crucial to our embodiment and its inextricable relation to our subjectivity, and to our successful functioning as agents in a potentially threatening natural world (something Descartes acknowledges clearly). When such non-materialist philosophers as Kant call it "the most fundamental sense" (Kant 1978: 63–4) and describe how "I am myself at my fingertips"—if not transcendentally, at least anthropologically (*Traüme ein Geistesehers* [1764], Ak II. 324),[12] they are noticing the irreducibility of proprioception. This was undoubtedly why, for example, Berkeley rejected Descartes' description of the blind man "seeing through his staff": because vision could not deliver to us the spatial properties of objects, for which we need touch (*An Essay Towards a New Theory of Vision*, 1709; 4th edn, 1732). In addition, he felt that the program of mechanistically explaining our sensory functioning was doomed, because each of our senses evolves through experience, and the resulting totality is not something that can be arrived at mechanistically (*Alciphron*, 1732, IV. §11ff.).

Interestingly, both the reductionist and the holist conceptions of touch can be turned into a metaphysics, with different results (and one could map out where various figures fit: Galileo, Hobbes, and Descartes in one corner, Lucretius, Harvey, and Gassendi in the other, with in-between cases like Willis). Most significant in our view, not least because it is the boldest reversal of the "nobility of sight," preserving its valuative dimensions, is the latter, holist approach, which is Epicurean-Lucretian. Recall that for Lucretius, touch was the sense of the body itself, its self-possession. This was often used against the skeptical fear of the senses as "deceivers," asserting in contrast the "infallibility of sensitivity," that sensitivity "cannot lie." Epicurus held that reason was dependent on sensation, which was irrefutable; various separate perceptions guarantee the truth of our senses, and "if you argue against all your sensations, you will then have no criterion to declare any of them false."[13] In the Lucretian version, this becomes infallibility: "there is no error in sense-perception" (Sextus Empiricus, *Adversus Mathematicos*, VIII.9; Lucretius, *De rerum natura* IV.474–99). Even Locke held that "This notice by our senses, though not so certain as demonstration, yet may be called knowledge, and proves the existence of things without us" (Locke 1975: IV.xi.3). Many of the clandestine manuscripts of the seventeenth and eighteenth centuries repeat these Lucretian topoi on how sensations cannot—or rarely—deceive us, sometimes with an extra hedonistic flourish (how could we be experiencing pleasure from something illusory, as in Diderot's "There is no pleasure felt that is illusory [*chimérique*]").[14]

The emergence of materialism brings with it a valorization of touch, notably in Diderot's 1749 *Letter on the Blind*. In Diderot's metaphysics of the senses, all the different senses "are just a diversified touch" and sight, the eidetic sense, is the idealist sense: "How deceptive the eye would be, if its judgment were not constantly corrected by touch." In contrast, touch becomes "the deepest, most philosophical sense,"[15] reversing the order of priorities in which the hands are "despised for their materialism." Yet this new respect for embodiment is not a mystification of "being-in-the-body": a materialism of touch is different from a phenomenology of body which often, as in Novalis, identifies touch with "the mystery of transubstantiation" (Novalis [1798] 1987: 622).[16]

When reflecting on the shift from a metaphysics of sight to a materialism of touch, one can ask *under which historical conditions such transformations occurred*—from the eye, divine and "like the sun" (from Plato to Grosseteste, Du Laurens and Goethe) to the praise of touch as more powerful (Harvey), exquisite (Ross) and excellent (Willis). And one could study currents and cross-currents of religiosity and secularization (including in the mechanization of vision), of profanity and transcendentalization (whether of sight, hearing . . . or the flesh). One could, as we have, strongly emphasize the central place of the *via medicorum* in this revalorization, and more metaphysically, point to the displacements effected by a modern Epicureanism, ultimately in the materialist reversal of the hierarchy of the senses. But our point was not that a sixteenth-century Italian miller saw or "touched" differently than we do (Ginzburg 1980), although we hope to have described some of the variety of sensory regimes, but to investigate the gradual inversion of the privilege of sight into a materialism of touch—without which "nature remains like the delightful landscapes of the magic lantern, light, flat and chimerical," in Henri Focillon's words:

> The possession of the world requires a kind of tactile flair. Sight slides along the universe, whereas the hand knows that the object has weight, is smooth or rough, and is not welded to the bottom of the sky or earth with which it appears to be joined . . . Touch fills nature with mysterious forces; without it, nature remains like the delightful landscapes of the magic lantern, light, flat and chimerical.
>
> Focillon 1943: 108, translation ours

ACKNOWLEDGMENTS

Thanks to Tawrin Baker, Benny Goldberg, and Brian Keeley for reading and critiquing an earlier version of this chapter; to Delphine Bellis, Guido Giglioni and Evan Ragland for their kind assistance.

CHAPTER SIX

Medicine and the Senses: Physicians, Sensation, and the Soul

STEPHEN PENDER

In 1497, the Strasbourg physician Hieronymus Brunschwig claimed that Galen "was aferede to touche the brayne" (1525: sig. Giiiv). Not so for seventeenth-century physicians, who not only touched, but tasted. The physician and controversialist Richard Boulton assures his readers that, should they "compare the Taste of the Brain, with the Tast of the Blood," it will be "evident" that the "sweet Substance" is *spiritus*, animal spirit. We learn by taste that spirits are the purest, most refined part of blood; on the tongue, they are "oyly, sweet, and mucilaginous" (1698: 84, 91). The English physician Sir John Floyer seems to have tasted blood frequently, confirming its acidity by the tongue (1696: 154ff., *passim*), having earlier organized the entire *materia medica* by taste and smell, drawing on the "*Tastes of all sorts of Persons*" in order to clarify the healing "virtues" of plants, to free medicine of "the common Scandal of being Conjectural." Physicians' central task is to "*chuse, and apply* Tastes" (Floyer 1687: 1.A5r-v, A6v, a3r, a4v, a5r, *passim*).

Chemical physicians, including the Leiden doctor Franciscus De le Boë Sylvius, embraced investigative tasting with enthusiasm. This is a change from the sixteenth century, as Evan Ragland argues, when the reluctance to treat excreta, and strident Galenic authority, meant the "devaluation of tasting and smelling for diagnostic signs." Of course Galen, too, had recommended various kinds of investigative tasting, especially of the sweat, but other qualities, like heat and moisture, were more indicative of a patient's condition in his and his followers' thought. Yet, by the mid-seventeenth century, Sylvius and others, following the Flemish chemical physician Jan Baptist van Helmont, lauded taste, vision, and touch as essential to both pedagogical and clinical medical practice, and engaged not only in conventional, tactile inquiry, like feeling a patient's body for temperature and pulse-taking, but in smelling the humors and even tasting cadavers (Ragland 2012). Even the well-respected English physician Thomas Willis tasted urine (1684, 167: 3.1, 7).

Tasting bodies, touching brains, smelling plants and fluids: this chapter focuses on the senses in Renaissance medical thought. How were the senses mobilized in medical theory and practice in sixteenth- and seventeenth-century Europe? What roles do the senses perform at the bedside, in the laboratory, as indications of health or illness? How were the external and internal senses taxonomized, treated, restored? What were their roles in the "animal economy," in the network of forces and functions that enable sensation and movement, apperception, passion, and thought? What was their epistemological purchase? The latter issue has been explored thoroughly in natural philosophical, "scientific," and theological cultures of the sixteenth and seventeenth centuries (see, for example, de Boer and Göttler 2012). As Barbara Shapiro notes, the "interplay between the necessity of sense-derived data and the weakness of the senses was a frequently expressed theme" in various disciplines and practices in the period (1983: 22).

The "medicine" of my title is a broad church. I use the term to denote not only the work of physicians and, occasionally, surgeons, but a range of writers, including philosophers, theologians, and popularizers of various sorts, concerned with hygiene and regimen, therapy and healing, physiology and anatomy, between the early sixteenth and the late seventeenth centuries. The eclecticism of medical thought is now proverbial (Wear 1995: 161), and its pan-European scope established by recent scholarship, including work that treats *epistolae medicinales* in the Republic of Letters (Maclean 2008). It was variously responsive to the ferment of philosophical inquiry: figures like Pierre Gassendi and Walter Charleton advocated a distinctly Epicurean program in both medicine and ethics, while skepticism, revived in the works of Galen, Celsus, and Sextus Empiricus, contributed significantly to the development of medical semiotics, the theory and practice of interpreting symptoms and signs. Available largely through Galen and Cicero, stoicism underwrote the adequacy of the senses (Hankinson 2003), and offered *pneuma* as solution to various problems of vitality; its influences are felt in most physicians' treatment of the passions of the soul, even though many rejected its strongest tenets. Unsurprisingly, the vast majority of medical theory and practice relied on various forms of Aristotelianism, even if it was unevenly acknowledged, but philosophers and physicians of every denomination, school, and sect essayed the senses, often with a confected mix of early Christian learning, scholasticism, and the "new" philosophy (see Rutherford 2006). The well-known physician Daniel Sennert, for example, compares Epicureanism with Augustine and academic skepticism in his examination of the sensorium ([1618] 1661: 371).

Throughout the period, physicians and philosophers thoroughly probed the structure and function, form and use of the senses. In order to explore these habits of thought, first I offer a glimpse into the Renaissance soul-body relationship, into the general depiction of the thinking, feeling human composite, in order to suggest that the senses do not have a history entirely their own. Second, I explore specific treatments of the senses themselves—both internal and external—as they appear in medical, philosophical, and popular texts. By examining medical thought, we learn that Renaissance physicians and philosophers were as anxious as they were celebratory about vision's capacities. "Unreason and instability never disappear from visual cultures," Stuart Clark writes, "and no amount of intellectual effort could have banished them during the seventeenth century" (2007: 331). Clark's wide-ranging, erudite work offers a signal lesson: in recent scholarship, the senses have experienced a renaissance, not unlike that which resuscitated bodies in the 1990s and the passions in the last ten years, but very few scholars turn to medical thought to ballast or test their views, a neglect most evident in treatments of vision (see, however, Harvey 2002; Heller-Roazen 2007; Jütte 2005).

The third part of this chapter examines the ways in which physicians employ their senses in Renaissance bedside encounters, their conceptions of their patients' distempered sensoria, and, briefly, the ways in which the senses are mobilized in medical experiment. While it seems that only rarely were physicians required to perform clinically as part of their education (Brockliss 1987: 395; Risse 1987–8), since antiquity the central medical task was to arrive at knowledge of patients' bodies, no matter how conjectural, using the senses and reason. But the delicate empiricism of bedside encounters—profound rituals of transformation, in which illness becomes disease, men and women patients, and disciplinary wisdom and comportment are pressed into service—demanded especially keen, active, refined senses, particularly sight and touch.

Inquiry concerned with the senses might be seen as part of a general anthropological programme, begun in the sixteenth century—evidenced, for example, in John Barclay's frequently reprinted 1614 taxonomy of nations, *Icon animorum*—and well underway by the 1640s. In the work of the French physician Marin Cureau de la Chambre, who treats, in detail, dispositions and passions, spirits and the soul, or in John Bulwer's ambitious "Muscular Philosophy" (1649: sig. A8r), we might see the ways in which Renaissance anthropology builds on the ancient dictum that the lineaments of the body "disclose the dispositions and inclinations of the mind in general" (Bacon 1857–74: 3.368). Physicians and philosophers in the period devoted significant efforts to reading the signs of the living body in order to identify not only illness, as in the *facies hippocratica*, but passion, will, intention. A renewed interest in gesture arose, at least by the twelfth century, only to intensify and spread by the sixteenth and seventeenth (Knox 2007), in which some argued that bodies disclose "Moral Actions" (Evelyn 1697: 332).

At the center of such anthropological and medical-moral concerns is the body as a "field of powers and forces," explained in the period as the "animal economy" (Pittion 1987: 120), the interconnected archipelago of animal functions—sensing and feeling, thinking and willing. During a period of increasing commitment to physiology as an explanans in a number of human sciences, the senses received sharp scrutiny. Indeed, "the reduction of psychic phenomena to somatic states ... became increasingly explicit in medical writings" (Henry 1989: 90). Divergent thinkers exhibited an interest in physiological explanation, even for moral states, sometimes thought to be predicated on habit, regimen, "second nature," and the senses. These were clearly the concerns of medical practitioners from the late Middle Ages through to the seventeenth century. An exploration of the senses in medical thought, then, must account for the ligatures between sight, hearing, smell, taste, touch, and the "inward wits," reason and the common sense, memory and imagination—all agents in the animal economy. Neither can the passions be neglected, since they too "color" sense (Pender 2010).

GALEN'S WOOL-WINDER

In the throes of illness, "all pleasures be painefull ... strength turned to feblenes, beauty to lothsomness, sences are dispersed, eloquence interrupted, remembrance confounded," Sir Thomas Elyot's assessment of the effects of moral and physical lassitude on the senses—they are dissipated, diffused—exemplifies Renaissance thought about the relationship between health and regimen, sickness and sensation: distemper vexes the soul, sours beauty, strength, and the senses themselves. While repletion dulls understanding and perception, for Elyot there are cures: moderate exercise, for example, "cleanseth the sences, and maketh them more quicke" (1595: 78, 81).

In *The Castell of Helth*—reprinted frequently, still cited in the eighteenth century—Elyot follows Galen's *De sanitate tuenda*, translated into Latin by fellow physician Thomas Linacre in 1517. The book inaugurated a glut of vernacular medical-moral advice manuals (Slack 1979: 250). Twenty years later, in 1561, the Dutch physician Levinus Lemnius summarizes contemporary medical thought in a text meant for those disposed to "perfectly and thorowly know the habit and constitution" of their own bodies: seasonable sleep, merry company, moderate exercise, calm passions, wholesome food, and sweet smells all nourish the spirits, and thus "marveilously comfort and clarify the instruments of the Senses, and enable them to doe and peforme all their proper actions" ([1561] 1633: 1, 13–14). Perfect health is in part defined by "fresh and perfect" senses, "every of the faculties natural, duely doing his office and function without stop, impediment or grievance" (54).

"Cleansing," enlivening the senses by exercise or diet, depends upon a broad agreement, shared by most Renaissance physicians and philosophers, that the disposition of the soul, the strength and health of its faculties, follow the "temperature" of the body—the balance or imbalance of the qualities hot and cold, moist and dry, conditioned by a balance or imbalance of the four humors, black bile, yellow bile, phlegm, and blood (Siraisi 1990). As the Spanish physician Juan Huarte argues in 1575, "*Galen* writ a booke, wherein he prooveth, That the maners of the soule, follow the temperature of the body, in which it keepes residence." Thus, according to their temperature, some people are "blockish, some wise: some of woorth, and some base: some cruel, and some merciful." Both ancient authority and experience demonstrate that the dispositions of the soul "spring" from somatic constitution: the "groundplot" of his treatise, Huarte explains, is the interrogation of the "differences of the habilities which are in men" with respect to arts and sciences, disciplines and practices (1959: 22–3).

Huarte's broad project—mooring inclinations to diverse "sciences," detailing necessary capacities for the pursuit of specific professions, including medicine—commits him to this widely accepted medical apothegm, drawn from Galen's *Quod animi mores*. In Thomas Walkington's rendition, "the soule sympathizeth with the body and followeth her crasis and temperature." What made "the minde of *Orestes* so out of temper that hee kild his owne mother," Walkington asks, "but the bodily *Crasis*?" (1607: 18–23). The term *krasis*, for Galen, is a "mixture" of the qualities of hot, cold, dry, and moist in bodies, on which depend apprehension, cognition, and passion. Such a view allows physicians to comprehend loss of memory, feeling, motion, or intelligence as "impairments of the soul's abilities to employ its natural functions," especially in cases in which sufferers see things which are not there, hear things that no one said, or make "meaningless utterances." If the soul were not some "quality, form, affection, or faculty of the body," if there were no "communion" with the body, how might the noble, immortal, and immaterial soul sicken? The "overwhelming effect on the soul of the ills of the body is clearly demonstrated by . . . melancholy, phrenitis, or mania," Galen concludes (1997: 159–60).

These notions—that the soul "follows" the temperature and disposition of the body, that this relationship is frequently revealed during illness—were repeated and interrogated throughout the period, and well into the eighteenth century, even as widespread investment in strict Galenic medicine waned (recalling that "the fall of the Galenic science of medicine" does not describe the waning of Galenic practice—Temkin 1973: 135, 165). Yet Galen, avowing that the soul functions according to the body, refuses to "infer that this invalidates moral judgment" (Temkin 1973: 45). This is especially pertinent for any inquiry into the history of the senses, for they are frequently moralized, especially in relation to their role in the animal economy, and increasingly impugned for their inaccuracy. Indeed, the senses bear a double burden: as means for apprehending and thinking the world, for *nihil est in intellectu quod non prius fuerit in sensu*, and as emblematic of the frangibility of knowledge itself. While Aristotle maintains that sensations are always true, or at least almost always true (*De anima* 428a11, 428b18), perhaps the legacy of the Renaissance is to introduce doubt into processes of perception and cognition.

This is what I shall call "the paradox of sense." On the one hand, the senses were essential to discovery and diagnosis, prognosis and treatment; practitioners and patients devoted significant energies to reading faces and bodies, their own and others, for signs of distemper, and for indications of recovery, even if physicians were often cautioned to be circumspect in their predictions, lest they impugn their reputations or their patients' confidence (Demaitre 2003: 776–80). On the other hand, there was an increasing awareness, in contradistinction to much ancient thought, that the senses were fallible, labile, unreliable, characteristics most evident when they tested themselves, as it were, probing their own functions and roles in thinking, feeling, often sick bodies.

In part, this paradox is responsible for medicine's reputation as an uncertain, low science; indeed, arguments about the uncertainty of medicine, its perils and promises, the incommensurability of medical theory and practice, the character and conduct of its agents, and its professional status—a discipline that trafficked in urine and blood, faeces and decay—flourished in medical and non-medical texts and contexts in the sixteenth and seventeenth centuries (Pender 2006). Although medicine was frequently lauded in university encomia and *paragoni*, physicians and surgeons were impugned in both learned and popular fora for atheism or incompetence, lucre, or their truck with the sensual. Central to learned criticism is the notion that healing is "oftentymes done more by chaunce, then by any certayne Methode or Reason" (Securis 1566: sig. Biiiir). Physicians merely "guesse at their physicke" (Goodman 1616: 97). In the preface to *The Passions of the Soul* ([1649] 1989), Descartes writes that "nowhere is our need to acquire new learning more apparent than in things that concern Medicine." Practitioners are unsure even about common illnesses, for medicine ignored physics, was poor in theory, and even the most "prudent" physicians were content with maxims and rules gleaned from experience alone ([1649] 1989: 6–7, 17). While physicians had little but sensation through which to ascertain types of disease and offer prognosis (the *doctrina prognosticationis*), sensation itself grew more suspect as the sixteenth and seventeenth centuries unfolded.

The recovery of skepticism, in its various forms, spurred these challenges to sense perception (Pittion 1987). In 1606, for example, Pierre Charron rehearses typical arguments for fallibility: illness and vehement passions, failures of vision at a distance, sensory contradictions that must be adjusted by reason, sensory superiority of animals (Charron n.d.: 39–42; Hatfield 1998: 956). Before Charron, Michel de Montaigne, sharply attentive to the uncertainty of medical thought, argues forcefully that it is the "privilege of the senses to be the extreme limit of our perception," and thus there is "nothing beyond them that can help us discover them; no, nor can one sense discover the other." Of course, he draws on the Aristotelian notion, mentioned above, that "there is nothing in the mind that is not first in the senses," or, in his own words, "all knowledge makes its way into us through the senses" (1958: 443–4). Whether in fevers or cases of sensory impairment, delirium or melancholy, the ways in which physicians apprehend effects *ante oculos*, hunt for hidden causes, or suture one to the other, sign to syndrome, all involve the senses, external and internal, and thus are dependent on the soul "following" the body, on the paradox of experiential, perceptual knowledge versus the *scientia* that characterizes demonstration from certain first principles.

As Harvey has argued, since the Middle Ages physicians were concerned with the senses, with faculties essential to the functioning of imagination and cognition, and with the brain, insomuch as they are subject to distemper arising from "bad complexion" or distress, as we shall see below (1975: 23–4). The ways in which distemper reveals relationships between cognition and sensation are available in an often-repeated example from Galen, his "wool-winder," an anecdote that also affirms an engagement with patristic thought in the early seventeenth century.

Nemesius, Bishop of Emesa, wrote *De natura hominis* with his Galen to hand: his forays into anthropology, his views of the function of the senses and of the relationships between bodies and souls, were important enough to be Englished by George Wither in 1636 (see Harvey 1975: 2–3, 31–5; Nemesius 1975). His exploration of the internal and external senses is, for the seventeenth century, remarkably current (1636: 268ff.), and he draws on a wide array of sources in addition to Galen. His attention to pathology and impairment leads him to argue that, while one sense might discover the faults of another—"by the *sense* of *touching*, the error of *sight* is discovered" (1636: 314)—patients experiencing psychic distemper are most instructive. Such a "frantick man, is mentioned by *Galen*," Nemesius writes,

> who being in a place wherein a *wool-winder* was at work by him, rose up, and taking certaine glasse vessels which hee found in the roome, ran to the window, and asked such as passed by, whether they would have such or such glasses cast downe until them, calling every vessell by the right name: And when they would have it so, hee threw them all downe, one after another.

Then the frantic asked if passers-by "would have the *wool-winder* throwne downe also; they (thinking he had but jested) replyed *yea*: whereupon he tooke up the *wool-winder* and hurled him headlong from a high place." Nemesius concludes that this man "had his *senses* whole enough; for hee knew which were the *glasse-vessels*, and which was the *wool-winder*; but his *cogitation* was diseased" (1636: 338–40). This anecdote, from *Quod animi mores*, demonstrates a frequent move in Renaissance treatments of the senses: pathologies disclose relationships, impairment or incapacity reveal function. In Nemesius' rendition, Galen epitomizes attempts to apportion malfunction along what we shall see below is called "the chain of cognition."

These notions underwrite the vast literature concerning regimen and care of self, largely present in self-help manuals like Elyot's. One among dozens of examples must suffice. Pierre Charron, for instance, directly linked sensory disorders with immoderate passion: the "*Soule* being stirred with Choler, Love,

Hatred, or any other passion, our senses doe see, and heare every thing other then they are ... the eye discerneth not that which is before it, and which it seeth" (Charron n.d.: 41). Explorations of the senses—mooring their soundness to regimen, habit, and counsel—speak to strong Renaissance investigations of the intersection of rhetoric, medicine, and moral philosophy. This "medical-moral" habit of thought sustains Renaissance inquiry, from the paeans to the senses as divine organs that preface many anatomical treatments to the ways in which the senses are essayed in divergent conceptions of the Renaissance soul. The faculties and the senses were central not only to medicine and moral philosophy, but often determined metaphysical disputes as well (Hatfield 1998: 953).

SENSE IN THE ANIMAL ECONOMY

Recent scholarship has demonstrated the various ways in which souls were held to "follow" or "sympathize" with bodies in Renaissance thought, while at the same time interrogating the maladroit dualism that governed mid-twentieth-century inquiry (French 1969; Wright and Potter 2000). In fact, the period "played a vital role in the transition from medieval to modern accounts of body, soul, and mind" (Michael 2000: 147). Even though the rational soul was sometimes seen as outside their purview, physicians made significant contributions to new conceptualiztions of body-soul interaction, for all faculties "only performed effectively when the bodily parts were correctly materially structured," as Galen's wool-winder anecdote exemplifies (Brockliss 1987: 401). But how were these faculties of the soul depicted and explored? Here, I offer a brief sketch of the complex, subtle, sometimes sharply divergent, conceptions of souls, faculties and powers, senses and feelings, governed by the sensitive ("animal") and rational souls (Park 1988; Siraisi 1990).

From antiquity through to the Renaissance, with much variation, accounts of the soul were largely Aristotelian (Du Chene 2000). As it was transformed by both medieval Christian and Arabic influence, ancient thought nevertheless yields a tripartite schema of souls to which most subscribed. Organs and functions were understood to be informed and actualized by three souls—the vegetative (or "nutritive," "generative"), the sensitive (or "animal"), and the rational (or "intellective")—which governed, broadly, nourishment, reproduction, and growth; sense and motion, perception and passion; and estimation, cognition, and judgment. Each soul ("power" or "faculty"; the terms are interchangeable, and denote the capacity to actualize potential) was seated in a major organ—the liver, the heart, the brain (see, for instance, Fernel 2003: 305ff.). Until anatomists, chemists, and others offered new explanations of several organic processes, from reproduction to the manufacture of heat, Renaissance medicine embraced this broad outline. By the seventeenth century, as is well-known, Descartes confined the soul to its intellective capacities, while others, including the physicians Sennert and Willis, revitalized the notion of the sensitive soul, widened its province, and reasserted its primacy in medical theory and practice (Willis 1683: 41ff.). To be sure, the sensitive soul was the locus of motive and perceptual faculties—appetite and motion, external and internal senses, respectively. Fernel describes the sensitive soul and its "animal faculties" as means by which we see, smell, hear, taste, touch, and "handle," but it also moves us, assists in discrimination, imagines, dreams, and remembers. As the seat of perception and sensation, in medicine the sensitive soul is king, even arrogating some functions which were earlier assigned to other souls or faculties; in Sennert's formulation, for example, the roles of the scholastic *vis estimativa*, usually confined to the rational soul, were re-distributed, mostly to the imagination as the faculty devoted to the reception and evaluation of images, species, or sensibles. As Sennert writes, the sensitive soul is composed of three faculties, "*the knowing, desiring, and moving.*" The sensitive soul is the "Primary Efficient" of the body, which is "sensitive" by means of the soul, the "sensator or perceiver of things by the senses" ([1618] 1661: 368).

Part of the sensitive soul, Willis writes, is "Co-extended or equally stretched forth with the Organical Body, and almost with all its Parts" (1683: 56). In these and other excursi, the sensitive soul's substantial powers rest in sensory function and capacity: we know and act based on the data offered our internal senses—imagination and memory, reason and the common sense—by sight, smell, touch, hearing, and taste (Harvey 1975: 41ff.). Its seat was traditionally the heart, but, more and more, thinkers settled on the brain as the locus of sensitive function, laying open the mind to medical care.

The brain supports three or four localized, internal senses, all participatory in most kinds of perception and reasoning: in Robert Burton's terms, again, the common sense, imagination, and memory "perceive the sensible species of things to come, past, absent, such as were before the senses." The powers of the sensitive soul, then, are distributed amongst the internal and external senses, the mediator of which is the common sense. For Burton, the common sense is the "judge or moderator of the rest," by which we discern differences in objects; the imagination executes gathering, storing, and estimative powers by examining the species "perceived by the common sense, of things present or absent"; and memory has the same object as imagination and "lays up all the species which the senses have brought in, and records them as a good register"

([1621] 1927: 1.1.2.6; 139–40). Burton's account differs slightly from the conventional, for usually the common sense, or *sensus communis*, is a receptacle for the data from the five external senses, or perhaps a sense in itself for motion, rest, number, shape, and size, or qualities not specific to the other senses. Burton takes the *sensus communis* for reason, understanding or, narrowly conceived, cogitation, the latter often the source of innate ideas, divinely imprinted, and the faculty that evaluates, judges, and commands the will. Whether these functions are ascribed to the common sense or to reason, they fund perception: by the faculty of "discernment," Fernel's term, we know what a sense senses, we combine sense data, and we know we are sentient (2003: 335–7; see Harvey 1975; Wolfson 1935).

Among the internal senses, most physicians agree with Fernel: the imagination "grasps the emanations [images, phantasms, *simulacra*] presented to it," but also engages in *effictio*, producing images not presented by the external senses (2003: 339). These images are, at first, "lightly imprinted in the brain" (the analogue of inscription is usually a wax tablet), and then stored, more durably, in the memory. The latter has two functions: storage itself, and recollection, "to reproduce the thing itself by grasping an image," the first an experience, the second an action. Fernel summarizes: "the phantoms of outside things derived from the senses" are presented to the imagination, which in turn presents such images to reason and to memory; if the imprint is strong, in various ways, including those marked by passion, we remember. To the French physician, all of these faculties belong "to the whole brain," over which the "main sentient soul" extends (2003: 341). But the influence is reciprocal: to the Anglo-Italian physician John Cotta, the imagination "is misstresse and great commander of all the senses" (1612: 63).

To accomplish their ends, to fulfill their capacities, both the sensitive and rational souls depend on *spiritus animalis*, rather a less familiar substance than the humors, at least in contemporary scholarship. What is animal spirit? The answer is controversial, but most philosophers and physicians agreed that spirits are attenuated matter, "subtle, invisible, and . . . exalted," produced by the thinning and aeration of blood, first in the heart, then in the ventricles of the brain (*Anthropologie Abstracted* 1655: 100). Elyot explains spirit as an "ayry substance subtyll" that, in its animal form, "maketh sence or felynge" ([1541] 1595: sig.12r). Fernel agreed (2003: 297–9). On Galen's authority, its functions, if not its etiology, were common store, and had been since the late Middle Ages (Bono 1995). Spirits appear in most medical treatises, and were frequently the subject of medical dissertations concerned with psychological illness (Diethelm 1971).

In Sennert's authoritative view, spirits are "the bond by which the body and soul are united, ... and being wrought in the principal parts of the boy are conveyed through channels [nerves] into the whole body, and are joined with Innate heat, that they may help the powers and faculties perform their actions." Although animal spirits "perform internal and external senses," Sennert is careful to insist that the soul is the faculty itself and merely "useth" the spirits as instruments ([1611] 1656: 12–13). Burton, too, argues that spirit is "a most subtle vapour, which is expressed from the *blood*, and the instrument of the soul, to perform all his actions; a common tie or *medium* betwixt the body and the soul." The animal spirits, formed from the vital, "brought up to the brain, and diffused by the nerves, to the subordinate members, give sense and motion to them all" ([1621] 1927: 1.1.2.2, 129). Attention to the spirits reveals the "entire chain of cognition from the external senses through internal senses to the intellect," subject to extensive debate, particularly in commentaries on Aristotle's *De anima* (Hatfield 1998: 955–6).

Thus the sensitive soul is, in Burton's terms, "an act of the organical body, by which it lives, hath sense, appetite, judgement, breath, and motion." The apprehending and moving faculties define the sensitive soul, the former responsible for locomotion and the "inward" movement of the spirits and the pulse, while by the latter power "we perceive the species of sensible things, present or absent, and retain them as wax doth the print of a seal." Apprehension is internal and external, and in *The Anatomy of Melancholy* (1621 and after) Burton begins his section on the sensitive soul by offering a typical account of the senses ([1621] 1927: 1.1.2.6, 137–9). As in most accounts, each sense is explored via its object, its organ, and its medium. The eye, for example, has as its object the visible (color and luminescence), its medium light, and its organ the eye itself, "chiefly the apple of it," its crystalline humors, its optic nerves, which convey, as we have seen, images to the internal senses (1.1.2.6, 138; Willis 1683: 75–86). Anatomy, function, and faculty are seamlessly intertwined, often celebrated as divine; the eye is most frequently the model for other senses, since God's hand could be found even in retinal displacement (Riskin 2011). The care and enthusiasm with which the eyes were explored is captured nicely in du Laurens' *Discourse of the Preservation of Sight . . .* ([1594] 1599), which celebrates vision almost ecstatically as the sense "of our blessedness," as the "most infallible sence," in what he himself calls a mix of medical, philosophical, and poetic discourse ([1594] 1599: 13, 17, 20). Other scholars offer full accounts of vision and its conditions in Renaissance culture, noting that as frequent as the paeans to the eye's superiority are realizations that vision, when impaired or subject to distemper, easily deceived or impaired (Clark 2007);

increasing complexity underwrites sharper concern. Briefly, I offer one sense, smell, as an epitome of medical thought in the period.

Smelling's organ is the nose, "or the two small hollow pieces of flesh a little above it," and "by avoiding bad smells, as by choosing good," we "as much alter and affect the body many times as *diet* itself." Its medium is air, and its object a "quality, fume, vapour, or exhalation" (Burton [1621] 1927: 1.1.2.6, 138–9), "drawn up along with spirit through the nasal passages" (Fernel 2003: 333). In fact, the majority of physicians thought odors were material—as does Juan Bravo in his 1583 *De saporum et odorum differentiis*—a notion which accounts for the tradition of smells being not only appetizing, but nourishing and therapeutic (Palmer 1993). But the operation of smelling is controverted "betwixt the Physicians and the Peripateticks," as Sennert points out in a passage worth examination, not least for its shrewd navigation of inherited opinion and its employment of empirical effort. The peripatetics hold the organ of smelling "to be the Nerves dilated in the Nostrils," while Galen suggests that the ventricles of the brain are olfactory organs. Others suggest that "from the Brain neer the Cavity of the Eyes, two Channels are derived to the bored bones of the Nose, whose ends seem like teats (whence they are called the mammillary or teat-like productions) and that in them as the proper instrument odors are discerned." Most physicians, he claims, adhere to the latter view: the brain is not a "proper organ" of any external sense, but simply supplies animal spirits; furthermore, experience confirms that, since we do not smell all the time, the perception of odor does not reside in nerves in the nostrils. Instead, the "examiners" of smells are "those mammillary or Teat-like productions," for smell is interrupted by diseases of the head, like catarrh. We cannot perceive smells without breathing, so smells cannot reach the "mammillary processes," the protrusions which make smell an "external" sense, without air ([1618] 1661: 377). Sennert adumbrates controversy, courts experience, and asserts, definitively, that the organ which judges odors is the brain. Willis more or less agrees, insisting that the nerves of the mamillary process are those that convey smells for judgment, on which depends, in part, the discovery of "agreeable and wholesome Aliments" (1683: 88), food one of the non-naturals.

The "non-naturals" were essential to securing and conserving health, to maintaing the liveliness of the senses. In fact, Renaissance medical practice is fueled by the knowledge and experience of distinctions between between "Thynges Naturall" (elements, complexions, humors, members, faculties, operations, and spirits), things contra-natural (sickness, its causes, effects, and accidents), and things non-natural: "Ayre, Meate and drinke, Slepe and watche,

M[o]vinge and rest, Emptinesse and repletion, and Affections of the mynde" (Elyot [1541] 1595: sig. Bir; see Pender 2010). While the soul and its acts are never fully determined by complexions and temperaments, the opportunities for regulation of interactions with the world that affect the soul and its faculties multiply as the period unfolds. Thus, the cases in which our senses may be "deluded" include the indisposition of an organ, as the eye suffers from jaundice; an alteration of the medium specific to the sense, as with, say, refraction; or by distance. So the evidence of "one single Sense" may be "undemonstrative and fallacious," and corrected by one's other senses and by the senses of others (Nourse 1686: 84–8; cf. Nemesius 1636: 314). Mentioning these three problems, Sennert argues that the senses may err by mistaking sound for smell, color for sound; by taking one quality for another, as in salt for sweet; or in their application to an object, as when we taste meat as bitter due to an abundance of choler, "wherewith the tongue is infected" ([1618] 1661: 371–2). These misprisions are sometimes those of the common sense or the external senses, but are most often those of the imagination in its league with sensation: as "Imagination follows the reports of Sense, so the Will with its Passions follows the Bent of the Imagination" (Nourse 1686: 103). Paradox appears again.

From the sixteenth through to the late seventeenth century, then, the functions and roles of the internal and external senses grew ever more complex, as did their relationship with one another, with *spiritus*, and with cognition. But, as we have seen, the senses were mobilized as objects of inquiry and remediation in various contexts; one is the Renaissance bedside.

ENTER THE SENSES

Since antiquity, conduct at the sickbed has received ample guidance. As the Hippocratean *On Decorum* specifies, at bedsides physicians should be serious and graceful in speech and disposition, comforting patients with "solicitude and attention" (1923: 3.281–2, 298–9). Renaissance practitioners emulated ancient physicians and counselors, who enlisted *to prepon* (decorum) in "clinical" speech and conduct, insisting, after Galen, that confidence and trust in a physician are essential to healing. "Bedside manners" were explored thoroughly in the Middle Ages and, by the Renaissance, physicians were urged to embrace propriety (see Bylebyl 1993; McVaugh 1997). A good opinion of a physician makes a patient "more capable to entertain the Medicine" (Nourse 1686: 99–100).

Such confidence-building was secondary to the identification and collection of symptoms via the senses, a process, as we shall see, combined with inferring proximate and remote causes of disease. At the bedside, external causes of disease are discovered by "the inquisition of the Physitian," but also by "the relation of the patient" (Holland 1633: 13). "Inquisition" was accomplished by mobilizing the senses, as we have seen: doctors palpated bodies, smelled their patients' breath, listened to their histories (Wear 2000: 120–2). Issues of prudery, privacy, and mendacity aside—the diarist Samuel Pepys mentions a mendacious fellow who posed as a physician in order to catch sight of a woman's "thing below"—the sickbed was the site of discussion and debate as well as physical examination (Porter 1993: 187). In conversation, patients told physicians "what was wrong: when and how the complaint had started, what events had precipitated it, the characteristic pains and symptoms, its periodicity." Patients would describe "key lifestyle features," like "eating and sleeping habits, his bowel motions, recent emotional traumas, and so forth." Physical examination consisted largely of looking, perhaps percussion and auscultation, frequently pulse-taking, listening to coughs, "wheezings and eructations," smelling the putrefactive (Porter 1993: 182–3). In this intimate scene of inquiry and remediation, as I have argued elsewhere, both patients' and practitioners' activities are rhetorical: praying, detailing symptoms, reading self-help manuals, chatting with visitors and physicians, receiving counsel, occasioning or assuaging emotion (see Pender 2002). Of course, physicians attended to a myriad circumstances, principally organized by the categories of the non-naturals and prognostic signs, but some indications were available only in discursive form, in sufferers' narrations or in case histories. *Historia*, in this case, is not the narrative presentation of inquiry, one of the antique meanings of the term, but "accounts of specific cases encountered in medical practice," sometimes termed *observationes*. Frequently occasioned by a rote ensemble of questions, and thus somewhat restrictive of both the patient's and the physician's expression, *historiae* and *consilia* (edited and therefore not direct records of consultations) nevertheless pose questions concerning the relationship between particular cases and general remedies, evidence and narrative, discourse and practice (Siraisi 1997: 196, 77; see also Pomata and Siraisi 2005). Their history is complex, and several accounts note the similarities between the *historia* and Galenic *curatio*, often self-congratulatory reports of successful cures (Hess and Mendelsohn 2010).

   A physician "visit[s] a patient, and by meanes of his sight, his hearing, his smelling, and his feeling, he knoweth things which seem impossible," as Juan Huarte puts it in 1575. About one hundred years later, in a rebarbative text that impugns a rival physician's diagnosis of a young girl, "Alius Medicus" details bedside consultation. First, physicians must establish "*Who* the Patient is," via the naturals, non-naturals, and contra-naturals. The naturals, at least here, include parentage, age and temperament, sex and complexion, disposition ("whether he be morose, or affable, weak or pettish and angry"), and "*Habit of Body*," including the hair and skin. The writer then considers the non-naturals, including "transpiration," or sweating, citing Sanctorius. Perhaps most interesting is the inclusion of other *historiae*: has the patient suffered any other sickness? What were the causes? What were the patient's complaints, the former physician's prognostications? The final topic of inquiry is symptoms, which are divided into animal, vital, and natural, the former consisting of principal actions, such as reason and imagination, and "*Less-Principal*," such as those belonging to sense and motion. The latter category includes pain and "all Gestures and Postures" of the body, while the "involuntary Natural" consists of heredity and nutrition, the vital of respiration and pulse. All the alterations of the patient's body can be divided into compounds of primary qualities—hot, cold, moist, dry—as well as texture, color, smell, taste, and sound, all of which "belong to the Physician's Judgement" (Willis 1683: 4–9). The results of these encounters are *historiae*:

> Now he that hath but half an Eye must necessarily discern, that much of judgment, much of contrivance is requisite in these Cases; and indeed so much, that it is well know many (and I hope that it may be affirmed of most) Physicians, make a History of the Patients condition, or Case; and then after due Consideration of all circumstances, determine to proceed after a certain Method from which they do not recede without great occasion given them, as intervening of some accidents, which Humane Wisdom, and Care, could neither foresee, nor prevent.
>
> Coxe 1669: 86; see du Laurens [1594] 1599: 20

Ideally, then, *historiae* embody not only observation, but circumstanced judgment, both of which foster care, both dependent on medical *phronesis*.

But perhaps Roy Porter is correct to label most physicians "thinkers" not "touchers," at least as opposed to barbers, surgeons, and midwives (1995: 185). The Huarte passage cited above continues, and he enlists another sort of seeing, something Hippocratic physicians call "mental sight" or reason and imagination (Hippocrates 1950: 87–9; Temkin 1973: 16). Thus a physician visits a patient, and "by meanes of his sight, his hearing, his smelling, and his feeling, he knoweth things which seem impossible." If we ask that physician, "how he could come by so readie a knowledge," he would not know, "for it is a grace which springeth from the fruitfulnesse of the imagination, which by another name is termed a readinesse of capacitie, which by common signes, and by uncertain conjectures, and of small importance, in the twinckling of an eye, knoweth 1000 differences of things, wherein the force of curing and prognosticating with certaintie consisteth." Curing and predicting depend on signs and conjectures, which are apprehended by the imagination, the "readiness of capacity" that Huarte singles out as essential to medical practice (as opposed to cognition, required for theory). As he claims, this "spice of promptness," *solertia* or shrewdness, clarity of *oculus mentis*, is part of the imagination: "men of great imagination, are not altogether deprived of understanding, nor of memorie. Wher-through, by having these two powers in some measure they are able to learn the most necessarie points of Phisicke: for that they are plainest, and with the good imagination which they have, can better looke into the disease and cause thereof, than the cunningest doctors." For Huarte, a physician is a "finder out of occasion," assessing place, time, circumstance via the "worke of the imagination" ([1575] 1959: 180–2).

This was certainly true of Giovanni Battista da Monte's clinical practice in the sixteenth century. Besides asking the patient about habit, food and drink, and exercise, da Monte's physical examination focused on the senses of both patient and doctor: he essayed the sufferer's senses, internal and external, his or her "animal functions," and by means of "the natural and animal functions, and whatever else is apparent to [the physician's] senses," made what he called "universal" judgments from his apprehension of particulars. From the "manifestly apparent" signs, following Galen, he perceives "those that are hidden within," by asking what is the affected part? Of what kind is the disturbance? What is its cause? Although no empiricist, it seems da Monte was intimately attentive to his patients' bodies, but also frequently mentions the internal senses as indications of disturbance (Bylebyl 1993: 45, 51–4).

Such was the case of Caspar Barlaeus, Dutch poet, scholar, and physician (though he seems not to have practiced), for whom we have a rather complete record of suffering in his correspondence. He experienced four serious episodes of hypochondriacal melancholy in the 1620s and 1630s, the second of which arose from fatigue "by too much exercise in my studies," occasioning "obstructions," feelings of anxiety, delusions. Barlaeus, by his own account, was rendered "almost dumb and speechless," "a motionless lump of stone," void of feeling, by what his biographer calls "depression" (Blok 1976: 40, 127). He was unable to fulfill his duties as lecturer during this period, because pressure in the hypochondrium affected his breathing, making his speech "curt," passionless (47; cf. 56). But his most troubling affliction is delusion, caused, as Barlaeus himself claims, by "vapors" of melancholy rising to cloud his mind: he is blind, he writes, but not actually so; he suffers psychically, and imagines his case as a footnote to one of his friend Constantijn Huygens' poems (128). In this rich correspondence, in which Barlaeus shares and documents his suffering, his interlocutors suggest several remedies for distress and delusion: noting that Barlaeus' own medical knowledge might be unnerving, Huygens urges "matter be found for laughing and joking," while others suggest changes in diet and moderate exercise as prophylaxes (58, 69). But, apropos "animal powers," while his physical health recovered, variously, after each episode, his mental health often lagged. Like other melancholics of the period, he sees things, his thinking suffers, he endures prolonged inactivity, and he imagines his body made of glass, a condition that Descartes uses to impugn the senses at the beginning of the *Meditations*. One late seventeenth-century scholar worries that we "infuse" melancholy into our children, which "may serve to discolour" objects meeting their senses in the common course of life (Temple 1681: 181). Here, in relief, is the anxiety about the verity of sight: vision cathected with meaning, the "vogue" for melancholy not only derived from the reception of Aristotle's *Problemata*, but from the ostensible but contested dominance of real and abstract "seeing."

EVIDENCE AND SENSIBILITY

Testing patients with one's senses inspires the testing of the senses themselves and their epistemological purchase. Above, I stressed the importance of *spiritus* to the animal economy, in part because the existence of the spirits themselves becomes one of the grounds on which the controversy about sensory evidence unfolds. To conclude, I return to taste, and explore the senses as they were used in the "laboratory," and finish by emphasizing their place in a fully functioning human being in order to argue that the moralizing common to anatomical and medical texts tends to be submerged in more profound concerns about the functioning of the animal economy as the period unfolds.

Recall that Richard Boulton tasted blood to confirm the existence of *spiritus*: we learn by the tongue that spirits are the purest part of blood, for they taste oily, sweet. Famously, and rebarbatively, William Harvey disagreed, and impugned his predecessors for freighting the spirits with overmuch power: "like bad poets" physicians and anatomists have offered dubious and conflicting notions of *spiritus* as the grand explanans in the "little world." While physicians admit three kinds of spirits, "the natural spirits flowing through the veins, the vital spirits through the arteries, and the animal through the nerves," Harvey demurs. "[We] have found none of all these spirits by dissection, neither in the veins, nerves, arteries, nor other parts of living animals." In particular, those "who advocate incorporeal spirits have no ground of experience to stand upon" (1965: 115–16). Efforts to distinguish and isolate the volatile, spiritous, or motile qualities of the blood are "uncertain and questionable" (117). The spirits are chimeras, merely "specious names" (502). While conventional anatomical wisdom asserted that the blood was too thick to "possess a substance intermediate between body and faculty" (Fernel 2003: 297), Harvey disproves the existence of spirits by the "simple senses" alone (Harvey 1965: 503). In his work on both circulation and generation, he routs out falsity from medical study "by dissection, by multiplied experience, and accurate observation," as he notes in the preface to *De motu cordis* (1628: 9). He deepens and refines his Aristotelianism by claiming that universals are apprehended in "the perception of individual things by the senses" (154). Harvey insists that some "weak" persons cling to argument with respect to areas of inquiry that should proceed only "on the evidence of the senses." Sensory investigation courts assurance: who would "pretend to persuade those who had never tasted wine that it was a drink much pleasanter to the palate than water?" The circulation of the blood, he continues, is shown through experiment, by proofs "cognizable by the senses . . ." No one has "apt scientific apprehension" who has no experience; they are likely to rely upon "sophistical reasonings" (130–1).

Experience, reason, and inference share governance in the examples of medical theory and practice, and of the paradox of sense, found in this chapter. As we have seen, medical thinkers explore the senses as they appear to function in animal economies—again, the senses rarely have a history entirely their own. Central to these histories, as I have emphasized, is the notion that the soul "follows" or "sympathizes" with the body, a notion to which I return, briefly, here. Recall Huarte's assertion in 1575 that "the maners of the soule, follow the temperature of the body, in which it keepes residence." While endorsing the broad outlines of Galen's assertion, Huarte complicates this notion, and reserves a place for regimen, and thus for volition. Dwelling in the body, the "reasonable soul" must use different instruments in order to accomplish contrary operations; his example is sense:

> This is plainly seen in the power of the soule, which performeth divers operations in the outward sences, for every one hath his particular composition: the eyes have one, the ears another, the smelling another, and the feeling another; and if it were not so, there should be no more but one sort of operations, and that should all be seeing, tasting, or feeling,

for the instrument determines & rules the power for one action, and for no more.

Huarte reasons from this point that the brain, too, must have several instruments—for the internal senses—and mentions that dissecting the brain reveals four "hollownesses," three for the imagination, memory, and understanding (he rarely mentions the common sense), and a fourth for "digesting and altering the vitall spirits" into animal ([1575] 1959: 51–4). The physician's commitment to both reason and experience yields a picture of one soul activating several capacities, each with distinct instruments, organs, or functions; and Huarte continues to speculate on the ways in which various kinds of complexions and temperatures affect them all, as, for example, his assertion that "he who hath a greate understanding cannot enjoy a good memorie," for the qualities that enable one, dryness and coldness, impair the other (63). A strong recognition of the conditions under which the soul must operate leads Huarte to conclude that its "sympathy" with the body is widely variable, frangible, uneven. Huarte alights on sense to exemplify this problem, perhaps because sensation itself discloses the relationship between active and passive functions of the same organ: as sensation is comprised of "receptions of species," it is a passion, and thus this function is passive; but sensation cannot occur without an activity of the soul, since it is "a kind of discerning and knowing of the Object by the Senses, received into the Sense, and so it is an Action" (Crooke 1616: 658; see Spruit 2008). In precisely this context, a mid-seventeenth century physician's conceptualization is germane: most accept that the mind's inclinations "do more frequently confess their subjection to the influence of the constitution of the body; but this is done *actu morali*, by *inclination* and *disposition*, not by *impression* of any *real, Physical, miasme* or *pollution*; by the same way whereby the stars rule us, and God the stares" (*Anthropologie Abstracted* 1655: 40–1). "Moral acts" alone determine the ways in which bodies impinge on souls; as the physician Walter Charleton avers, if we fall into error, "the defect lieth in our own act, or in the use of our *liberty*, not in our nature" (1674: 169, 171).

Just as this same cluster of ideas animates Descartes' assertions for the autonomy of the will, so the paradox of sense organizes his famous conclusion to his *Meditations* (1641): the senses exist to "inform the mind of what is beneficial or harmful for the composite of which the mind is a part; and to this extent they are sufficiently clear and distinct." But we are wrong, he continues, to trust their apprehension of the world, since they offer "only very obscure information" (1985: 2.57–8). Descartes resolves this paradox with regimen: in his letters to Elisabeth, princess of Bohemia, in the mid-1640s, and in his final work, *The Passions of the Soul* (1649), a neo-Stoic psychology of assent, as well as an investment in habit, govern human conduct, expressed in the ways in which he reconfigures scholastic accounts of volition to offer, as it were, a poetics of internal persuasion. His position is well known (Gaukroger 1995: 394ff.). He turns our attention to regimen as a way of supplementing the deficiencies of the senses. As he wrote in the *Treatise of Man*, "the mind is so dependent on temperament, and on the dispositions of the organs of the body, that if it is possible to find some way to make men wiser and more clever than they have been thus far, I think it must be sought in medicine" (1972: 86, n. 113). Perhaps that is why his contemporary, the physician Sanctorius, recommends that a physician should be a *sensatus philosophus* (quoted in Maclean 2002: 198). Those seeking wisdom through medicine must examine the roles and functions of the senses.

CHAPTER SEVEN

The Senses in Literature: Renaissance Poetry and the Paradox of Perception

HOLLY DUGAN

Shylock's famous rebuttal to his Christian tormentors in Shakespeare's imagined Venetian Rialto posits a theory of sensation that is at once both common and specific. He asks them:

> Hath not a Jew eyes? Hath not a Jew hands, organs, dimensions, senses, affections, passions; fed with the same food, hurt with the same weapons, subject to the same diseases, healed by the same means, warmed and cooled by the same winter and summer as a Christian is? If you prick us do we not bleed? If you tickle us do we not laugh? And if you wrong us shall we not revenge? If we are like you in the rest, then we will resemble you in that.
>
> *Merchant of Venice*, 3.1.49–61

His is a stunning articulation of likeness in a play known for its reliance on turgid early modern notions of embodied difference, particularly of gendered, ethnic, and racial differences. Shylock's claim, and the theory of sensation upon which it depends, feels almost modern, even as it works to justify a distinctly early modern notion of revenge. It seems to offer a model of liberal tolerance based on shared sensations: if affect flows from embodied perceptions that we all share, then our differences must matter less than we think.

Shakespeare's play, of course, does not enact this theory of sensation. Shylock remains a villain throughout: by the end of the fourth act, he has lost his daughter, his bond with Antonio, his property, and even his status as a Jew. He is forced to convert to Christianity in a Venetian court and he is lucky to escape with his life, though he expressly wishes for death (4.1.369). In seeking to apply a physiological theory of affect to Venetian social and economic bonds—arguing that "hands," "organs," "dimensions," and "senses" shape "affections" and "passions"—Shylock ironically ends up alone, exiled from almost every vector of identity that matters in the play.

What, if anything, does this English literary representation of an imagined "Venetian" Jewish merchant and his ramblings about theories of affect offer to those seeking to historicize sensation in the past? After all, the eponymous Venice of Shakespeare's play bears almost no connection to its historical counterpart (Platt 2009: 128; Tanner 1999: 45). Nor does "Jewish," for that matter, especially since England formally expelled its Jewish residents in 1290, defining itself as a space without a Jewish presence (Shapiro 1996: 13–55). On the one hand, it is a powerfully evocative literary representation, whose relationship to the material realities that shaped social meaning in the past is complex at best. And yet, Shylock's synecdoche of senses, affections, and passions, articulated in an imagined moment of charged confrontation, provocatively suggests that theories of sensation were inextricably linked to social identity. In doing so, it raises questions about the role of evolving medical theories of sensation on shared experiences of social reality.

Shylock's eloquent defense of his truly awful desire for revenge asks his tormentors a profoundly evocative question: what moves us? Shylock posits a shared material environment. But Shakespeare's play also asks that of its audiences, who for at least a short period of time were heated and cooled not only by the same air but also by their experience of hearing the play (and perhaps also subjected to the same affections and passions because of it). The details of his argument—its metonymic association of hands, organs, dimensions, senses, affections, and passions—are also theories of matter, raising questions about how large-scale sensory shifts were understood and described by ordinary men and women in their everyday lives.

In this chapter, I argue that metaphor is an intrinsic part of understanding sensation, and because of this, literary representations have much to offer scholars working on its history. Artistically idiosyncratic yet also intrinsically linked to broader notions of genre and form, literary works like Shakespeare's play usefully remind scholars of the methodological challenges of historicizing sensation even as they offer a way to navigate around such challenges. This is particularly true of the Renaissance—a period defined by medical breakthroughs, a burgeoning global culture of trade, new technologies of print, political upheaval, and religious controversy: all of which influenced not only theories about sensation but also material experiences of embodiment.

Consider, for example, the role of literary sources in the history of ambergris, a material whose scent remains hard to describe precisely because it is so unlike any other. Described in early modern English as "sweet," "sweet-smelling," "sweet in itself" and a "sugared smell," ambergris emerges through what we might term synaesthetic metaphors of taste ("Taming of a Shrew," sig. F2 r, Lloyd sig. Y2 v, Kendall sig. Avii v). But it was its "curious" smell that fostered these associations (Nicholson sig. G3v), lending its perfume to food imports (as well as other luxury goods). Ambergris and its distinctive scent briefly became a key component of every kind of luxury imaginable—from chocolate and tobacco in Spain, medicinal curatives in France and the Netherlands, sauces in Belgium, and rosewater, tobacco, and perfumed gloves in England (Duerloo 2012: 240; Dugan 2011: 49, 107, 148; Kemp 2012: 59; McCabe 2008: 39; Norton 2010: 18, 87). Such linguistic imprecision fueled metaphoric descriptions; these descriptions connected its smell with a host of cultural, economic, and political arenas of Renaissance culture. As I have argued elsewhere, its salty, musky scent dominated the new smellscapes of European markets, a scent implicitly connected with global trade and growing luxury consumption. It was also a scent associated with profound paradoxes: unlike any other Renaissance scent ingredient it thus seemed profoundly novel, even as it became overly associated with luxury. It was identified as a divine smell, yet mostly by religious zealots who seemed untroubled by its association with classical theories of medicine and with the Muslim legacy of Al-Andalus (Constable 1999: Ch. 2; Donkin 1999: 25; Feinberg 2002: 55). It was believed to be a curative for melancholy but was also considered a dangerous aphrodisiac (Dugan 2011: 115; Feinberg 2002: 55); it was by its nature foreign, yet it had no clear provenance and flouted the logic of trade that depended on such origins. Its scent was thus all of these things at once, its sensory history comprised both of large-scale cultural shifts as well as the idiosyncrasy of individual sensation.

That ambergris is mentioned as evidence in such varied historical approaches to the period speaks to the ways in which sensory history has contributed to scholarly knowledge about the Renaissance. The "sensuous turn" in scholarship has galvanized Renaissance literary studies, producing both new understanding about the role of sensation in the past as well as new approaches for studying literature (Dugan 2011; Gallagher and Rankin 2010; Howes 2005a; Milner 2011; Newhauser 2010; Quiviger 2010; Sanger and Walker 2012; B. Smith 2008; M. Smith 2007a). Literary studies has also galvanized sensory history: what Bruce Smith provocatively termed "historical phenomenology" over a decade ago (to describe a promising approach to study sexuality in the past) is now a thriving critical mode of historical and literary scholarship, expanding well beyond sexuality studies, connecting with almost every major facet that defines the Renaissance (B. Smith 2000; cf. B. Smith 2010).

Phenomenology, whether cultural or historical, emphasizes a sensuous scholarly approach as well as a critical language that captures the complexity of studying relationships between "ideas, bodies, and objects" (B. Smith 2012: 479). It is, as literary scholar Stephen Connor argues, a research practice that "aspires to articulate the worldliness and embodiedness of experience" (Connor 2000: 3). It has, since its inception, focused on the ways in which literature and history intersect and, for this reason, it has made a significant contribution to sensory history through its sustained and scholarly engagement not only with cultural theories about perception, material culture, or the history of embodiment, but also with the ways in which these relationships were articulated in the past.

A kind of zygote formed from the philosophical traditions of Maurice Merleau-Ponty and the practices of a Marxist-inflected historical materialism, historical phenomenology emerged as a robust way to research sexuality and embodiment in the past. Early work expanded this focus on embodiment to consider perception, including each of the individual faculties of sensation (Bloom 2007; Craik 2007; Dugan 2011; Harris 2007; Harvey 2002; B. Smith 2000; Stanev 2012); more recently, scholars seek to understand sensation in comprehensive and cross-modal ways (Curran and Kearney 2012; Milner 2011; Stanev 2012; Waldron 2012). Because literature is often a formal articulation of affect, its metaphors offer a powerful interface between the senses and the social. As such, historical phenomenology as a literary methodology continues to resonate with new research on sensation emerging in other disciplines, research that extends the study of sensation well beyond the model of the five senses to include global approaches, sensory archeology, extrasensory perception, invisible materiality, and synaesthesia (Blackman 2012; Drewal 2012; Helmreich *et al.* 2012; Howes 2009; Hsy 2012).

Understanding the role of the senses in Renaissance literature has led to new kinds of questions about what counts as archival evidence of sensation.

Literary representations not only bear the trace of what we might identify as embodied sensation—the sights, sounds, tastes, touches, and smells experienced in the past—but also of embodied experiences no longer coded as sensory modalities—of inner passions, humoral fits, disembodied visions (Farina 2012). As Kevin Curran and James Kearney recently argued, historical phenomenology offers both "a language of speculation and inquiry dynamic enough to accommodate both historicism and theory, a common language that can speak as compellingly to questions of law, ethics, performance, and hospitality as it can to questions of feeling and sensation" (Curran and Kearney 2012: 353).

It is this emphasis on a common language that I hope to exfoliate in this chapter. Including Renaissance literary allusions within sensory history may seem to emphasize all too familiar claims that the sensate is too subjective, fleeting, or ephemeral to properly historicize. Michel de Montaigne himself queries something similar in his essay on experience: what is the best approach to study the world? Is its knowledge esoteric or embodied? Montaigne stylistically posits that to feel is to know: "In this universe of things I ignorantly and negligently let myself be guided by the general law of the world; I shall know it well enough when I feel it; my knowledge cannot make it change its path; it will not modify itself for me" (Montaigne 1958: 815). This haptic learning process is rough; the body is bruised by its encounters with the laws of the world and it is through these encounters that knowledge becomes experience.

Montaigne's elegant articulation grounds itself in the interface between physics and metaphysics, between the somatic realm of the body and that of the mind. Scholarship that seeks to explain how the human body has adapted and developed new modes of perception over time needs to ground itself in this interface. Though Aristotle famously proposes the traditional five senses as a theory of perception, Augustine posited a sixth sense that perceived not only external sensation but also the senses themselves (Howes 2005a, 2009; Nichols 2008). Contemporary science now posits nine senses, expanding what we traditionally think of as the sense of touch as different modalities that process heat, speed, pressure, and pain (Geurts 2003). Such varied beliefs raise important questions about the coherence of the field even as it argues for its importance. One salient way to do this is to focus on language—especially literary language.

Such an emphasis on literary language provides a way to trace what David Howes has described as "culturally patterned 'loops' through the environment" (2005a: 5). Though recent breakthroughs in neurology and biomedical engineering seemingly corroborate the important role of metaphor as itself a kind of sensory way of knowing (Lakoff and Johnson 1980), these fields have yet to grapple with the way in which cultural modes of perception might alter perception (Howes 2005a). For example, though recent studies suggest that the same areas of the brain used to produce a sensory-motor action are also used when that action is conceptualized abstractly (Aziz-Zadeh and Damasio 2008) and that smelling a lily, watching someone smell a lily, and even reading a description of someone smelling a lily all rely on similar areas of the brain (Aziz-Zadeh *et al.* 2006), we don't yet know whether this might also be true in cultures that have radically different cultural "loops" through a sensory environment than those who participated in the study (Howes 2005a). Likewise, distinctions between these different kinds of action blur when remembered, confusing memories of what we've seen with what we've done (Lindner *et al.* 2010). Metaphors of sensation, even clichéd ones, can trigger sensory memories— hearing a friend complain about a "rough" day engages the same areas of the brain that process tactile sensory data (Lacey *et al.* 2012)—yet such data only amplifies Proust's famous meditation on the powerful cultural pull of certain sensory memories. If technologies like fMRI are believed to offer an objective way to "view" how language influences sensory modalities, then literature surely offers another, challenging the essentialism of biology through emphasizing the cultural processes through which one learns to process relevant sensory data (those sensory clichés mentioned above) and describe it.

All of this suggests the potential of literary sources within a broader archive of sensation which is amplified when applied to early modern reading practices (Craik 2007). To read literature in the Renaissance was a multi-sensorial affair. Poets, sharing their work in discrete côteries, often preferred more intimate, epistolary connections; that ink was often mixed with sugar provided a gustatory and olfactory resonance of the affective literary bonds between poets (Masten 2004). Yet Renaissance technologies of print, so critical to our tales of large-scale sensory shifts towards the predominance of vision, were also more tactile and auditory than we think (Dugan 2009). Books allowed readers to flip easily between disparate parts. Modern missals, for example, with multicolored ribbon bookmarks hint at the dexterity needed to navigate liturgical services in the past. Protestant readers of the Bible often used all available fingers to quickly move between specific passages when reading aloud (Stallybrass 2002: 42–3, 47). Likewise, reading aloud was the norm: Catholic reading practices in early modern France, for example, emphasized communal listening, connecting pious devotion with earlier traditions of the *veillée* or storytelling (Davis 1965: 201; Rendall 1996: 39). So, too, did Jewish communities in Italy: in 1611, an

English visitor to Venice's Jewish ghetto commented on the "sober, distinct, and ordered" readings and the loud volume at which they were read (Coryat 1611: 294–6). Recent scholarship has focused on the ways in which religion influenced theories of sensation (Milner 2011), yet despite radical differences in specific configurations, early modern reading practices were decidedly multi-sensorial, emphasizing links between sensory perception and textual representation. Across the early modern period, in places as distinct as the multi-cultural environment that defined al-Andalus (Kimmel 2012), the patronage cultures of northern Italy (Cohen 2011: 21) or the contentious political climate of northern Europe (Mader 2012), reading was a vexed and sensuous affair.

The sensuousness of Renaissance reading practices was not limited to books themselves. Even the most quotidian of material objects—a wool-winder, a cheese trencher, a brass ring—were often inscribed with aphorisms, meant to jog other kinds of literary associations when utilized. Rather than representing two opposite poles on a scale of materiality, words and things were inextricably linked in Renaissance reading and writing cultures (Richardson 2011), revealing mutually constitutive links between the materiality of the world, early modern men and women's perceptions of it, and the language they used to describe it. These practices connect with our own sense of archival materials such as the smooth tactility of leather binding, its sharp tang utterly distinct from the sweetly vanilla-like scent of decaying paper. But they also resonate across literary representations, such as Hugh Platt's description of ink made of rosewater and ambergris (Platt 1609), or Thomas Dekker's harrowing invocation for a pen that echoes the cries of Renaissance plague victims (Dekker 1603).

Such descriptions remind us that material and metaphoric evidence is not always mutually exclusive: synaesthesia, for example, is both a neurological condition and a long-established literary device. It is both a process in which one sensory modality triggers activity in an area of the brain associated with another, and a poetic trope used to signal an aesthetic of disorientation, of divine, erotic, or natural intervention. A loud noise is experienced as a sweet smell, or, as Sir Toby quips in *Twelfth Night*, "to hear by the nose is dulcet in contagion" (2.3.52). To state that synaesthesia is only a metaphor blithely ignores the fact that others perceive the world in vastly different ways than we do (Hsy 2012). But to insist that its somatic iteration is more important than its metaphoric expression risks delimiting sensation to pre-fixed models and discounting the ways in which metaphoric expression reveals alternate modes of inhabiting the sensate. The noise that Sir Toby heard sweetly through the nose may reflect a unique material reality within an early modern understanding of olfaction already vastly different from modern ones. Synaesthesia—as both an embodied condition and a metaphoric trope—reminds us of Howes' point that sensory history, at its best, offers not just a field of study but also a methodological approach (2005a). Synaesthesia offers a useful reminder that sensation is a cultural interface between the body and the world at large (Howes 2011); as such, it reveals how poetry might offer a way to approach the history of sensation without insisting on ahistorical, trans-historical, or universally able-bodied experiences of embodiment.

In the following pages, I explore how certain literary allusions, in their complex relationship to broader conventions of literary form in the Renaissance, provide a model for how to grapple with that which remains most ephemeral and subjective within traditional histories of the senses—individualized, embodied experiences of sensation. What follows is not meant as an exhaustive argument about Renaissance literary devices or even about theories of sensation; rather I hope to demonstrate how a literary approach to the history of sensation and a sensory approach to the study of Renaissance literature invigorate both fields. The three literary devices traced here—the blazon, ekphrasis, and aposiopesis—are important in the Renaissance in that a number of poets working in different locations experimented with them and each is hinged to an important poetic form that developed or redeveloped during this period. The blazon was perhaps the most influential component of Petrarchan desire more broadly and of sonnets specifically: in a blazon, the poetic narrator adopts the persona of a besotted lover, cataloguing his beloved's beauty through obsessive poetic praise of each body part. In contrast, ekphrasis—in which the visual beauty of an art object is recreated through poetic description—offered a more expansive view, identified by Renaissance poets as an integral part of classical epic poetry. Finally, aposiopesis, in which a speaker interrupts him or herself in order to indicate a new thought mid-sentence, drew attention to the process of writing poetry. Its visual iteration on the page, through diction and a range of punctuation, reveals a broader poetic trend towards what Castiglione's *Il Cortegiano* described as *sprezzatura*, the masterful performance of elaborate artifice as seemingly effortless (Castiglione [1528] 1976: 67). Though any attempt to describe a cohesive "Renaissance" is already limited in its usefulness, given the diversity of works clustered underneath such a tag, these three devices each reflect a poetic desire to express something that cannot be adequately captured in language. For this reason, they capture the complex ways in which language can—and cannot—express sensations in the past.

RENAISSANCE INFLUENCE

If metaphor influences how we process sensory phenomena, then perhaps it also influenced how early modern men and women understood their sensory worlds. Influence, material, and metaphoric, defined Renaissance literature; in one sense, a renewed emphasis on form enabled certain patterns to emerge across the sixteenth century, even as its practitioners stemmed from vastly different geographic and political realms. Likewise, humanist ideals of education provided a kind of shared platform that connected across great divides, including emerging theories of geohumoralism, like the one articulated by Shylock that grounded sensation in the particularities of shared environments (Floyd-Wilson 2006). Yet this emphasis on form also produced startlingly original descriptions of sensation—of pleasure, longing, pain, religious fervor, and grief—precisely the kinds of metaphors that scientists now suggest trigger sensory recognition when read by others. Though it might seem paradoxical that a work of literature bears the imprint of influence even as it attempts to articulate a unique perspective, this is an intrinsic part of many of its forms.

Sonnets, for example, are exercises in just such a paradox. Though the literary traditions they drew upon were vastly disparate, sixteenth-century sonneteers like Garcilaso de la Vega, Joachim du Bellay, Pierre de Ronsard, Luis de Camões, and Philip Sydney shared an investment in its Petrarchan form (Fineman 1986: 193; Navarrete 1994: 143; Warley 2005: 2–12). Put simply, their poetry is as much about writing sonnets as it is about the content of each individual poem. As such their work demonstrates the complex ways literary representations do—and do not—archive sensation. Representations like Shakespeare's sonnet 94 that rely on a description of "lilies that fester" to capture an ambivalent desire for a fair youth (line 14), or Ronsard's "*Quand vous serez bien vielle*" that imagines the poet buried under the shade of a myrtle tree ("Par les ombres myrteux je prendrai mon repos," line 10), stem from—and speak to—vastly different cultural modes of production, even as they are inextricably linked through their form and their Petrarchan influence. When Luis de Góngora, for example, describes a "viola truncada" (line 12) in his *carpe diem* sonnet "Mientras por competir con tu cabello," he achieves a poetic sense of urgency: the beauty of violets, cut and rendered limp, will soon turn to dust just like the beloved's visual beauty. The point of his poem—and of Shakespeare's and Ronsard's—is that the beauty of the poetry will outlast all other. But in making this overarching point, each poet dwells differently in the quotidian details of everyday life. The poem documents the smell of rotting lilies, the cool shade of myrtle trees, and the flaccid texture of day-old violets in order to insist that all but the beauty of poetry fades. These sonnets thus offer useful reminders of the ways that sensory experience is both visceral and constructed, both idiosyncratic and formulaic.

As such they are subjective, but such subjectivity whispers of sensory worlds of the past; the most poignant metaphors in Renaissance literature are those that connect with phantom traces of embodied experiences now long lost. The cliché of love's blindness, for example, may seem an empty metaphor, but as Shakespeare's Romeo reminds his friend Mercutio (and us), "he jests at scars that never felt a wound" (2.1.44). So too does Mary Wroth's poetic narrator, Pamphilia, whose "stage of woe" in Sonnet 42 is entirely too visible to everyone but her "blind" lover: "For had he seene, he must have pitty show'd" (11, 12). Metaphors of the pain of love's blindness and its smarting wounds take on added material dimension when one connects these sonnets to a broader cultural history of blindness in this period and before. Read against, say, a description in a late medieval French chronicle of a theatrical "entertainment" that pitted four blind men against one another under the guise of attacking an animal, love's blind wounds resonate not only with classical tropes of Cupid and his famous arrow, and of medieval courtly traditions of love at first sight, but also with more insidious theatrical performances that turned on a tactile embodiment of the bodily wounds of blindness (Wheatley 2010).

Likewise, relationships between metaphors of darkness and material experiences of it are equally complex. Which is meant when a poem makes use of this convention? Does it matter if the poet himself was blind? For example, John Milton's "On His Blindness" reconfigures the Petrarchan sonnet to express a fervent religious desire: blindness in the poem is every bit as metaphorical as in Wroth's poem. Musing on how his light is spent in this "dark world," the poet's narrator begins by connecting encroaching blindness with broader questions of religious faith (2). The temptation, of course, is to read into the poem an additional material resonance, a trace of an embodied experience of darkness. But the poem famously ends with anticipation, connecting physical blindness to spiritual awakening: those also serve God who stand and wait (14). How then is one to make sense of this invocation within a broader archive of sensory experience? Elsewhere in his poetry, Milton reminds us that poetic darkness is paradoxical: "darkness visible" is both a trick of poetry (63), an oxymoron that captures both the lofty, impossible aim in his epic *Paradise Lost* to "justify the ways of god to man," but also perhaps a more quotidian experience of darkness that resonates through both Sonnet 16 and *Paradise Lost*.

DESIRE AND SENSATION: THE BLAZON

For Milton, the absence of light conjures forth a darkness that can be seen; as such, his allusion also connects with evolving discourses of race in the seventeenth century (Habib 2008; Hall 1995). Darkness, as a Petrarchan conceit, of course confers a difference that is seen. Shakespeare's sonnets to the "dark" lady (Sonnets 127–54), for example, describe what some scholars identify as an emerging discourse of racial difference, mapped through both the blazon and its progeny, the counter-blazon (Hall 1995). His mistress's eyes are, famously, "nothing like the sun," and her breasts as "dark" as "dun," yet he insists her beauty is "as rare as any other belied with false compare" in other sonnets (Sonnet 130, lines 1, 3, 14). Shakespeare's Sonnet 130 insists on a material reality that punctures such poetic fantasy, yet it is still in service of the sonnet's turn: what is false compare? His, too, employs poetic devices that allow an articulation of sexual desire that is more than the sum of its parts, so much so that scholars have used these allusions as a starting point for re-examining English archives for evidence of a significant black presence in early modern London that has been for too long ignored (Habib 2008; Salkeld 2012).

Such schematic descriptions of beauty reveal the ways in which the blazon tradition was part of broader cultural shifts in medical knowledge, particularly anatomical science (Friedman 2012). Traditions like the blazon and the counterblazon, where a beloved's beauty is catalogued and metaphorically compared to other kinds of beauty, natural or otherwise, can seem effusive. And it is easy to dismiss such effusiveness as excessive, as Shakespeare's counterblazon in Sonnet 130, yet these traditions emerged in tandem with technological breakthroughs in distillation, botany, anatomy, and dissection (Dugan 2009; Sawday 1995; Vickers 1985). For example, the sheer number of roses that metaphorically capture visual, olfactory, gustatory, and tactile beauty documents one of the ways in which these histories collide (Marot "du beau tetin," Shakespeare "Sonnet 130," Herrick "To the Virgins to Make Much of Time," and Góngora "Sonnet 23" and "Fábula de Polifemo y Galatea"). The Renaissance blazon is thus one way in which the body is rendered knowable through its discrete parts. A poem such as Clément Marot's "Du Beau Tetin" ("the beautiful breast") extends synecdoche to the point of incredulity, a fact acknowledged by the poet's own answer to it in the "Du Laid Tetin" ("the 'ugly' breast"). The beautiful breast is imagined as white as an egg, as soft as satin, and as firm as marble (1–2); the beauty of its nipple shames even the rose. Its counterpoint has a long, black nipple and is both haggard and flaccid (1, 5, 9). Such uncomfortable myopic detail also collapses into metonymy: the beauty of the breast hints at other sexual parts not on display (Persels 2002).

Marot's good and bad breasts are metaphorical, of course. The blazon tradition was a display of wit, reflecting masculine poetic prowess more than anything else, yet that is not to say that it is wholly imaginary. Its emergence in early sixteenth-century France connected the visual arts of heraldry with poetry: the blazon of old French—literally a shield of armor—became a literary form through poetic skirmishes of wit in the sixteenth century (Sawday 1995: 191–2). Its popularity in France, and quickly after that in England, stemmed in large part from broader cultural investments in rendering bodies as texts and texts as bodies (Bates 2007; Kritzman 1991). The influence of the French *Blason Anatomique*—printed seven times in France between 1536 and 1572 (Persels 2002: 32)—was part of a broader Renaissance investment in connecting poetic desire and literary form to shifting understandings of embodiment, including sensation. By the time Shakespeare writes of his "dark" lady, the tradition has come full circle: her breasts, when compared to white snow, "be dun," her dark skin materially invoked not through metaphor but through the failure of the conceit itself in his Sonnet 130 (line 3).

To question the precise meaning of a "darkness" that is also "visible" is to engage with the poetic traditions of the Renaissance, especially sonnets and blazons, but also with the cultural meanings of embodiment and sensation. In describing what is seen, these poets also query what it means to see. Read in its harshest light—as a masculine tradition of scopophilic pleasure based on objectification of women—the blazon rendered poetry as part of an eroticism of visual control (Vickers 1985). An objectified body, with its metaphoric pieces, comes into view through a kind of poetic gaze; yet even this highlights the odd ways in which language functions to create an experience of vision. The blazon creates a synecdoche across bodies; neither is rendered whole.

This point is brought home by Louise Labé's Sonnet 23, when she writes from the perspective of the beloved, questioning his desire written through her own body yet ultimately sympathizing with his pain:

Donques c'estoit le but de tal malice
De m'asservir sous ombre de service?
... Mais je m'assur', quelque part que tu sois
Qu'autant que moy tu soufres de martire.

[so the goal of your malice
was to subjugate me under the guise of service?
... But I am assured that wherever you are
Your suffering and pain are as great as mine]

Lines 9–14 in Yandell 2002: 8

What might be described as the objectified lists of beautiful or ugly parts inspires an experience of desire or revulsion in the poet that must stand in for his whole. It is a sensuous desire that can easily collapse into revulsion: the full or flaccid breast, the soft or wiry hairs, the sweet or stinking breath that threatens to overwhelm another. In Herrick's poems to Julia, the poetic blazon devolves into epigrams upon various parts, no longer purporting to signify the beloved's whole at all, only a perverse, myopic pleasure in the details of her body—her nipples, the pomanders between her thighs, her sweat-stained silks (Sig. X2 r-v, Sig. E7v, Sig. N7r). It is an uncomfortably intimate articulation of desire, rooted in sensuous detail.

VISIONS OF THE PAST: EKPHRASIS

And what of ekphrasis, the formal trope of such verbal descriptions? How might it connect to a broader investigation of what it meant to see in the Renaissance? Renaissance authors delighted in ekphrasis (Bearden 2011). Like the blazon, it was an attempt to display poetic prowess. But these verbal descriptions of material arts also connect with broader issues of representations and with shifting understandings of vision itself. Ekphrasis is an experiment in translating one artistic medium into another (Mitchell 1995); but how can one connect the aesthetic pleasure experienced from viewing a painting into the pleasure of reading a poem? Renaissance literature seems to offer an endless configuration of ekphrastic experiments in narrative: it can be disruptive (momentarily halting the action of the narrative to describe the work of art), informative (describing the work of art's origins), allusive (merely citing but not describing the work of art, leaving the reader to imagine its visual details for herself), even meta-theoretical (in which the narrative describes in detail another ekphrastic narrative) (Armas 2005: 22). All turn on the pleasure that emerges from querying whether or not we "see" the same thing.

But these ekphrastic moments are also the work of epic poetry (Becker 1995). Homer's description of the shield of Achilles is answered by those described in Ariosto's, Spenser's, and Milton's epic poems: phenomenological doubt about vision is productive, especially in the Renaissance, as medieval models of the passions began to merge with anatomical models of sensation. These theories of vision troubled clear and bright distinctions between the material realm and what one saw with one's mind's eye. When Boccaccio, in the opening of the *Amorosa visione*, offers his beloved a vision of his lovesick dreams, he engages with poetic allusion, an inner fantasy, and a vision: "Mirabil cosa forse la presente / vision vi parrà, donna gentile, / a riguardar, sì per lo nuovo stile, / sì per la fantasia ch'è nella mente" (1–4) [A wondrous thing to behold, perhaps, the present vision will seem to You, noble lady, as much for its new style, as for the phantasy stored in my mind] (Castells 2000: 21). The poetic vision offered to his lover is of his own lovesickness, which was thought to be both an embodied state of passion but also a communicable disease, transferable through eyesight (Castells 2000: 22). Lovesickness affected external and internal sight.

So, too, did religious faith. When Richard Crashaw, in the "Flaming Heart," queries what he sees "Upon the book and Picture of the seraphicall saint Teresa, (as she is visually expressed with a Seraphim beside her)" he offers a corrective strategy, commanding the poem's audience to "transpose it quite" and "spell it wrong to read it right" (10). In short, the audience is to "*read* Him for her and her for him" (11). Crashaw's ekphrasis exposes the poem's paradox of faith, in which the subject longs for an experiential, embodied knowledge of a divine ravishment that cannot fully be represented artistically. Yet the poem's invocation of an almost dyslexic reading practice suggests how language was integral to an evolving theory of vision. As Kathryn Mayers argues, "ekphrasis not only reflects history but produces it," and "it functions not merely as a passive literary expression of a historical period, worldview, or scopic regime, but as a nexus between aesthetic and semiotic formal boundaries and figures of social difference" (Mayers 2012: 8). What Mayers locates as the tension between aesthetic and semiotic difference also raises questions about the relationship between metaphoric and material realities, a point upon which Crashaw's poem depends.

If ekphrasis purports to describe a visual realm, but the delight lies in the fact that the visual realm may or may not exist, then how does this artificial construction of "visions" resonate with other, semiotic, fields of meaning? Put more simply, when Gertrude, for example, describes in *Hamlet* the image of Ophelia, drowned in the river:

> Her clothes spread wide,
> and mermaid-like a while they bore her up

which time she chanted snatches of old tunes,
as one incapable of her own distress . . .
But long it could not be
Till that her garments, heavy with their drink,
Pulled the poor wretch from her melodious lay
To muddy death.

4.7.146–54

How did Renaissance audience members interpret this significance? How does this aesthetic description of Ophelia's corpse connect with other ghastly sights of London? As both Bearden and Mayer argue, ekphrasis was a key factor in shaping emerging discussions of social differences both in Renaissance England and in Baroque Spain. Master Peter's puppet show, "the Liberation of Melisendra," in the second part of Miguel de Cervantes' *El ingenioso hidalgo don Quijote de la Mancha*, offers one such example: its complicated doubling—of disguised characters, of its chivalric plot, and of its puppet and animal performers—strains incredulity, especially when the eponymous Don Quijote breaks the narrative frame and attempts to rescue Melisendra from her Moorish captors (Cervantes 1605, 2: part 27). Yet as critics such as Haley, Smith, and Mayer argue, this minor episode connects to broader aspects of framing throughout Cervantes' novel. That Don Quijote mistakes puppets and apes for the characters of chivalric romance, a mistake that echoes across the novel's many complicated framing devices, raises questions about the relationship between literary description, "mimetic norms," and realistic sensory worlds. It is ekphrasis at its most complicated form: Don Quijote's ridiculous destruction of the puppet theatre is ironically rendered in believable detail. Cervantes thus playfully interrogates how certain details matter—semiotically or discursively—shaping sensory perception. These ekphrastic descriptions also resonated in multi-sensory ways, reminding us of how vision connected with a broader sensory world. Ophelia's muddy death is sonic: the sound of songs slowly replaced by the gurgling of mud. Do such details matter? As Catherine Richardson argues, Gertrude's description begs such a question: "if Gertrude or someone else had seen so much, watched so long and carefully, so filled with the strange slow beauty of Ophelia drowning, why did they not intervene?" (Richardson 2011: 179). Likewise, Master Peter's performance involves both a narrator and wooden puppets; it is the confluence of both sound and sight that inspires Don Quijote to destroy the wooden puppets, which he believes are Melisandre's "Moorish villians" (M. Smith 1995: 50).

AESTHETICIZED FAILURE: APOSIOPESIS

Gertrude's vision and Don Quijote's violent outburst thus resonate with the question posed by Crashaw's poem: what are the limits of ekphrastic description? Are these moments merely purple patches—overblown descriptions that obscure the materiality of vision—or do they offer insight into how sixteenth- and seventeenth-century men and women grappled with the nexus between the material world and their unique sense of it? Read amidst accounts of the rise of print culture and its influence on shifting sensory hierarchies in the seventeenth century, it is easy to interpret these as yet more examples of the triumph of vision over other sensory modes, yet we might also read these ekphrastic descriptions as part of an evolving literary history of affect. Gertrude's language aesthetically dilates the moment of death in a spectacular vision, yet it hints of a grief that cannot be adequately expressed in language, connected to Ophelia's insanity, and perhaps also Hamlet's.

Grief, in *Hamlet,* is marked by overblown language about it and by that which remains unspeakable even in such moments. Gertrude's aestheticized grief at the sight of Ophelia drowning recalls Hamlet's critique of her failure to properly mourn his father:

> A little month, or ere those shoes were old
> with which she followed my poor father's body,
> Like Niobe, all tears—why, she, even she—
> O God! A beast that wants discourse of reason
> Would have mourned longer.
>
> 1.2.146–50

Though Gertrude's grief may be false, Hamlet's grief over her betrayal is not. His broken speech betrays his emotions. Read in this way, Gertrude's ekphrasis marks an aestheticized failure of language, as does Hamlet's aposiopesis.

The rhetorical device of aposiopesis has a long history, but its use in seventeenth-century poetry emphasizes the complex relationship between the history of affect and of print culture (Woudhuysen 2004). In classical rhetoric it was a deliberate device, a pregnant pause meant to connote restraint rather than failure (Henry 2005). Yet Renaissance writers engaged with it as a trope of affect as well: Henry Peacham, for example, quite literally defined it as a trope of affection: "the Orator through some affection, as either of feare, anger, sorrow, bashfulness, or such like, breaketh off his speech before it be all ended" (Sig. R3v). Such affection could be interpreted as a defect: George Puttenham, for instance, in his *Arte of English Poesie* (1589) posits aposiopesis as a visual blemish on the text (cited in Henry 2005: 54). Aposiopesis, usually defined as a tool of self-interruption, becomes a placeholder for Puttenham, a way to represent an embodied experience of emotions like anger, shame, embarrassment, even forgetfulness: "We begin to speake a thing and breake off in the middle, as if either it needed no further to be spoken of, or that we were ashamed, or afraide to speake it out. It is also sometimes done by way of threatening, and to show a moderation of anger" (cited in Henry 2005: 54). What Puttenham interprets as a defect provides a useful way to approach the relationship between language, affect, and sensation. These spaces in the text required the reader to draw upon their own experiential knowledge of affect; lost in such pauses are the threatening gestures of anger, the blushes of shame, the hush of silence.

Poets like Philip Sydney, for example, utilized aposiopesis as a tool of productive silence, calling for the reader to connect to the text on the page in specifically embodied ways (Alexander 2006; Sherman 2011: 85). This connection was so strong that the device was often deployed to represent death itself. When the "earthy and cold hand of death lies" on Hotspur's tongue, for example, it stops his life before he can complete his final thought, "thou art food for—" allowing Prince Hal to finish it for him: "for worms, brave Percy" (*1 Henry IV*, 5.4.85–6). The printing of playscripts, for instance, required such a code; the em-dash provided a way for readers of *Henry IV* to understand what would have been heard in the theatre (Woudhuysen 2004). The space it marks on the page does not quite suggest silence, given the materiality of decay with which Hal emphasizes. Yet the em-dash as an evolving visual code and the silence it engenders comes to signify not a poetic mark of failure but an embodied limit to language.

Aposiopesis, as a trope of death, is, of course, now itself a cliché (Neill 1997: Ch. 6). Yet the link between drama and poetry reminds us that death silences, but it is not necessarily silent. Aposiopesis was visually marked in a variety of ways—em-dashes, semicolons, ellipses—to code a host of emotions (Sherman 2011). Though its use was increasingly standardized in the mid-seventeenth century, we might retain its capacious, earlier definition as a reminder that traces of the past remain embedded within literary sources. Read in this way, aposiopesis emerges as a nexus between the sensory worlds of the past and the archive, offering an experience of language that is both productive and frustrating.

For example, when aposiopesis appears within a blazon, it is generally thought to enact an erotic extension of the poet's praise of a beloved's visible body parts to those that remain unseen. In *Orlando Furioso,* for example, Ludovico Ariosto pauses in the midst of his description of Alcina's enchanting (and visible) body to muse on those parts that remain unseen (Taylor 1992: 9). In between a poetic description of her hair, eyes, mouth, breasts, and her arms, hands, fingers, and feet, the poet interrupts himself, musing: "Non potria l'altre parti veder Argo: / ben si può giudicar che corrisponde / a quell ch'appar di fuor quel che s'asconde" (7.14) [But Argus self might not discern the rest; / Yet by presumption well it might be guessed / That that which was concealed was the best] (Ariosto [1516] 1607). The space created by such a diversion is meant to represent Alcina's genitals and the desire they might engender in the reader: the poet lingers in a space metaphorically located beneath a description of her breasts yet before description of her appendages.

Such a poetic display of rhetorical restraint is meant to invoke power, a point that Nancy Vickers uses to explain similar strategies of representation in Shakespeare's *Rape of Lucrece*. Aposiopesis, like the trope of the blazon, is "a legacy shaped by the male imagination for the male imagination" (Vickers 1985: 96). Thus, when Tarquin surveys Lucrece's body, comparing the beauty of it to her husband's boasts about it the night before, aposiopesis marks a violent desire born of such complex comparisons: "Now thinks he that her husband's shallow tongue, / the niggard prodigal that prais'd her so, in that high task had done her wrong" (78–80). Lucrece is evaluated by Collatine, by Tarquin, and by the reader, who may marvel at the poet's ability to connote what Collatine cannot. Yet aposiopesis also marks the failure of that legacy, capturing, albeit temporarily, an embodied experience that is not easily rendered into language. When Tarquin rapes Lucrece in Shakespeare's poem, aposiopesis denotes the violation:

> So let thy thoughts, low vassals to they state—
> "No more," quoth he.
>
> 665–6

It is only two stanzas later that the reader learns why: that Tarquin "pens her piteous clamours in her head" with her "nightly linen" (681). One step removed, the poet "pens" her revolt even as he silences it ("pens"). But the space of her violation marked by aposiopesis remains for a stanza or two, even if it is explained moments later. It is there, in the poem's visual performance of Lucrece's silence, that we might begin to hear echoes of past sensory worlds, if only we learn how to grapple with such devices as tropes of synaesthesia.

CONCLUSION

As I have tried to demonstrate here, Renaissance literary representations offer a unique and complex contribution to the archive of sensation. These literary devices are all tools used to describe a phenomenon that beggars description—an erotic desire that is more than the sum of its parts, the pleasure of visually poring over a work of art, or an emotion too powerful to articulate fully in language—yet they also connect with evolving theories of sensation that defined the period. Renaissance poets utilized these tropes masterfully, dwelling in what we might term as discursive lack and supplementing it with beautiful language. In doing so, these poets and writers provide a trace, albeit a highly stylized one, of how medical models and theories of perception intersected with the details that concerned everyday life. These traditions, I suggest, argue for a way to historicize ephemeral sensations, despite their status as feint, suspect, and subjective evidence because, as literary texts, they also participate in much broader histories about genre and form. To return briefly to the allusion with which this chapter began, Shylock argues for a world in which our perceptions are grounded not only in a shared experience of our social realms but also in the language we use to describe it. Renaissance writers grasped this joint desire for an individuated commonality, seeking words that could make sense of the paradox of perception and that could describe it.

CHAPTER EIGHT

Art and the Senses: Representation and Reception of Renaissance Sensations

FRANÇOIS QUIVIGER

Following the philosophy of Aristotle, the Renaissance valued and treasured sight more than any other sense because, thanks to it, images can awaken our multisensory experience of the world. Indeed the Renaissance is also the period of history in which a visual tradition of representing the senses as personifications was first created and subsequently broadcast.

This chapter deals with two very different aspects of the relationship between art and the senses during and after the Renaissance. It begins with iconography: the history of identifiable types. It then moves on to explore the more vexing question of sensation in representation, as representation and record of sensory culture. Here "sensory culture" is taken broadly as the sum of experiences, habits, and assumptions necessary to apprehend and empathize with images.

The chapter discusses the allegorical tradition as a point of entry to the role of senses and sensation in the visual arts of the Renaissance; then focuses on religious art, and then on secular art. The latter division is artificial, since both fields constantly interact within the painter's workshop: indeed Venus and the Virgin are painted with the same brushes and pigments. Yet, as we shall see, Renaissance secular art inherited its sensory language from medieval art, which developed in response to the demands of religion.

THE ALLEGORICAL TRADITION

Scholars have identified three ways of representing the senses: by means of animals reputed for the acuity of a specific sense; by means of figures experiencing sensation; and by means of sensory organs. It was in the fifteenth century that the senses made their first noted appearance as female allegories in the tapestry set of the *Lady with the Unicorn* (Nordenfalk 1976: 26–7). By the sixteenth century, series representing the five senses had become an iconographic type disseminated across Europe through prints. Most of the time these consist of a series of five plates, such as those of Georg Pencz (1540) or Cornelis Cort (1561), featuring female personifications experiencing the sensation they represent and accompanied by related animals (Ferino-Pagden 1996: 26–7).

Five cycles of the five senses printed between 1570 and 1603 by the prolific Antwerp artist Maerten de Vos (1532–1603) expanded this type by associating narrative subjects to each sense (see Figure 8.1). These prints, alternatively engraved by Anton Wierix, Raphael Sadeler the Elder, and Adriaen Collaert, follow the same compositional pattern: in the foreground, one personification surrounded by animals and objects; in the background, one or two biblical stories related to the sense described (Nordenfalk 1985: 143–5). Each figure experiences the sensation it symbolizes: Sight looks at herself, Hearing plucks a lute, Smell smells a flower, Taste is about to bite an apple, Touch feels a spider's web and experiences the bite of a bird clawing her hands. The animals placed at the foot of each personification are proverbial, each for the acuity of a single sense: the eagle for sight, the dog for smell, the tortoise, the lizard, and the scorpion for touch, and the monkey for taste. Natural and artificial objects associated with one or several senses also serve as attributes: flowers for Smell, a mirror for Sight, musical instruments for Hearing, and food for Taste. The main innovation of Maerten de Vos' series is the addition of biblical stories in the background. The stories are as follows:

Sight: God showing Eden to Adam and Eve—Christ healing the blind man
Hearing: God calling Adam and Eve—John the Baptist preaching

Smell: Adam animated by the breath of God—Mary Magdalene anointing the feet of Christ

Touch: Adam and Eve expelled from Eden—Christ rescuing Peter from drowning

Taste: Adam and Eve eating the apple—Christ multiplying the loaves and fishes

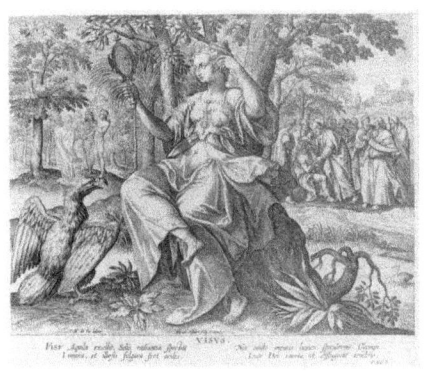
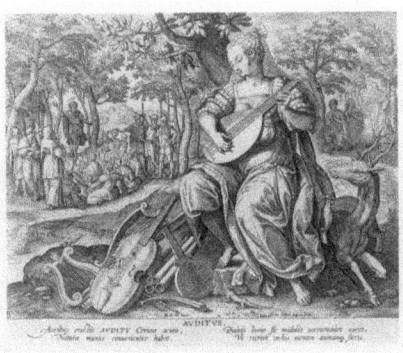
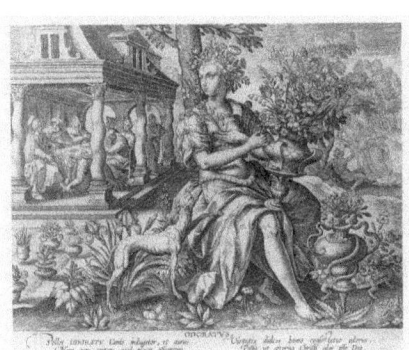
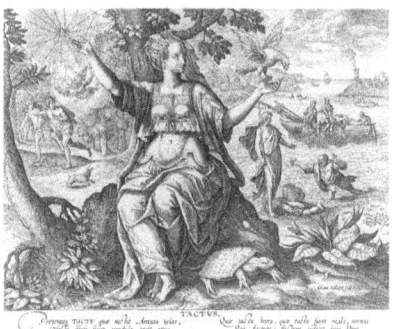
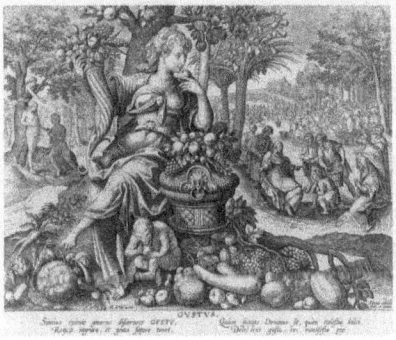

FIGURE 8.1: Maerten de Vos, *The Five Senses*, Antwerp, 1570s. Courtesy of the Warburg Institute.

This arrangement is in fact a familiar compositional formula reminiscent of many medieval and Renaissance paintings where accessories and attributes occupy the foreground, serving as hints to identify the scene featured in the middle ground. Among the most common attributes are lilies and roses for the Virgin and instruments of the Passion of Christ for scenes of the Deposition. In the present case, however, the image in the foreground invites the viewer to imagine the background scenes within a specific range of sensations.

Furthermore, four of these five allegorical figures have roots in Christian art. The ancestors of Hearing tuning or plucking a stringed instrument are the angels and musicians of medieval Psalters and Renaissance altarpieces. Those of Smell are Madonnas smelling flowers presented to them by saints. The hand of Touch seized by the claws of a bird has a precedent in the iconography of the bird pecking the fingers of the Christ child, and Taste about to bite an apple is undoubtedly evocative of the Fall. Sight looking into a mirror is the only sense allegory with no precedent in Christian iconography—but a secular equivalent, the allegory of Prudence, is generally shown holding a mirror.

The five senses series by Maerten de Vos not only enriched the iconography of sensation with narrative subjects, they also provided a synthesis and a celebration of several centuries of sensation in images. Nevertheless, even if these allegories alert us to sensory meanings in the visual arts, they also involve a certain falsification of reality since in fact we always perceive with several senses at the same time, rather than with one.

WHICH SENSES?

The first step is to disentangle the relationship between early modern and present conceptions of the senses, for by modern standards the Renaissance anatomies of the brain and the senses are fanciful, to say the least.

Humans always engage with the world through multiple senses. Moreover, while the five senses are still referred to in everyday language, present-day science acknowledges the existence of many more. Touch itself is now a broad conceptual umbrella embracing finer categories, such as thermoception, alloception, and bodily senses such as proprioception. These channels of perception were certainly active in the early modern period, but the language of science had at the time no specific words for them.

Early modern humans only had Aristotle and his commentators to rely on. Aristotle's *Treatise on the Soul* offered the most durable classification of the senses into five ascending categories: taste and touch, which perceive only by direct contact, hearing and sight, which perceive multiple information at a distance, and somewhere in the middle, smell. This traditional division of the sensory system in five broad categories has remained in common language and popular culture up to the present day. Nevertheless Aristotle believed, like neuroscientists today, that our perceptions are in fact multisensory. The long lasting impact of the "five senses tradition" has overshadowed a sixth sense which Aristotle described as a faculty that joins various sensory perceptions into multisensory mental imagery: the *common sense*. Thanks to this sense we perceive what Aristotle calls *common sensibles*: figure, size, movement, and rest (Aristotle 1975: 418a). Indeed, for Aristotle, sensations are the building blocks of the multisensory images by which we see and anticipate the world.

For the early modern era it is the faculty of the imagination which represents sensory perception of the outside world and through which higher faculties can deliberate on the world. As we shall see, the imagination is also the primary faculty which early modern European artists sought to train, cultivate, and represent, and "common sensibles" are the subject of the visual arts.

Early modern anatomical cuts of the brain offer a standard and straightforward account of this theory (see Figure 8.2). They frequently display lines linking the sense organs to the common sense placed in the first ventricle of the brain. From there, sensed images pass to the *fantasia* and imagination, located in the second ventricle of the brain, before being stored in the memory, located at the back of the brain. Thus the Renaissance is at the heart of the multi-secular reign of the Aristotelian conception of the mind as a processor turning multiple sensations into mental images.

This theory of the mind, which combined Aristotle's faculty psychology with a fanciful anatomy of the brain dating back to the Roman physician Galen (129–200 CE), dominated Europe from the twelfth century until the seventeenth century, when the philosophy of Descartes and the observations of Thomas Willis eventually made it redundant. It has, however, survived far longer in popular culture. It is also the foundation upon which Renaissance art theory is built, a theory which states the primacy of the image in the mind of the artist over the image on the canvas. Such a claim was in fact intended to highlight the intellectual status of the arts of drawing. But detaching the images from the hand does not necessarily imply detaching the senses from the images: Renaissance conceptions of the imagination and the mind suggest on the contrary that the visual arts sought to represent the multisensory universe carefully imagined and reproduced by artists and artisans.

It is not particularly useful, therefore, to think in terms of individual senses. Such an approach is a misreading of the early modern and modern traditions. It would be more accurate to envisage Renaissance art in terms of "common

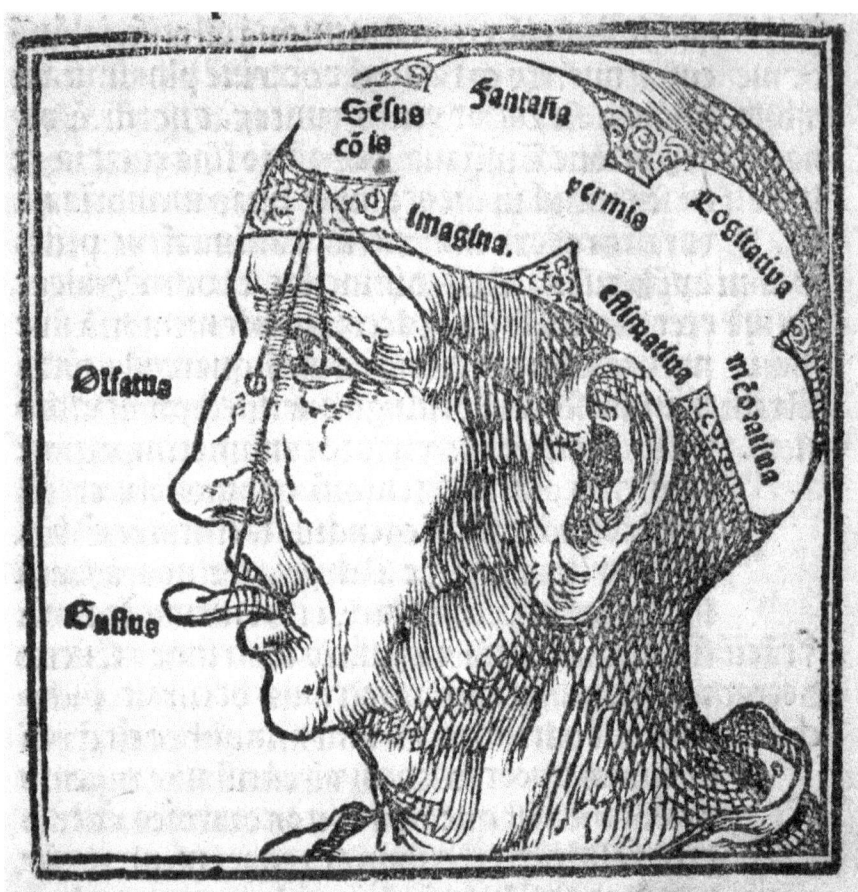

FIGURE 8.2: Anatomical cut of the head from L. Dolce, *Dialogo . . . nel quale si ragiona del modo di accrescere e conseruar la memoria* (Venice, 1562). Courtesy of the Warburg Institute.

sensibles" and to set the importance of sight in relation to its ability to provide the ground for multisensory anticipations of the world. Following these leads we should examine how clusters of non-visual sensations were signified visually, in which contexts and for which purpose.

THE SENSES IN RELIGIOUS ART

From the Middle Ages onwards the Church was the main patron of the arts, and so its requirements necessarily shaped the art it commissioned. Medieval religion actively sought out lively images, with Pope Gregory the

Great (540–604) setting the tone when he wrote that images are the books of those who can't read—with the implication that images should address the lowest common denominator, as well as the lowest mode of apprehension: sensation. The eight-century Byzantine controversy, eventually won by the partisans of images, led to another consequential claim: the argument that by making himself human Christ also made himself visible and could as a result be depicted by artists. This controversy also imposed a long-lasting theory of the tripartite function of images according to which they should be mnemonic, didactic, and inspirational.

From roughly the twelfth century onwards, Western European monastic ambiences extended the image of the human God to that of a suffering God and developed an imaginative piety requesting worshipers to empathize with Him. This aspect is perhaps best exemplified by the section on the Passion of Christ in the *Golden Legend* of Jacobus de Voragine (c. 1230–98), one of the most popular medieval accounts of the lives of the saints. The text describes in five short chapters how Christ suffered through each of his senses (Voragine 5.1–5). Such a model of empathy was very common in the religious sphere, especially in the writings and meditation methods of mystics, but it also trickled down to lay audiences by means of particularly influential textual traditions promoted by monastic orders, in particular the Dominicans and the Franciscans. The most important text is undoubtedly the *Meditationes Vitae Christi*, attributed to Bonaventure until the nineteenth century. The text not only survived and circulated through over 200 manuscripts, it also had a considerably long afterlife in the age of European vernacular printing well into the seventeenth century, thereby providing a model for countless other devotional retellings and their representation. In fact, the 400 years when the *Meditationes* and similar texts were most influential coincide with a period of considerable stylistic change in Western art, from the medieval to the Baroque era. In the history of devotional literature, the *Spiritual Exercises* of Ignatius of Loyola (1542), the founder of the Jesuit order, relay the *Meditationes*. Its relevance here is that it systematizes the art of visualizing into a straightforward method for imagining multisensory images as a preparation for prayer and meditation. Such images are built through five sensory layers by imagining how a scene and its actors look, sound, smell, taste, and feel. Here is how Loyola recommends apprehending hell:

> The first Point will be to see with the sight of the imagination the great fires, and the souls as in bodies of fire.
>
> The second, to hear with the ears wailings, howling, cries, blasphemies against Christ our Lord and against all His Saints.

The third, to smell with the smell smoke, sulphur, dregs and putrid things.

The fourth, to taste with the taste bitter things, like tears, sadness and the worm of conscience.

The fifth, to touch with the touch; that is to say, how the fires touch and burn the souls.

Loyola [1542] 1923: 41

Images, and especially paintings, were deemed particularly helpful in this process. This is confirmed by the *Directory of the Spiritual Exercises* of 1588, a manual intended for those monitoring the daily practice of the spiritual exercises. Here the outcome of Loyola's method, the so-called "composition of place," is compared to the reminiscence of paintings, and those who have difficulty imagining are advised "to remember mentally the painted stories which they saw on altarpieces and in other places such as for instance pictures of the Last Judgement, of the Passion" (*Directoria* 1955: 449).

In order to assist these devotional practices, artists developed a range of signs prompting viewers to apprehend images in terms of their own sensory experience. From the age of Giotto onwards, artists treated these signs with increasing realism, shifting from a vocabulary of signs to representations evoking textures and tactile sensations. It is possible to examine the impact of this approach through two themes encompassing opposite sensory experiences of gentleness and violence, namely the Madonna and Child and the Flagellation.

Emphasis on empathy is considerable in the sections of the *Meditationes* on the infancy of Christ. The text encourages worshipers not only to imagine the scenes such as a Madonna and Child, but also to imagine themselves holding the Child. If taste is not apparent, smell, touch, and sight are particularly present (*Meditations* 1961: 38–9). The history of this theme in Italian painting from the thirteenth to the sixteenth century reveals that artists have expanded signs of tactile contact into sophisticated representations of volume and texture. One good example is the sub-theme of the Virgin holding the foot of the Child (Cannon 2010). Comparing for instance the flat rendering of a thirteenth-century Madonna and Child of Byzantine inspiration by the Magdalene Master with a late fifteenth-century version of the same theme, we can see that the visual signs are the same: an adult hand feeling the foot of a baby (see Figure 8.3). The Magdalene Master has also experimented with light and shade in order to highlight the volume of the hand and feet. But a comparison of his work with an early sixteenth-century anonymous version emphasizes how

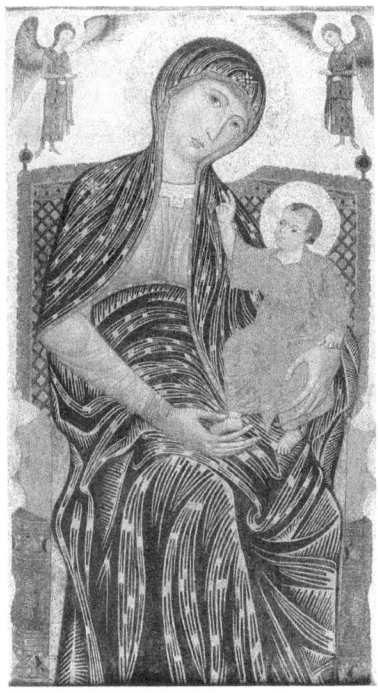 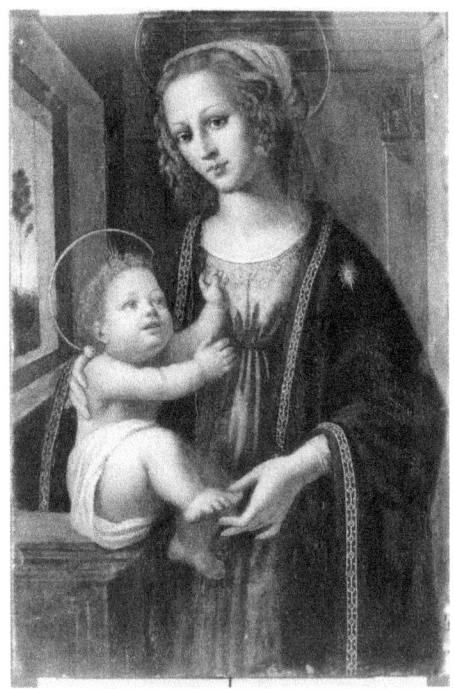

FIGURE 8.3: Magdalene Master, *Virgin and Child*, tempera and guilding on panel, c. 1260–70. Gemäldgalerie, Berlin.

FIGURE 8.4: Anonymous early sixteenth-century Italian, *Madonna and Child*. Walters Art Gallery.

conveying volume, expression, movement, and textures has become a central preoccupation of painters (see Figure 8.4).

As artists developed means of expressing volume, relief, and epidermic sensations they became increasingly reluctant to render the extreme violence imagined and described in the retellings of the Passion of Christ, at least in Italy. The episode of the Flagellation, the second theme of interest here, is a case in point.

The *Meditationes Vitae Christi* describe this episode at length. Notably, Christ is reported to have received innumerable blows (*Meditations* 1961: 379). The medieval textual tradition of such brutal imagery continues well into the Renaissance and even features in the most popular devotion of the age: the Rosary which counts 6,666 blows, an ordeal which no human body could survive (Castello 1541: 112r). Although literal illustrations appear throughout the fourteenth and fifteenth centuries in Northern European painting, blood and lash marks fade away almost completely from Italian art. Thus by the

1560s the Counter Reformation writer Andrea Gilio could complain that the painters of his time were too interested in representing beautiful and elegant anatomical figures, and recoiled from representing the pains and torments endured by Christ during the Passion (Gilio 1564: 87). Indeed, Gilio was partly right, although he probably had no knowledge of pre-Reformation northern painting which offers many examples. A comparison of two works on the same subject provides a useful contrast between North and South.

The Christ of the Flagellation in the painting of Michael Pacher is covered in numerous and distinct dripping wounds (see Figure 8.5). This rendition is a fine illustration of the *Meditationes* text which explains that the "royal blood flows all about, from all parts of His body" (*Meditations* 1961: 328). Indeed each wound is meticulously painted and together they appear to form a pattern over the body, both enhancing its volume and at the same time inviting the viewer to count the whip lashes. Furthermore, the entire body of Christ is forced into a deliberately awkward and uncomfortable position. This Germanic Christ figure could not be more different from that of Sodoma's Flagellation, painted only a

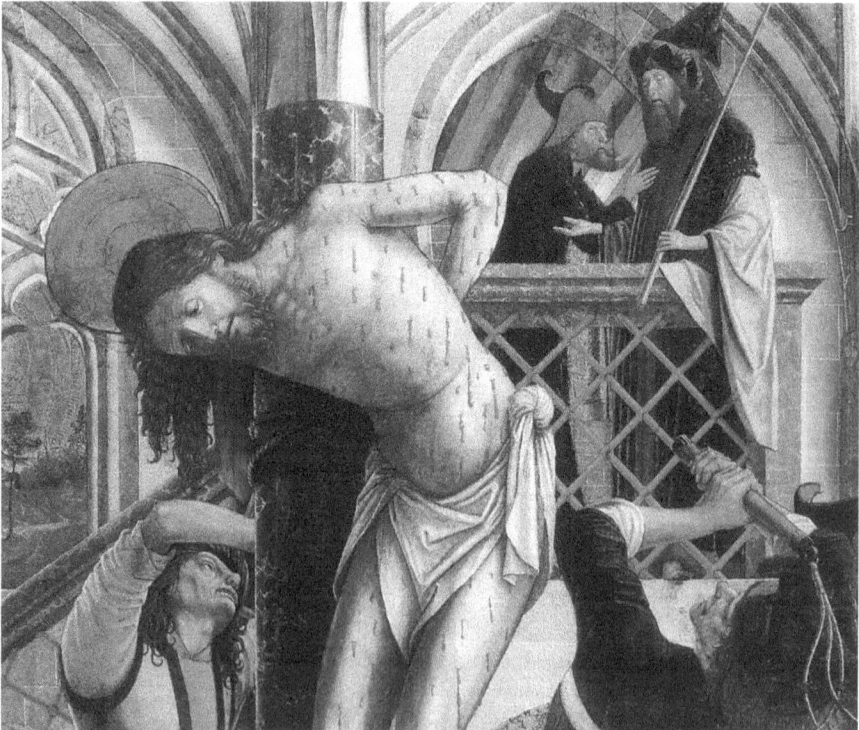

FIGURE 8.5: Michael Pacher, *Flagellation*, c. 1495. Österreischische Gallerie Belvedere.

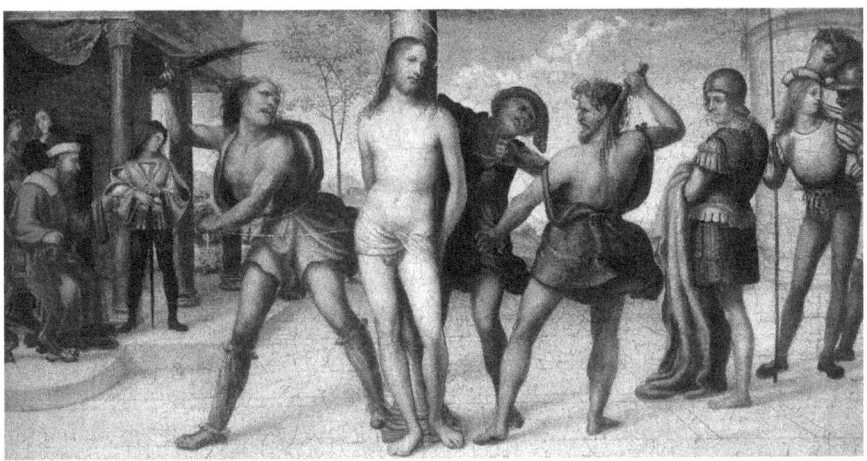

FIGURE 8.6: Sodoma, *Flagellation*, c. 1510. Budapest Museum of Fine Arts.

decade later (see Figure 8.6). Christ poses in an elegant contraposto, with two executioners preparing to whip him while a third one ties him to the column. Here Sodoma is following a formula adopted by numerous Italian painters including Michelangelo and Sebastiano del Piombo. In this interpretation, the body of Christ is always shown intact. In this way, artists are able to suggest that the Flagellation is about to begin, thus leaving the horror of the whip lashes to the anticipatory imagination of the viewer. For a writer like Gilio, however, such representations are inadequate, since the whipping appears to be carried out with soft cotton ropes unlikely to produce either pain or wounds. In fact Gilio's criticisms apply to most Italian depictions of the main episodes of the Passion. Such remarks from a minor writer like Gilio would have only little interest if he had not added: "I have often discussed this point with painters. They all responded to me with the same voice, saying that [such depictions] would go against the conventions of their art" (Gilio 1564: 88).

The reluctance to depict pain deplored by Gilio was indeed defended by painters and stands out as very representative of the Italian pictorial treatments of the Christ of the Passion. His visible body remained mostly intact in the visual arts while equally authorized narratives, in the textual tradition, continued to cover him with wounds. This distanciation between the visual and textual traditions, far from implying a sensory loss, on the contrary placed emphasis on how sensitive the human figure in representation had become, to the point that the depiction of excessive pain and wounds was deemed so unpleasant as to become incompatible with the conventions of the visual arts.

By the last decades of the sixteenth century, the techniques of the visual arts had reached such fine ability to represent the world as to prompt the beginning of scientific illustration. This context is particularly useful to highlight the fact that while artists had the full command of their media to make the most detailed and graphic representations of extreme sensations, they did not do so. The emphasis on post-Renaissance religious art is on emotions rather than on sensations. Velazquez's *Christ at the Column after the Flagellation* (1628–9) provides a fine example of this general trend (see Figure 8.7). The composition illustrates an episode from the medieval retellings, nevertheless Velazquez engages the viewer's gaze to empathize with Christ's sorrow rather than with the pain one might surely experience after the 666 whip lashes listed by the *Meditationes*. The painting suggests that the blows fell on Christ's back and the only suggestion of blood is the tiny red dots on the whip placed on the foreground at the viewer's hand reach. While images of blood and wounds survive in Spanish polychrome sculpture, it seems that seventeenth-century

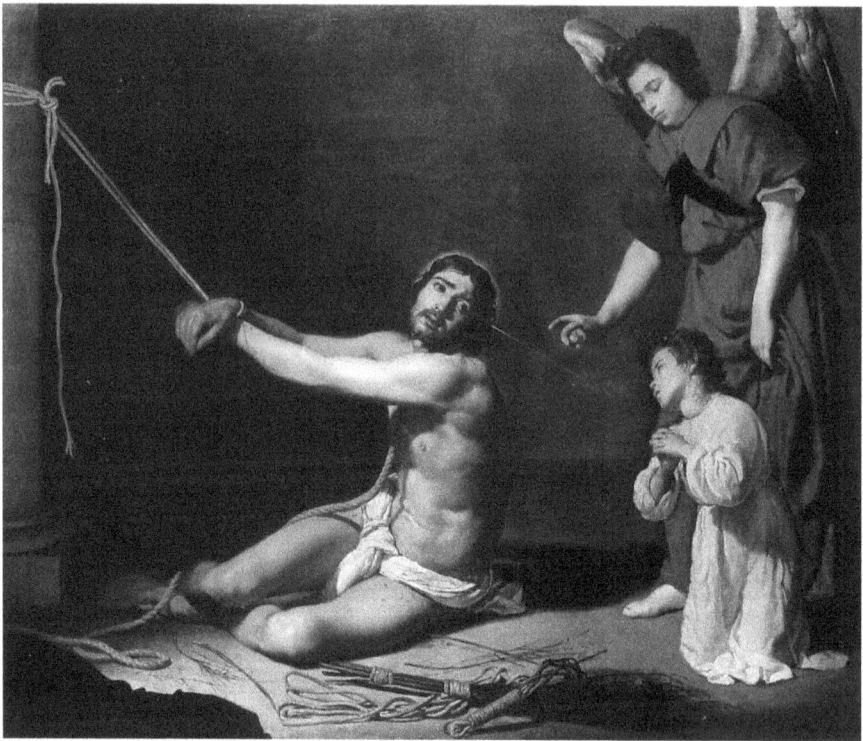

FIGURE 8.7: Diego Velazquez, *Christ at the Column after the Flagellation*, c. 1628, oil on canvas. London, National Gallery.

religious art elsewhere serves a religion which increasingly produced far more images of sensory pleasures than of pains.

This phenomenon appears nowhere better than in the unification of architecture, sculpture, and painting engineered by Gian Lorenzo Bernini whose art dominates Baroque Rome. In his *Ecstasy of Saint Theresa* all the arts offer a prelude to the flow of marble which expresses the intensely physical character of the vision experienced by the saint described as the mixture of intense pain and pleasure caused by an angelic arrow constantly entering and exiting her entrails (see Figure 8.8).

CHANGES AND SHIFTS

From the 1520s onward, north of the Alps and the Pyrenees, the Reformation brought much of medieval religious imagery to an end. Luther considered images neither good nor bad in themselves but felt that as a result they had to be controlled. The other Reformers were far more radical: Karlstadt, Zwingli, Farel, and from the 1540s Calvin, all thought that images ought to be eradicated from worship (Michalski 1993: 43–74). They based their arguments on the fact that the Old Testament forbids images and that no evidence of their use can be found in the New Testament nor in early Christianity. They dismissed as wishful thinking the notion of images as books for the ignorant. On the contrary they considered positive attitudes towards religious images as a survival of pagan polytheism. The intense late medieval cult of saints and relics confirmed their worries that images in churches were promoting idolatry and so they decided to wage a war against the idols.

Such convictions prompted heated controversies among theologians, eventually generating one of the greatest waves of iconoclasm ever to roll over Europe north of the Alps and the Pyrenees. In France alone, scholars have estimated that over 20,000 churches and 2,000 convents fell prey to iconoclastic zeal and fury (Christin 1991: 78). Religious leaders almost invariably advocated the peaceful removal of images but documentary evidence points to a more animated turn of events. Images were not only removed and destroyed, nor were they merely recycled when made out of precious metal, they were also attacked in their sensory parts. Surviving fragments confirm indeed that sculptures had their eyes gouged out and typically their hands, arms, and legs broken. Accounts of iconoclastic riots bring us one step closer to the sensory world in which these images participated. We read of crucifixes on which the Passion was re-enacted, of sculptures being whipped, beaten, humiliated, and frequently challenged to perform miracles before being burnt (Michalski

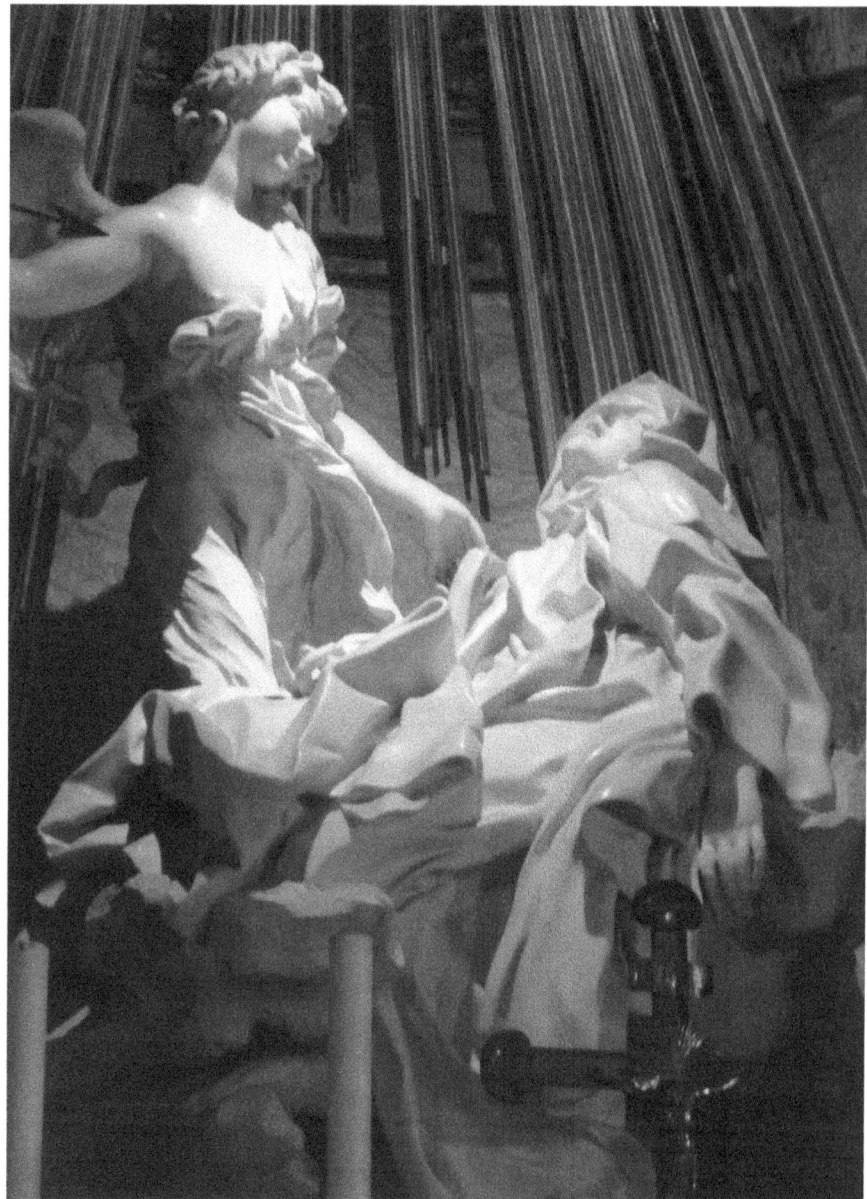

FIGURE 8.8: Gian Lorenzo Bernini, *Ecstasy of Saint Theresa*, 1647–52, marble. Church of Santa Maria della Vittoria, Rome.

1993: 75–98). Quite significantly, Catholic prints of the time speak of the patience of images. Their representation of iconoclastic deeds leaves no pictorial indications that would allow us to distinguish the living from the images (see Figure 8.9). In this illustration, showing soldiers pulling a crucifix

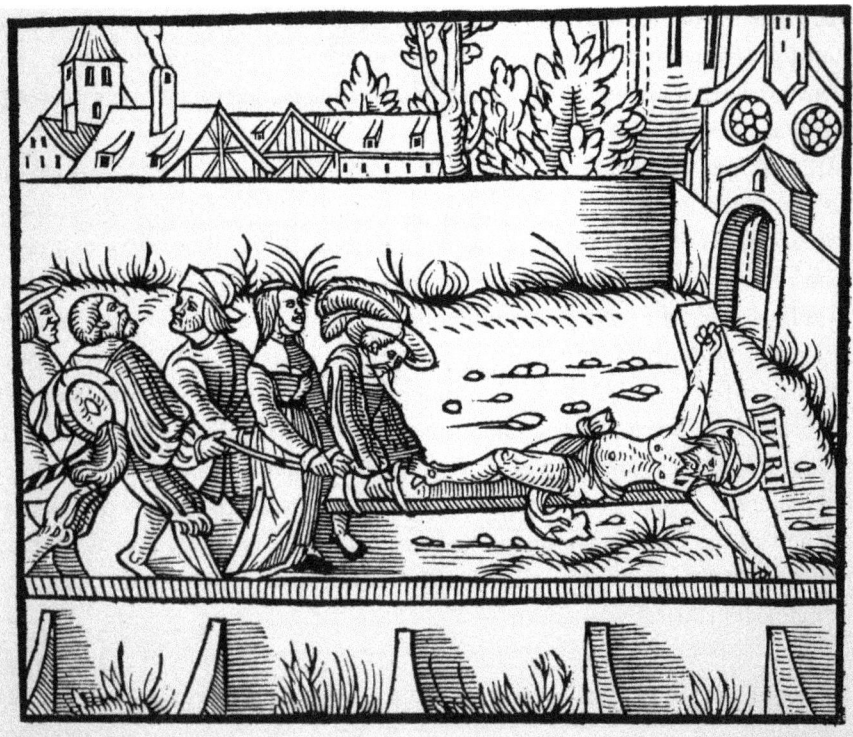

FIGURE 8.9: Scene of iconoclasm from a Catholic pamphlet: *Eyn Warhafftig erschrölich Histori von der Bewrischen uffrur so sich durch Martin Luthers leer in Teutscher nation . . .*, c. 1525–7. Courtesy of the Warburg Institute.

out of a church, the image of Christ on the cross is treated as a living figure rather than a sculpture.

The implicit assumption that holy images are "alive" is also present in Reformist thought, as something to exorcise. This attitude is best exemplified by a paragraph near the end of Karlstadt's treatise on the removal of images. Beyond the theological and philological arguments raised against images stands out a visceral fear:

> I should not fear any image, just as I should not venerate any. But I lament to God from my youth onwards my heart was trained and grown up in the veneration and worship of pictures. And a harmful fear has been bred into me from which I would gladly deliver myself and cannot. As a consequence, I stand in fear that I might not be able to burn idols.
> *Reformation Debate* 36

Such concern not only referred to images produced by artists, but also extended to the problem of relics and miraculous images reputed to move, bleed, or even grow a beard, many of which Calvin had denounced as frauds in his *Treatises on Relics* (1543).

Protestant ideas did circulate in Italy and Spain in the first half of the sixteenth century but were severely repressed from the 1550s onwards and never generated any lasting iconoclastic fervor. While Reformers exorcised their fears of images, the Catholics defended and multiplied them. The Church stood by its old doctrine of the mnemonic, didactic, and inspirational function of images and attributed abuses to the neglect of artists. The decrees of the Council of Trent (1545–65) considered the manifesto of the Counter Reformation Church, and pointed out that local bishops should control and eventually remove images with inappropriate content—a resolution at times implemented in Spain but very rarely in Italy. In answer to charges of idolatry, the acts of the Council stipulated that images should be adored for what they represent and that their material should not be considered to contain any virtue or magical property whatsoever.

MULTI-SENSORY CATHOLICISM: THE ROSARY

The Reformers were probably right in their assumption that the cult of images could breed idolatry. Images were not only seen, but frequently touched and kissed, and attributed supernatural powers (Johnson 2011: 64). One method of prayer which circumvented the dangers of idolatry inherent to image-based worship was the rosary. Introduced in the late fifteenth century, it disappeared from Northern Europe during the Reformation but was increasingly promoted in the South under the impulse of the Counter Reformation Church. The exponential proliferation of the rosary led to the foundation of a commission in 1593 destined to keep track of the hundreds of rosary confraternities—lay organizations practicing the rosary under ecclesiastical guidance, reciting innumerable Ave Marias and Pater Nosters each week (Duval 1988: 954–5).

A rosary is a cycle of prayers focusing on the life of Christ. It is divided into three cycles of five episodes each, generally referred to as mysteries. The joyful mysteries deal with the infancy of Christ, the sorrowful mysteries focus on the Passion, and the glorious mysteries extend from the Resurrection to the Assumption (Castello 1541: 29v ff.). Many of these scenes come from the *Meditations of the Life of Christ* tradition rather than from the Gospels. Described as a spiritual exercise (Castello 1541: Aiiij), rosary recitation consists in reciting ten Ave Marias and one Pater Noster while focusing on each of these fifteen mysteries. This practice bred a multisensory and material culture reflecting this mental itinerary. Rosary images are best described as a road map for the soul, comparable in some way to a Monopoly board. Instead of throwing the dice to move forward the recitant contemplates each scene featured in a medallion surrounded by five or ten roses for each of which he or she will recite respectively one or two Ave Marias. Prints provide endless variations on themes pertaining not only to sight but also to smell and touch (see Figure 8.10).

A rosary is also a crown of prayer, often compared to the crowns of flowers placed around images of the Virgin. The association was not only visual, however. Prayers were customarily compared to the perfume of roses ascending towards the Virgin and the depiction of Marian flowers in rosary iconography could well be allusive to this. Church incense and prayer beads did bring this olfactory dimension tangibly into the world. We know that rows of prayer beads devised to assist recitation often included a pomander, a hollow jewel containing scented matter (Falkenburg 1999: 39–40). Moreover, early modern books of domestic recipes frequently include instructions as to the preparation of scented pastes hardening into beads to make "sweet smelling Pater Noster" (Cortese 1604: 102, 168–71). The moisture and warmth of the hand and fingertips manipulating the beads would release their scent and leave an odor of church interior on the fingers of the recitant. Some prayer beads also include figurative images. One type of rosary features the instruments used to torment Christ. Another variation on the rosary set up by the Franciscans focuses on his wounds and even inspired rows of beads featuring stigmatized hands and feet. A late fifteenth-century engraving brings in fact flowers and wounds together. Flowers replace the Ave Maria beads, while a stigmatized limb signals the Pater Noster bead (see Figure 8.11).

This sensuous devotion, extremely common in Catholic lands well into the present, had the advantage of avoiding the pitfalls of idolatry while serving the mnemonic and didactic requirements of religious art as well as the pleasure of owning fine and inventive jewelry. The rosary generated a wide corpus of images and objects, from monumental sculptures to rows of prayer beads in a variety of metals and stones, from the most humble to the most expensive. Thanks to these, medieval retellings of the gospels survived well into the modern era.

THE SENSES IN RENAISSANCE SECULAR ART

While Reformers were attacking images, in the South, and particularly in Italy, they were being glorified and artists were being elevated to a high status. By the beginning of the fifteenth century, secular ideas on art were emerging among

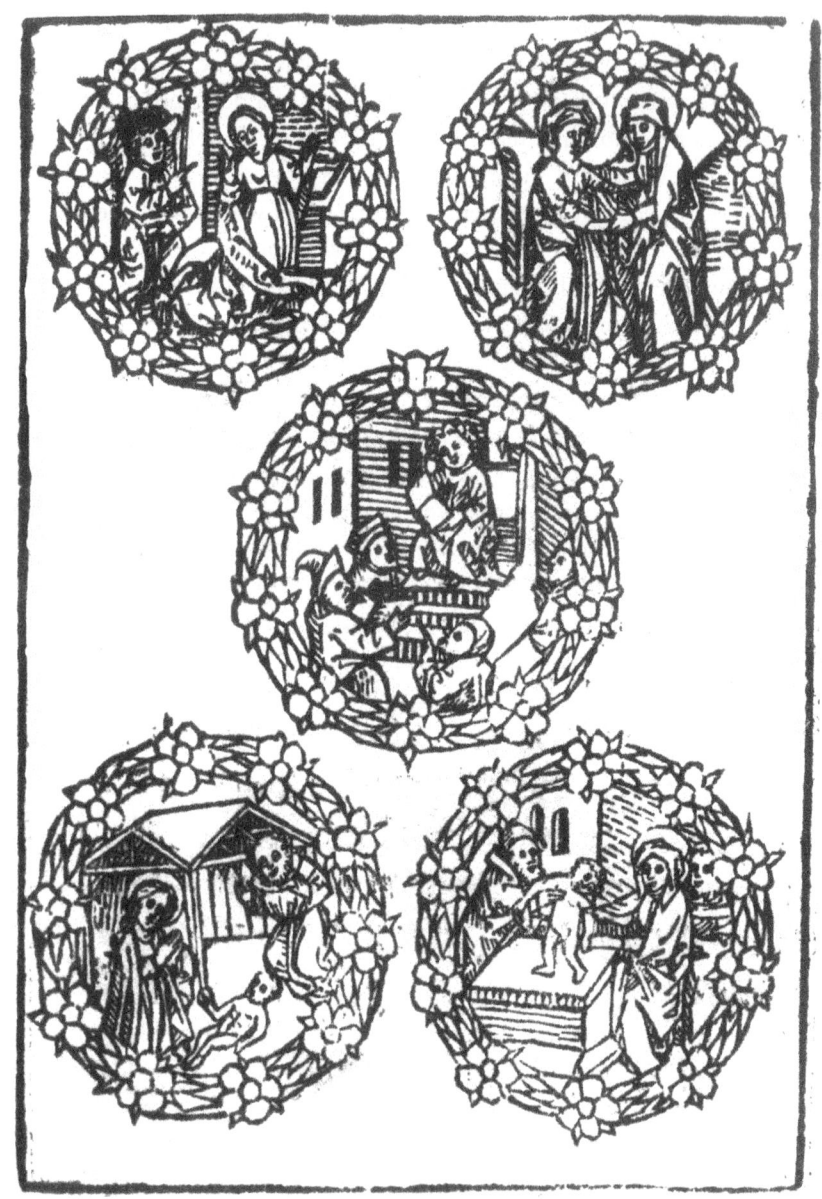

FIGURE 8.10: *The Joyful Mysteries of the Rosary*, from Unser Lieben Frauen Psalter (Ulm, 1483). Courtesy of the Warburg Institute.

Italian humanists; by the sixteenth century an all-encompassing humanistic theory of art had emerged.

At the core of the humanistic theory of painting is the concept of *disegno*, which in Italian means both *drawing* and *intention*. To paraphrase the most

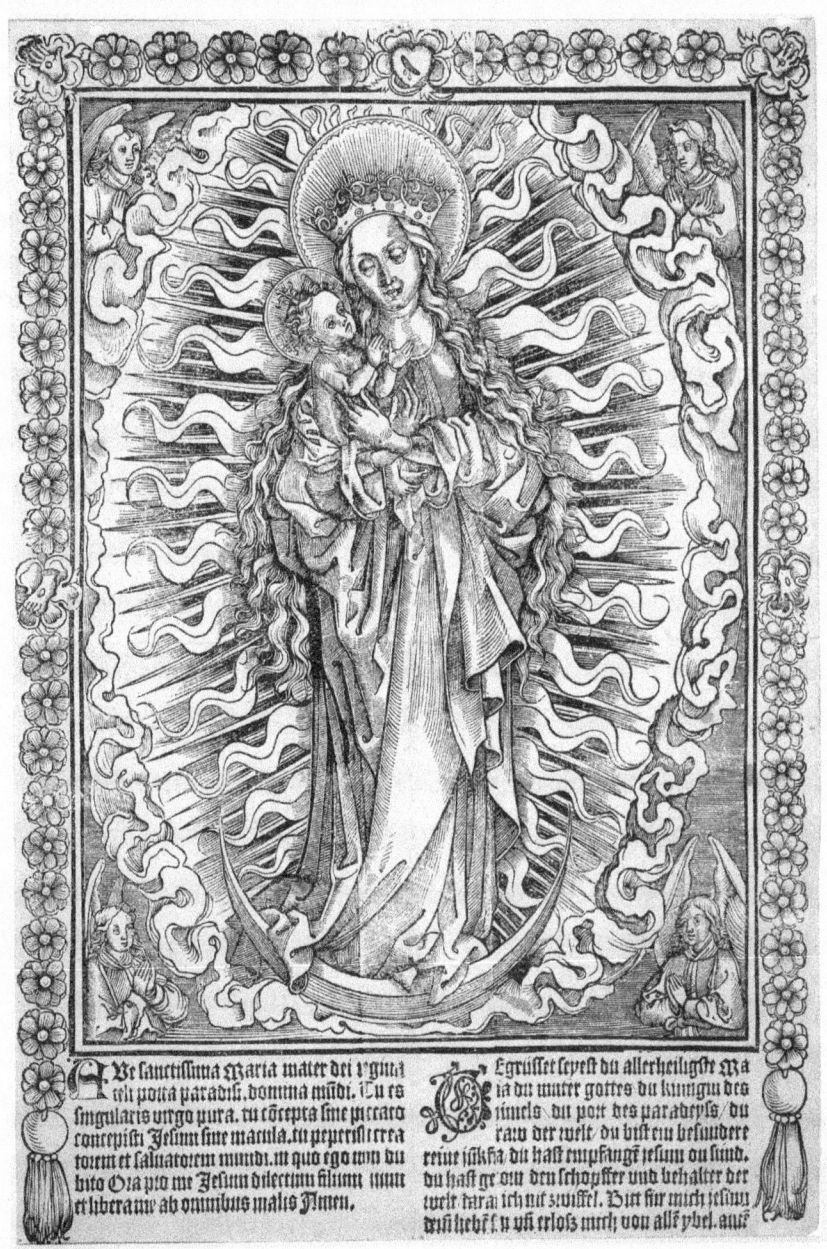

FIGURE 8.11: *Virgin of the Rosary*, German, late fifteenth century. Courtesy of the Warburg Institute.

famous definition, laid out in the introduction to Vasari's *Lives of Artists* (1568), *disegno* is nothing but a visible expression and declaration of the concept that is in the soul and that has been imagined in the mind (Vasari 1976: 111).

The most elemental unit of Renaissance art, and the principal vehicle of artistic expression, is neither line nor color but the human figure. Renaissance artistic education aimed at mastering *disegno* by means of training the imagination to represent the human figure and transcribing these mental images onto a solid surface. For this purpose Renaissance art education focused on the human body, proceeding generally in three consecutive steps. In the first, the apprentice learned to depict the sensory organs: eyes, mouth, nose, ears, hands. In the second step the budding artist would focus on anatomy to draw skeletons in order to understand bones and their articulation, learning to cover the bones with muscles, muscles with skin, and skin with clothes. Later, once the apprentice has reached fluency in the anatomical grammar of the human body and developed his own style by studying antique art and the masters of the recent past, he could move on to the final step: to draw from imagination without models in order to represent almost any figure in any position.

One central attribute of *disegno* was its intellectual character. *Disegno* was indeed the unifying concept devised to sustain the claim that painting, sculpture, and architecture were liberal arts, that is to say activities that could be performed without manual labor. This claim, essential for artists' promotion to a higher status at the time, has forcibly led scholars to approach Renaissance art from a strongly intellectual and somewhat disembodied angle. This need not be so, however, especially since the inner world of Renaissance artists was one of moving figures endowed with sensation. Furthermore, the concept of *disegno* is hardly more than an adaptation to image-making of the Aristotelian theory of the soul examined at the beginning of this chapter. This theory asserts that there is nothing in the intellect that was not previously in the senses and confirms that sensory data was part of the mental imagery which artists were trained to develop, control, and represent. Thus the art of Michelangelo and his followers, often referred to as Mannerism, should also be envisaged from a sensory perspective.

The works of Agnolo Bronzino, the leading mid-sixteenth-century Florentine Mannerist, provide particularly striking examples. His poem, the *Capitolo del pennello*, compared the painter's brush to the generative male organ, asserting that just as a skilful lover can perform in a wide variety of positions, so a painter can express figures in all possible and imaginable positions (Quiviger 2010: 60–3).

Bronzino's famous allegory—sometimes called *Luxury Unveiled by Time*—has generated many interpretations which have tended to overlook its intense sensory contents (see Figure 8.12). The postures of the figures, those of Venus and Cupid in particular, are typical of mid-sixteenth-century art: though the postures appear to look graceful, adopting them would require a level of flexibility barely attainable even through advanced yoga practice. But this is indeed the aim of *disegno*: to shape the human figure in ways that are pleasing to the imagination. Simpler sensations and straightforward sensory contrasts

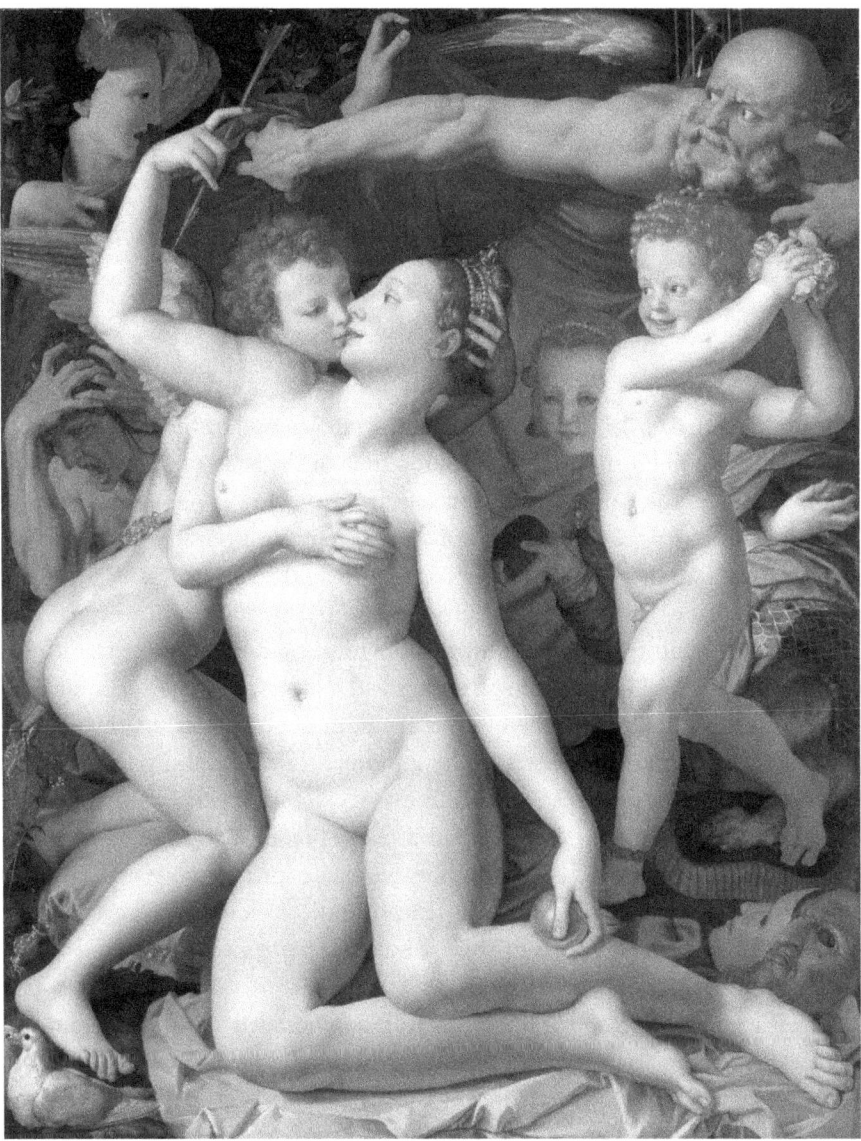

FIGURE 8.12: Agnolo Bronzino, *Allegory*, *c.* 1545. The National Gallery, London.

also abound in this picture. From left to right we have a man screaming and pulling his hair in rage, beside him Cupid exchanges a twin tongue kiss with his mother, Venus, while feeling her hair and diadem with one hand and her breast with the other. The golden apple which Venus holds in her left hand echoes the spherical shape of her breast, further defined by Cupid's pressing hand. The golden arrow in her right hand surely alludes to the poetic topos of the wounds of love. Here Bronzino has emphasized the sharpness of the acute and graphic metallic end of the arrow by setting it in relation to two further tactile ranges suggested by the tender fleshy inside of Venus's arm and the colorful feathery fluff of Cupid's wing.

On the left, further invocations of sound, touch, taste, and smell come in the form of a putto with bells around his ankles who rubs roses in his hand while a little girl with a dragon tail presents a honeycomb to the viewer. Bronzino's work is also tributary of classical art and its treatment of low relief figures through which he plays on images of sensations on marble-toned flesh.

AFTER MANNERISM

The period between 1550 and 1650 is at the intersection of three art historical time zones: Mannerism, roughly from the time of the Sack of Rome (1527) to the mid-1560s, the Counter Reformation from the 1560s onwards, blending into the Baroque which extends beyond the seventeenth century. By the 1560s Mannerist experimentations with proportions and anatomy gave way to a more naturalistic rendering of the human body. Artistic education also changed, progressively shifting from the workshop to the academy. The traditional apprenticeship based on drawing from the old masters, from nature, and from the antique eventually morphed into a program of study and art theory. The emphasis on composing images in the mind before representing them on the canvas eventually produced a hierarchy of pictorial genres and subjects formulated in France in the 1660s but already present and implicit since the Renaissance (*Conférences* 50–1). Genres requiring intellectual visualization—allegory, sacred and profane history—feature at the apex of the hierarchy while still-life, landscape, and portrait were less considered since they only required technical transcription of the visible.

The academic hierarchy of the genres downgraded naturalism, but the demands of the market led to a proliferation of still-lives and scenes of daily life, particularly in the Netherlands. By the seventeenth century, these traditions were blooming. They applied the full illusionist tools of painting to represent scenes evocative of social *sensorial*, ranging from the warm, cushy, and clean interiors of the Dutch bourgeoisie depicted by Vermeer, Ter Borch, and De Hooch, to the dense atmosphere of taverns made famous by the works of van Ostade, Brouwer, and the Utrecht Caravaggists, all precious documents of sensory history.

THE RENAISSANCE OF CLASSICAL ART AND THE SENSES

By the sixteenth century the place of the antique in artistic education had reached such importance that a trip to Rome was part of standard artistic education. Classical art was not only to be found in Rome, of course. It was disseminated by means of sketchbooks and above all by the prevailing reproductive medias of the time, in particular engraving, small format sculpture and casting. By the late sixteenth century, a repertory of the most important classical sculptures had crystallized, thereby providing one of the principal models of artistic education.

Renaissance rediscovery of classical art includes one particularly sensational item: the Laocoon. The image is so unusual that some scholars have even suggested that it might be a forgery by Michelangelo. Be that as it may, the sensory impact of the Laocoon was intensely felt during the era of its immediate reception (see Figure 8.13). The standard narrative has it that the sculptural group was discovered on January 14, 1506 in a Roman vineyard and soon authenticated by Michelangelo and Giuliano da Sangallo. Emotions and sensations dominate the sculptural group. The writer Pietro Aretino (1492–1556) composed one of the most compelling descriptions of the group, presenting it as a three-step sequence in time showing the distress and fear of someone about to be bitten by a snake, someone experiencing the bite of the snake, and someone languishing under the effect of the poison (Aretino 1538: I, 299, XCIIIv). Renaissance artists frequently recycled these figures (Bober and Rubinstein 2010: 166–8), and the motif of the biting snakes seems to have multiplied in Renaissance ornamentation, sometimes in a burlesque form, as in Agostino Veneziano's ornamental version where one bites the bottom of a hybrid figure (see Figure 8.14). Indeed, the revival of classical art not only introduced a new repertory of figures, as well as an anatomical type and a canon of proportions, it also provided a theory of ornamentation, which produced images more akin to surrealism than to arabesque: the grotesque.

Until the late fifteenth century, the main sources for antique ornamentation were sarcophagi, vases, and architectural fragments. In the early 1480s, artistic cravings for classical models found exponential and fertile relief in the discovery

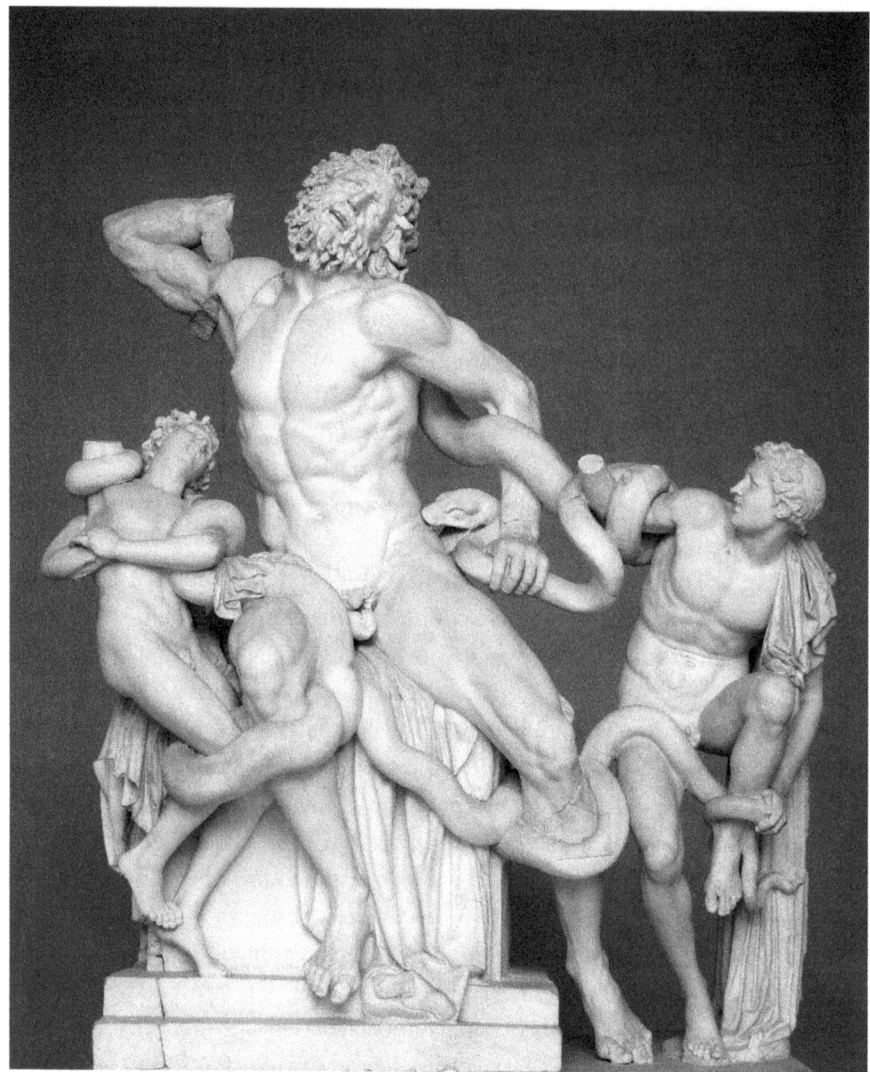

FIGURE 8.13: *The Laocoon.* Vatican Museum, Museo Pio Clemantino.

of the Domus Aurea, the former palace of the Emperor Nero (37–68 CE). The ornamental stuccos and frescoes of its inner vaults promptly came to the attention of the leading painters who had been brought to Rome by Pope Sixtus IV to decorate the Sistine Chapel. Rodolfo Ghirlandaio, Filippino Lippi, Pinturicchio, and Luca Signorelli assimilated the new ornamental style and disseminated it through their public works in Roman churches and later in Tuscany and Umbria. By the early sixteenth century, this new repertoire underwent further transformations under the talented and witty hands of

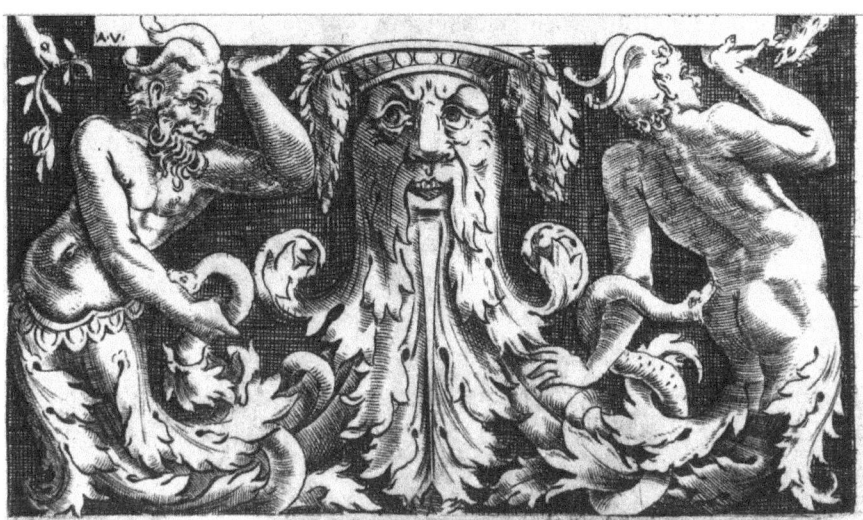

FIGURE 8.14: Agostino Veneziano, ornamental panel, engraving, 199 × 135 mm. *The Illustrated Bartsch*, Vol. 27, *The Works of Marcantonio Raimondi and of his School*, 579-II (399). Courtesy of the Warburg Institute.

Raphael and his studio, in particular Giulio Romano, Perino del Vaga, and Giovanni da Udine. They produced canonical models in Rome, notably at the Villa Farnesina (1510–11), the Vatican Loggie (*c.* 1517), and the Stuffetta (or bathroom) of Cardinal Bibbiena in the Vatican (1516). After Raphael's untimely death in 1520 and the Sack of Rome in 1527, the departure of these artists from Rome further disseminated the new ornamental style. By the mid-sixteenth century, *all'antica* ornament had spread to the minor arts and extended its presence to the borders of most genres and media.

These ornaments were called *grottesche*, after the grottoes in which they had been rediscovered. They matched the testimony of the Roman architect Vitruvius (born *c.* 80–70 BCE, died after *c.* 15 BCE) who disapproved of them but nevertheless provided an authoritative textual precedent confirming their appreciation in the classical world. Writing from the angle of architecture and engineering, Vitruvius criticized these images for showing impossibilities such as columns and temples supported by small and fragile hybrid animals. He compared them to those produced by imagination during sleep and called them *dreams of painting*. Renaissance writers enthusiastically picked up on this last aspect. The Florentine Anton Francesco Doni (1513–74), for example, fondly described *grottesche* as castles in the air (*castelli in aria*) and chimera, and associated them with figures projected by the imagination onto clouds, dust, and dirty walls. By the late sixteenth century, the genre was well enough established to command an entire chapter of Giovan Paolo Lomazzo's *Trattato dell'arte della pittura* (Milan, 1584), of Giovan Battista Armenini's *De'veri precetti della pittura* (Ravenna, 1586), and of Federico Zuccaro's *Idea dei pittori* (Turin, 1604), all of whom associated ornamentation with the multisensory imagery generated in the imagination.

Sonic and tactile themes proliferate in this population of animated hybrids touching, pinching, and sometimes biting one another. A plate of modest draughtsmanship by Nicoletto da Modena (*c*. 1506) stands out in the present context as an anthology where ornamentation has clearly outgrown its narrative function of describing some of the deeds of the god Apollo (see Figure 8.15). Starting from the top, we find a sonic contrast between the harp of Apollo and the bagpipe of Marsyas. The heels of the musicians are about to be bitten by tightrope-walking leopards. In the center two equine heads sprouting from a vegetal outgrowth bite the horn of a bovine skull which has a snake running through its eye sockets. The screaming floral sprouts and tightrope walking birds with open beaks at the bottom evoke still more sound and music.

Such intense animation, generally absent from classical art, is particularly common in Renaissance ornamentation and grows on about every surface that can accommodate images. It is a continuation of the medieval language of marginal ornamentation, but in contrast to the fixed media of the manuscript, ornamental border prints were frequently used and re-used in unrelated titles. Approached from the angle of the Aristotelian imagination, *grottesche* provides a plethora of playful allusions to multiple clusters of sensations, highlighting some continuity between medieval and Renaissance ornamentation, despite striking stylistic differences. The frontispiece of a collection of gems engraved by Enea Vico offers a fine example with the hybrid figure tickling the inside of the mouth of a mask whose expression seems to convey discomfort (see Figure 8.16).

The Renaissance was indeed the golden age of what we now call "ornament" because it saw ornamentation as a genre in which artists could freely display their imagination, to the delight of their patrons. This aspect of Renaissance culture came to an end largely as a result of the development of Renaissance art theory, which by the seventeenth century had established a hierarchy of genres based on the primacy of history painting thereby relegating ornamentation to the lower rank of craft.

With the rediscovery of classical art and culture came a new demand for mythological subjects in which artists could use antique models to represent ancient fables with modern means. This included not only commissions of mythological paintings, but also a strong demand for illustrations for works like Ovid's *Metamorphoses*, one of the most frequently edited texts of the

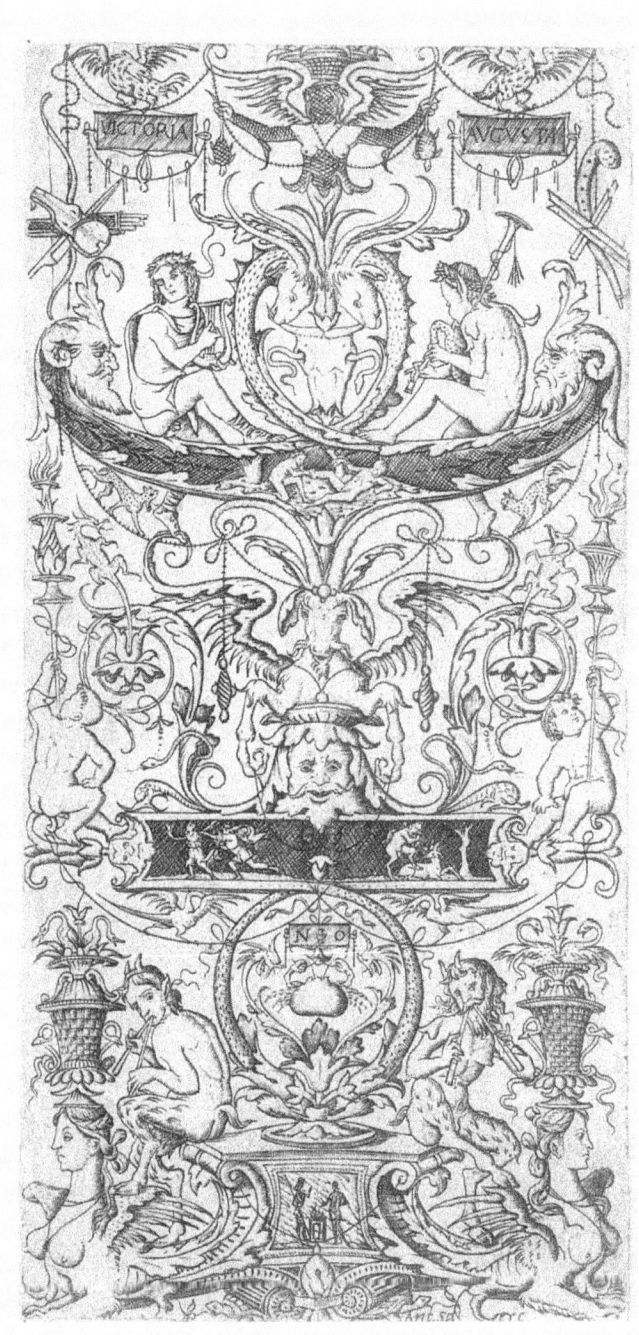

FIGURE 8.15: Nicoletto da Modena, ornamental panel with the stories of Apollo, c. 1507. Courtesy of the Warburg Institute.

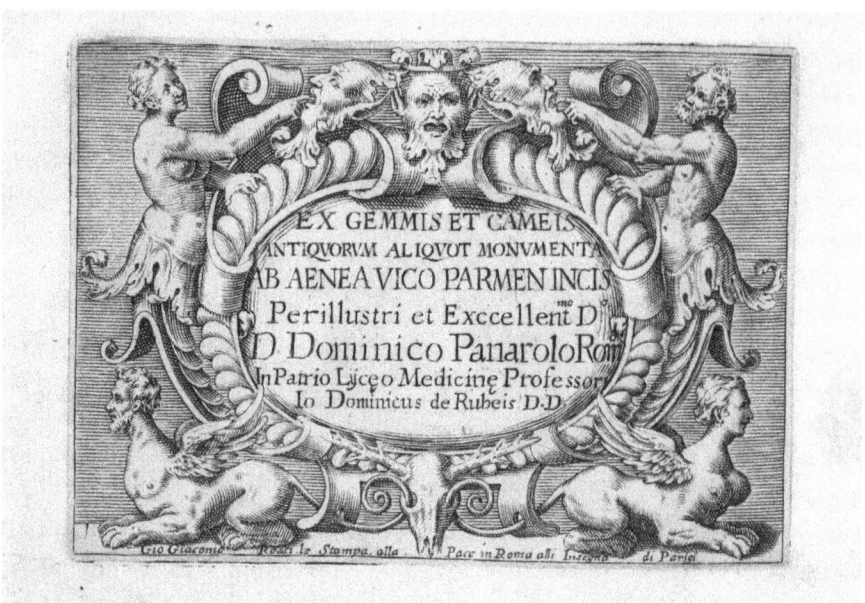

FIGURE 8.16: Frontispiece of Enea Vico, *Ex Gemmis et Cameis Antiquorum Aliquot Monumenta ab Aenea Vico Parmensi incisa* (Paris, n.d.). Courtesy of the Warburg Institute.

sixteenth century. Such images abounded in depictions of multiple sensations. The erotic deeds of the pagan gods or of the Labors of Hercules, displaying superhuman muscular strength, are just two of many examples. On a gentler register, representation of Zephyr, the sweet-breathed wind of spring, gave artists plenty of opportunities to represent scattered flowers in the air as in Botticelli's famous rendition of the Birth of Venus.

THE BACCHANAL

Taste is probably the least represented of all the senses in the Renaissance. Food of course is depicted in scenes of banqueting, but consumption, and the experience of taste, rarely are, with one exception: the Bacchanal. No survey of the senses in Renaissance art would be complete without some considerations on this particularly common, yet overlooked subject, displaying sensory abuses. Bacchanals essentially show the consumption and the effects of wine and often use *putti*, toddlers sometimes with wings, for this purpose. An anonymous Ferrarese engraving of the fifteenth century presents a fine example rehearsed through the sixteenth century and beyond (see Figure 8.17). From bottom to top children are harvesting grapes which two of them are trampling

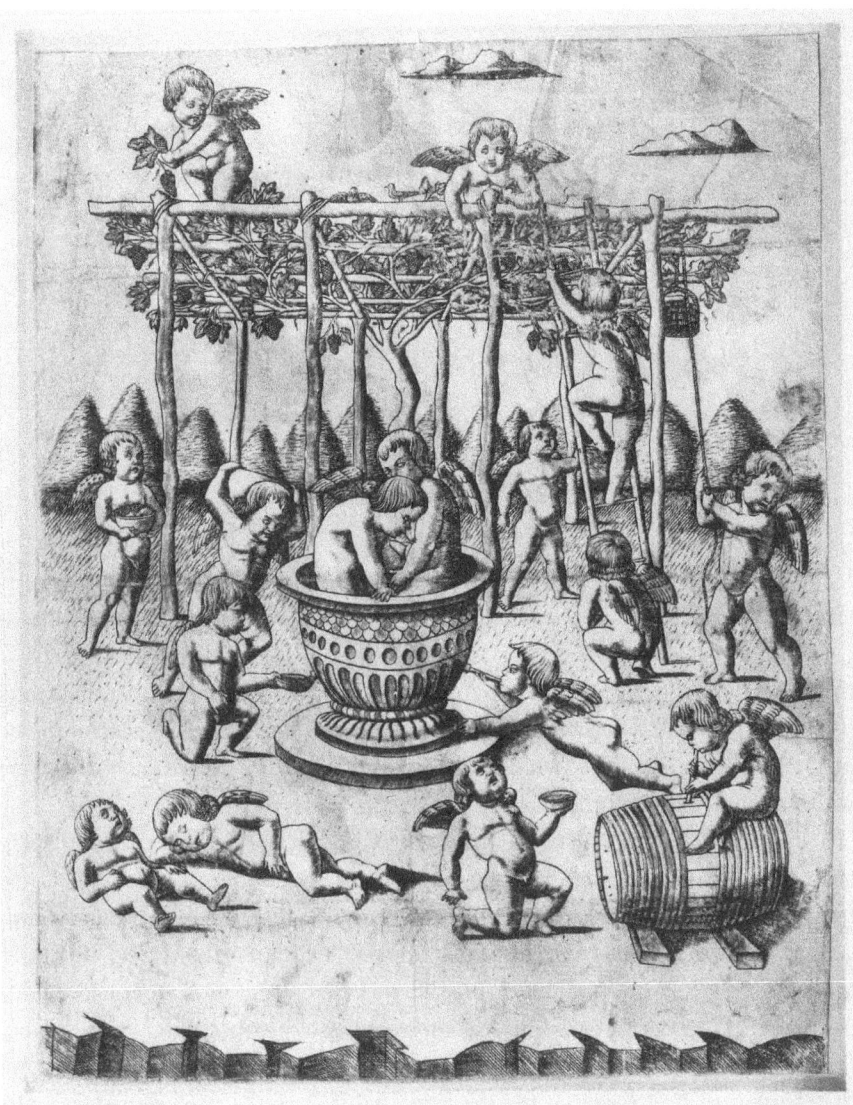

FIGURE 8.17: Bacchanal of children, Ferrarese print, late fifteenth century. Courtesy of the Warburg Institute.

in a large cup, another two are drinking with a straw (a well-known means of accelerating drunkenness), at the bottom one of these, a little winged angel, seems to express gastric discomfort, while two others are on the verge of collapsing. Depicting the divinities associated with wine challenged artists not only to suggest frenetic dancing and music-making but also bodily weight, a demand previously requested by themes such as the Descent from the Cross or

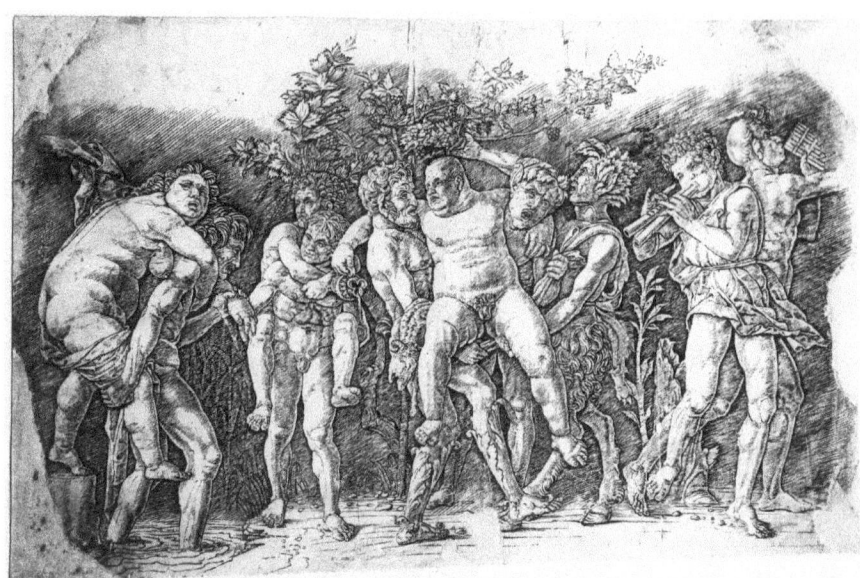

FIGURE 8.18: Andrea Mantegna, *Bacchanal*, c. 1470. Courtesy of the Warburg Institute.

the Entombment (see Figure 8.18). Another important theme of the iconography of wine is postural disorders: staggering and stumbling figures, a central theme of Michelangelo's well known Bacchus whose staggering unfolds as the viewers walks around the sculpture (see Figure 8.19).

Ancient Bacchanals survived mostly through sarcophagi, but do not display such excesses. One reason for the expansion of the modern Bacchanal can be found in the fact that wine consumption dramatically rose from the thirteenth century onwards. Early modern consumption averages about 300 liters per annum per person—about five times higher than present-day consumption (Martin 2010: 29). Yet early modern approaches to alcohol differ considerably from today's common knowledge. Wine was considered a medicine, containing the element of fire, essential for the inner balance of the four elements in the body, a core aspect of early modern medical wisdom. Thus, while drunkenness was frowned upon and condemned, both on moral and medical grounds, wine consumption was encouraged. The advices of the Platonic philosopher Marsilio Ficino are in this respect particularly representative. In his *Book of Life* (1489), a manual destined to help intellectuals to care for their health, he writes: "Take wine in the same proportion as light—abundantly, so long as neither sweat nor dehydration, as I said, nor drunkenness occurs" (Ficino [1489] 1989: 379).

Thus, although the Renaissance did not really appreciate or seek altered states, it regenerated the Bacchanal, a genre alluding to the effect of alcohol

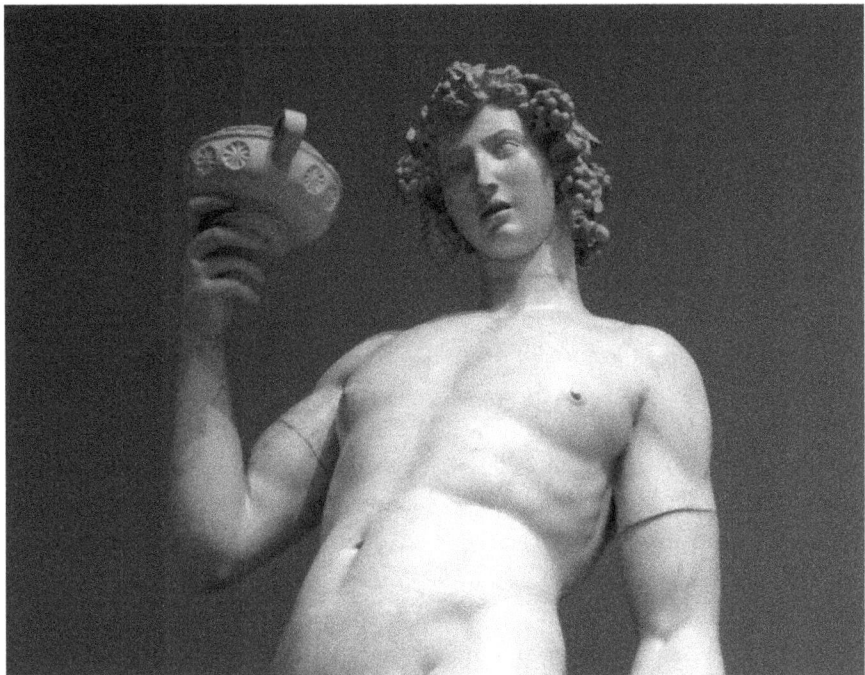

FIGURE 8.19: Michelangelo, *Bacchus*, c. 1496–8. Florence, Museo del Bargello.

abuse with some humor and little moralization. It remains to be seen how the high alcohol intake of this period could have exercised an impact on the early modern sensorium and its representation. Ficino, like Rabelais and many others, associated the mild effect of wine to a light and joyful style, and this might provide another key to understand aspects of the playful side of Renaissance culture.

CONCLUSIONS

The importance of sensation in Renaissance art reflects the ideals of a period in which the imagination dominates the theory of the visual arts and for which imagining amounts to reshaping and representing multiple sensory images. Renaissance artists inherited the demands for liveliness and empathic imagery of medieval religion to produce an art centered on the human figure. This aspect eventually became predominant, sometimes even at the expense of the narrative contents of images. In contracts, the price of paintings was set according to the number of figures to be depicted, while mastery of the human figure became the predominant focus of art appreciation. Many examples confirm this state of affairs, such as the Counter Reformation criticism of inappropriate artistic license. The Renaissance debate opposing painting and sculpture as reported by Vasari provides another instructive instance of focus on the figure at the expense of the subject (Vasari 1976, IV: 46). Partisans of sculpture asserted the superiority of their art on the grounds that a sculptor has to take into account the various angles from which his work will be seen. Painters replied that a good painting shows one single figure in all possible positions. In fact the concepts of variety and abundance, so central to Renaissance aesthetics, fully apply to the ways in which viewers delighted in seeing the human body arranged in unexpected and ingenious ways.

The fact that artistic training was focused on the human figure and its anatomy, invisible to the naked eye but necessary to convey volume and presence, should also be helpful in moderating the intense scholarly focus on linear perspective which characterizes so many surveys on Renaissance art. After a period of experimentation in the fifteenth century, perspective features only as one of the many means by which artists represented space. The central means was the human figure and indeed the most influential figure painter of the period, Michelangelo, hardly used any perspective—except of course when dealing with architecture. Two of his most important followers, El Greco and Caravaggio, used it so seldom that scholars have even suspected them of not knowing perspective at all. Space is conveyed primarily by means of human figures moving and touching each other and by means of prompts triggering the viewer's imagination. When sound is suggested then space is filled with sound in the imagination of the viewer. When smell is suggested through scattered flowers, or someone pinching his nose, again it is the viewer imagining the space between the flowers, or the air filled with stench, thereby reinventing space on the flat painted surface by means of seeing a familiar sign of sensory experience.

The early moderns believed in the ability of the imagination to make present what is not, and the ability of images to represent and stimulate the imagination. Today neuroscientists have the mirror neurons. Both theories explain the familiar multisensory discomfort of watching something painful being inflicted on someone else as if it was inflicted on us. The history of the uses and application of this faculty is the theater of the history of sensation represented in the visual arts.

It could be advanced with a broad brush that from the Middle Ages to the seventeenth century, Western painting acquired body, senses, movement, and emotions. At the center stage of post-Renaissance high art are emotions, actions, and passions which, whether contained or unchained, remained a subject in which sensation played only a subsidiary role. As a result scholars have rarely studied sensation in art outside the confines of the iconography of the five senses. Nevertheless, mental visualization of themes from mythology and sacred and profane history abound in implicit requests to represent the entire range of human sensory responses. In the seventeenth century, they were interpreted by artists of the caliber of Caravaggio, the Carracci, Bernini, Poussin, Velazquez, Rubens, Rembrandt, Vermeer, and Van Dyck to name but the most obvious. The sensory world of their work awaits scrutiny.

The introduction of classical themes in mainstream secular art also furnished some particularly striking sensory contrasts. The most obvious is the iconography of the rose, a flower well known in the Renaissance for its perfume, color, thorns, and even for its taste. The rose serves as the attribute of two diametrically opposed figures: Venus and the Virgin. Stench on the contrary is associated with the decay of the body as in the iconography of the Raising of Lazarus or in paintings related to plague and contagion, two sub-genres frequently featuring figures pinching their nose in disgust (Quiviger 2010: 132–6). This is precisely when the study of sensation in representation sets the textual tradition—which opposes Venus and the Virgin—at odds with its visual representation, thus opening a bridge leading from art history towards cultural anthropology.

But perhaps the most important and specific aspect of the senses in the arts of the Renaissance is the field of ornamentation. Ornamentation became a minor genre in the centuries following the Renaissance, and is still considered so by many twentieth-century scholars. Nevertheless Renaissance ornamentation, as we have seen, is a field set up by some of the leading artists of the time as a space "par excellence" where sensory imagination could expand without constraint.

The increasing demands for "sensory realism" also opened new pictorial avenues. One of them is the little known art of depicting randomness. In a first example we see the wounds on the body of the Christ of the Passion in the Northern traditions, here illustrated by Michael Pacher's version (Figure 8.5), a particularly common feature in late medieval Northern European painting. It is a part where artists enjoyed the unusual freedom of randomly disposing colors, drops of red signifying wounds, on a painted body. Equally bright is the topos of scattered flowers which features in countless banqueting scenes and Marian paintings where it indicates the presence of a pleasant perfume. It is also an attribute of the sweet breath of Zephyr, the springtime wind (see Figure 8.20). From the angle of the painter, depicting scattered flowers is a way

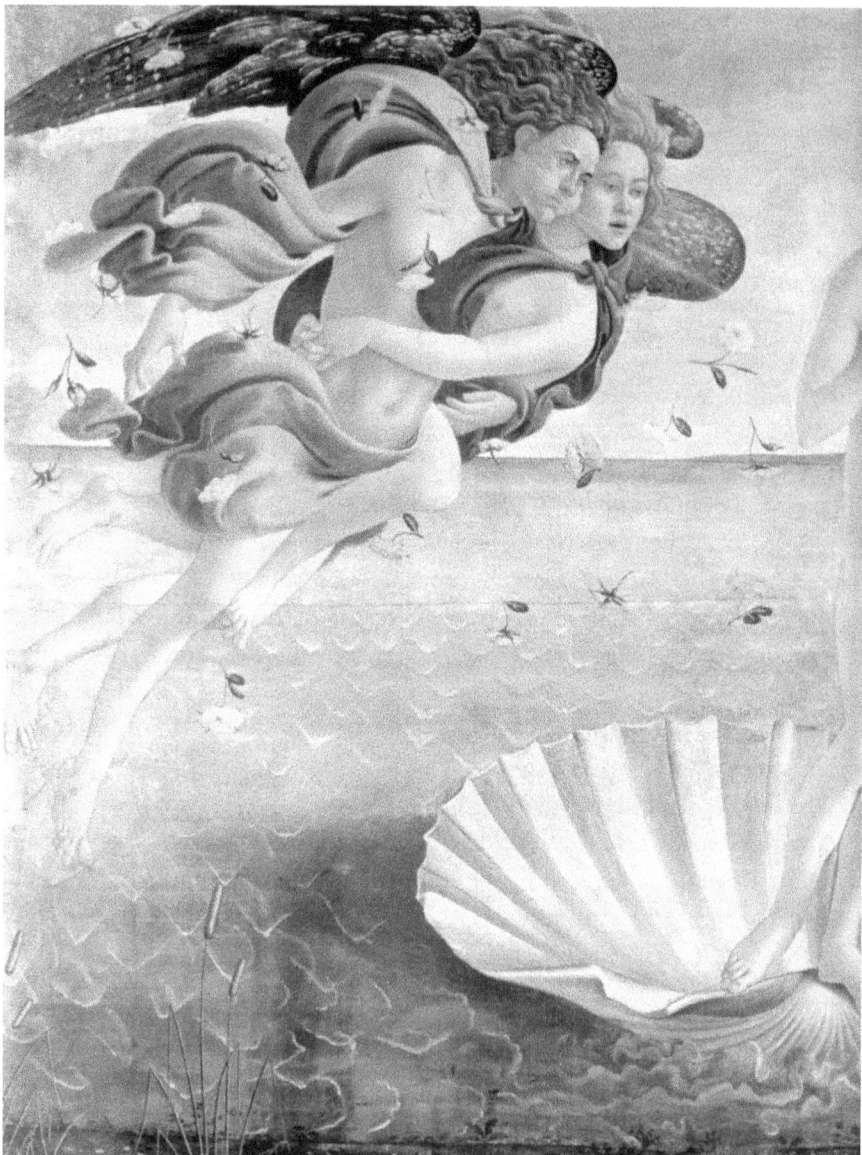

FIGURE 8.20: Sandro Botticelli, detail of *The Birth of Venus*, c. 1485. Florence, Uffizi.

of filling the space with random dots of color. In a profession dominated by the human figure such spaces, invented to prompt the imagination of scent, seem to have been, long before the beginnings of abstract art, one of the first channels through which painters would eventually shift their attention from figuration while focusing on the painterly expression of sensation.

CHAPTER NINE

Sensory Media: The Circular Links between Orality and Writing

FEDERICO BARBIERATO

On April 7, 1648 Guglielmo de Egregis, a gentleman from the region of Friuli, appeared of his own free will before the Udine Inquisitor. This was common practice for those who felt they had committed a crime or ran the risk of being reported. What Guglielmo revealed was not particularly striking: reading the odd prohibited book of anti-curial and libertine nature, which was far from unusual at the time. In fact, *Il Corriero Svaligiato*—a book by Ferrante Pallavicino, sentenced to death in Avignon in 1644—circulated widely. That it was one of the many *pasquinate* (mocking verses) against Pope Urban VIII Barberini was also unremarkable. But what is of interest in Guglielmo's deposition is the semantic ambiguity of his confessions. He declared that he read the *Corriero valigiato* "in the workshop of signor Giuseppe Fabris who read it to him." Also, when lodging at an inn in Venice, he came across a poetic composition, "which spoke ill of Pope Urban and of some cardinals." Again, he could not say "whether I had it or I heard it from a Ferrarese doctor." In other words, "I do not know if I heard it read aloud or else it was given to me to read" (Kermol 1990: 76–7). His was not an isolated case. In 1674, again in the Venetian Republic, Teodoro Paganin, having some heretical writing in his hands, declared he could not continue reading for long because "when I read as above, as I heard such things upset my mind."[1] Reading or hearing? Did Guglielmo read any pages or did he hear them read aloud by someone else? And in what sense did Teodoro "hear" what he was reading (the Italian *sentire* also meaning "feeling, sensing")?

Over the last few decades, reading, its relation with written texts and the many complex interactions between individuals, societies, and media have developed into an innovative field of research. It has been noted that from the late Middle Ages onwards the world of communication was to a large degree a multimedia world, striving "to build in its users mental structures located at the boundaries between words and images, between hearing and sight, in which knowledge of all kinds could be neatly inserted" (Niccoli 2011: 8). As is generally accepted now, communication processes involve intersensoriality (Howes 2003). They not only depend on speech and written texts but are also represented by actions, objects and by hearing, tasting, and smelling (Douglas 1978, 1999; Douglas and Isherwood 1996; Goody 1993). Since verbal language, written or oral, is not the only language that obeys contexts of meanings and sets of symbols, virtually every act can be interpreted as a communicative element within complex and diversified semantic processes. Even a landscape may be decoded as a text, considering that each of its elements contains the linguistic and cultural marks of the humans who have inhabited and transformed it (McKenzie 1985; Walsham 2012).

In this chapter I will be forced to omit a number of aspects of this world of communication. I will not discuss such media as food and drink, nor the symbolic use of, for instance, dress, flowers, perfume, or gesture: each of these aspects deserves to be treated on their own (Douglas 1978, 1999; Goody 1993). Acoustic codes will be left out as well—for instance the sound of church bells, so central to the Christian world, not only in providing a sense of time but also as a code of communication signaling either danger or rejoicing (Thompson 1991). Take the trumpet-calls or drum rolls accompanying the announcement of bans or official declarations by the authorities, and so on. Sounds could express social bonds and solidarities, emphasize force and power relationships, and recall or restate the presence of authority and of God. The very fabric of life manifested itself in a sensorially complex compound of gestures, words, images, odors, postures, and sounds. The faithful were raised in this compound from early on. As children they already learned that the act of prayer was wedded to the body and all its senses (Bayley 2009).

To follow a more homogeneous path, I will focus on the relationships between "images" and sounds, in particular between written text and orality.

For many years historiography has so much identified the period of the Renaissance with the technological "revolution" epitomized by the introduction of the printing press, that it almost forgot how the culture of the largest part of the population remained essentially oral. Overlooking the persistence of cultural codes relating to orality, it also undervalued the complex circular paths between orality and writing. Yet it is precisely at this intersection that we find communication processes which deeply affected European culture and society.

Today, historians of communication bear these questions in mind. They figure prominently in a variety of disciplines, from the history of the book to analytic bibliography and the sociology of texts, where scholars prefer to study the entire "communication circuit" (Darnton 1990) instead of merely tracing the material conditions for the production and circulation of texts. Some important insights were developed. For instance, one of the most innovative scholars in the field, the New Zealand sociologist of texts, Donald McKenzie, has suggested using the word "text" in a wide sense in order to stop its unwarranted identification with merely a written text or a book. Instead, "text" should refer to whatever form of speech or expression may find written codification or be registered on some kind of material support, or be reproduced. In addition, the act of reading has become an object of historical study. Its many forms and changes are now investigated, including the social attitudes and social boundaries involved. One of the issues this renewed attention raises is that of identifying reading as both a social phenomenon and an individual experience, a process of divergent modes of reception and attributions of meaning which not only constitute an intellectual act but are also embodied in gestures, postures, behaviors. They are acts calling upon the multiplicity of sensory experience, involving at least sight, hearing, and touch and occasionally, as we will see, taste as well.

In other words, the reader has been put under observation and, in his capacity of both actor and interpreter, has increasingly become the actual hero in the history of the book. Simultaneously, practices of reading are now observed and deciphered. "Reading, like any human activity, has a history. It cannot be assumed that the cognitive processes that enable today's reader to decipher the written page have been the same throughout the recorded past" (Saenger 1997: 1). The act of reading has altered through time, developing into a technology involving various of the senses and having a greater or smaller impact, depending on whether one measures it at a social or an individual level.

The reader or user of a "text" (whether codified in letters or images or else pronounced) always participates in the process of attribution of meaning. As several scholars have repeatedly demonstrated—in particular, and in different ways, Roger Chartier, Robert Darnton, and Carlo Ginzburg, all implicitly or explicitly referring to "reception theory"—it is impossible to establish a direct causal link between reading and inference. Reading is always an active process of reception and appropriation of meanings, sometimes even wholly independent from the text.² A text does not produce a single model of response. When readers appropriate a text, now or in the past, they tend to insert it in a socially informed horizon of meanings, a pre-existing cultural context. The meanings bestowed on it, precisely because they result from language, are social products, related to the readers' cultural codes. Even the most original interpretations are still part of what Stanley Fish described as "interpretive communities," the whole complex of codes, languages, and competences in which readers are inserted (Fish 1981).

If it is difficult to assess the users' intellectual affiliation with a text—and, frankly, the authors' as well—it is clearly impossible to establish precisely which criteria of appropriation were adopted by users of both different social origins and different intellectual backgrounds.³ As historians we do not even know exactly which words were pronounced or which texts were being used, including their material features and the reading paths suggested in these features.⁴ For example, John Locke already noted that the typographic disposition of biblical chapters and verses—while helping their pronunciation—favored their interpretation as autonomous particles, ready to use in controversy but losing the consequential argument. Such disposition allowed the use of Scripture as a repertory of examples, of fragments easy to bend to anyone's purposes. Anybody could pick and choose the verses they found most appropriate, either to reject them, or to call on them in favor of their own faith (Locke 1707).

The text disposition and its outlook, then, were far from neutral: they influenced the processes of appropriation of the given text, particularly when they resulted in influencing the senses involved, for example, when a text, through its pronunciation and verbal communication, came to be recoded in the process of memorization or public performance. Consequently, if we start from the presumption that the attributions of meaning to a text always to some extent depend on the forms and disposition of the text, it follows that the writer's choices played a role of some importance in directing the reading. This structuring of the writings shows in fact that the reader's "agressive originality" (Ginzburg 1980) was not totally anarchic, not completely disconnected from the text, but rather somehow channeled by the forms the text took. The publisher, in the widest sense of the person who gave the writing a form and circulated the text, intervened actively though perhaps unknowingly in the processes of constructing and attributing meanings. The format, the presence or absence of illustrations, the type and size of the characters, like the division in chapters, were all formal traits that to some extent oriented and guided, or at least affected, reading practices (Chartier 1991, 1995; Darnton 1990; McKenzie 1985, 1999). They did not do so in a binding way, but the intervention certainly left traces both of the traits of writers and of the readers a publisher expected. As Natalie Zemon Davis wrote, people "were not passive recipients (neither passive beneficiaries nor passive victims) of a new type of communication. Rather they were active users and interpreters of the printed books they heard and read, and even helped give these books form" (Davis 1975: 225).

If texts in McKenzie's definition are either material objects or sounds articulated, they clearly imply a complex sensorial involvement. According to the Aristotelian tradition adopted by Aquinas and long predominant in the Christian West, sight represented the most reliable form of knowledge: "spiritualior et subtilior inter omnes sensus."[5] It was even deemed more reliable than hearing despite St. Paul's postulate of "fides ex auditu" (Romans 10:17), which only Luther reclaimed in all its implications, almost reversing the hierarchy of sight and hearing.[6] His was a revolutionary act, not only in its religious but also in its wider, cultural consequences. It suggested a contrast between the two sensorial spheres, which had always converged in practices of access to written texts. The long domination of reading aloud was always based on particular textual dispositions that presupposed a certain oralization and pronunciation.

One could argue that from the late Middle Ages on, reading gradually abandoned a purely public, ceremonial or declamatory sphere to limit itself more and more to the private sphere. A technology of reading connected to pronouncing texts aloud (even for oneself, not necessarily for others) was increasingly replaced by silent reading, favoring processes of internalization. Practices of reading in silence first developed among monastic circles, to subsequently extend to universities, a literate laity and, with the introduction of the printing press, to ever broader sections of the population. The practices caused a change in what was considered the primary function of writing. According to the monastic model, writing played a predominantly instrumental role. It functioned, first of all, to preserve a text, and was not necessarily involved in the art of memory. With the establishment in the twelfth century of scholasticism and the emergence of the first universities, the text became an intellectual tool also fulfilling other roles and gaining in intersensoriality.

The model of university teaching introduced a lecturer (a *lector*, that is, a reader) giving *lectiones*, in which he read a text aloud and encouraged students to write it down and keep a personal copy. They could then read it silently in the common rooms and meditate on its contents (Hamesse 1999; Saenger 1997). For the medium term, it introduced a new relationship to reading: its practice became private, silent and mental, and made it possible to go through a text without following the system of reference between discourse and marginal annotations.

If reading aloud saw its nature and outcomes changed, it certainly did not disappear. During most of the Renaissance period the practice of reading by pronouncing the words, either for oneself or for a greater or smaller audience, remained a central element in all diffusion of information and knowledge. The oral reproduction of a text could accompany reading but could also occur separately. The text might be memorized and recited afterwards before various audiences, as for instance happened with the *cantari* emerging in late medieval Italy and deriving their subject matter from the *chansons de geste* (Roggero 2007). As we know, knowledge of literary texts was also widespread among the illiterate who heard them recited in public places—performances in which everyone could become an actor and, of course, an active interpreter. In fact, changes introduced in the reciting of the texts could be received in many ways and thus become the starting point for new traditions.

Despite the undeniable developments and concrete changes to be observed in the multiple practices of using texts, the relations between orality and writing and between hearing and sight remained essential. For a long time many intellectual histories of Renaissance Europe took it for granted that, after the introduction of movable type, orality and the oral transmission of knowledge lost most of their import. It was only in the 1970s that they were rediscovered in the study of what in nearly folkloric terms came to be defined as "popular culture," including fairy tales, *cantari*, and other popular tales. In the meantime, such exclusive pairing of the oral with the popular was no longer accepted. Even in intellectual history, the spoken word was awarded a new role: the oral dimension was still crucial (Goody 2010). To quote Robert Darnton: "we will never have an adequate history of communication until we can reconstruct its most important missing element: orality" (Darnton 2010: 2). Or take an early observation by Davis: "In short, reading from printed books does not silence oral culture. It can give people something fresh to talk about" (Davis 1975: 214).

Indeed, the learned elite accorded orality an equal importance as the book and even a higher cognitive value (Waquet 2003: 7–12). A case in point is the erudite discussion of rhetoric, which to the end of the seventeenth century and even beyond was still interested in the oralization of writing and how a written text, to be successful, should be constructed in view of an oral performance. In the phrasing of Giovan Francesco Loredan, "prince" of the Venetian Accademia degli Incogniti and particularly sensitive to these themes: "Letters in the end are letters. They are messengers, if not dead, at least lacking in warmth. The presence and voice, in my opinion, are that which binds men's will" (Loredan 1693: 333). At the time Loredan wrote these words, the spoken word still played a prominent part within the schemes of academic transmission. Only gradually, in the course of the eighteenth century, did the written word impose itself in its literary circles and institutions, though it saw a marked resistance on the part of orality (Chartier 1990).

Over the whole of European history the effects of writing on society have been dramatic, but during much of the Renaissance writing and reading were still confined to a small minority, that of the elite, while the majority depended on lecto-oral communication alone, especially in the sphere of "literature." In many cases the two traditions existed side by side (Goody 2010: 42–3).

Although one can speak of "oral genres"—for instance, in Jack Goody's listing of "folktale; song, comprising laments, praise and work songs; folk drama; myth; and the closely related legend and historical recitation" (Goody 2010: 46)—the circular links between orality and writing reveal themselves in different terms, in different environments and in different, highly variable and complex forms. Often the links not only involve the act of solitary reading, they also involve the act of reading aloud, of ritualized reading, and the unpredictable appropriations not just of written texts becoming oral, passing from sight to hearing, but also of texts that from an initially oral form happened to get written down.

In this way, sensory switching becomes a constant feature of the handling of texts in the Renaissance. A fine example is the close connection which since antiquity linked blindness to narration and song. The memory of Homer lasted for the entire period and with it the idea of a direct connection between the inability to see and the development of particular mnemonic-vocal capacities. With the rise of printing, the act of performance, which remained a market attraction and a most absorbing entertainment for audiences gathering around the blind actor, was sometimes flanked by the sale of popular songs, pamphlets, orations, and printed sheets (Carnelos 2012: 210). Such commercial activity, usually ensured by the authorities through specific privileges, was often undertaken by the blind, allowing them to survive without having to rely on alms only (Botrel 1973, 1993; Carnelos 2012).

The kind of relations with the world of communication maintained by those who lacked the main sense in the act of reading is also interesting for other reasons involving the sensory. In 1832 Henry Williams, a missionary in New Zealand, was visiting a Maori village. There

> my attention was called . . . to a blind man reading the Scriptures . . . He came to me some time since, and requested that I would let him have a complete book. I asked of what use a book would be to him, as he was blind. He replied that it would be of great use; for though he could not see, he could hear, and by possessing one he could let others read to him, until he should see with his heart.
>
> Quoted in McKenzie 1985: 18

To "see with one's heart" was a semantic and sensorial shift well known between 1450 and 1650. Preachers and orators relied on it abundantly. Such transfers from an outer eye to the mind's eye, from one type of inscription and representation to another, were already recorded in a sermon by the famous preacher Bernardino of Siena, held in Florence during Lent 1424: "Three are the forms of writing, one mental, one verbal, and one figural of grace. One in the heart, one in the word, and one in the exemplar, depicted or revealed. While often seeing it with the physical eye, you will show it to the mental one inside, and very often mention it for reverence, love and faith" (Bernardino da Siena 1934, II: 208). Three languages intersect in this passage: the image, the spoken and the written word, and finally meditation, three interdependent languages which support one another in the processes of perception and the construction of mental images (McKenzie 1985: 18). Such semantic shifts between languages were long present in the definition of texts. When Galileo Galilei, in a passage from his *Dialogue Concerning the Two Chief World Systems* (1632), praised the inventor of the printing press, he emphasized how printing allowed one to "communicate . . . deepest thoughts to any other person, though distant by mighty intervals of space and time." Above all, it made possible "talking" to people who inhabited the Indies, as well as "speaking to those who are not yet born and will not be born for a thousand or ten thousand years" (Galilei 2001: 119).

The senses of seeing and hearing, the two senses involved in the process of creating mental images, of evoking the same images in people remote in time and space, illustrate the intersensoriality of communication during the Renaissance, its multiple possibilities of access and its multiple modes of reception. Everyday experience, in other words, revolved around a series of multiple perceptions giving life to meanings, images, and visions, in which the senses were implicated simultaneously.

In a context like this, it is not difficult to understand how manuscripts, images, or books were not considered as mere containers of a text. They often represented simple points of departure or even pretexts. A striking case is that of the emergence, from at least the sixteenth century on, of political information among both the ruling and the subaltern classes. In all European cities, and to a smaller degree also in the countryside, the consumption of such information increased enormously. Printed and manuscript material reporting the news, war events, dynastic successions, or all kinds of curiosities started to circulate in ever greater numbers to reach their highest popularity in the seventeenth and the eighteenth centuries. This aroused the curiosity and scorn of observers, who felt both annoyed and amused about this devouring passion which an increasing portion of the population now manifested for questions they had not the slightest chance of influencing. Gazettes and newspapers circulated both in the hands of private citizens and in public places, where they were sold to read or to be read aloud and discussed. Often they were enlivened by iconographic elements such as maps, portraits of rulers, and representations of monstrous creatures or calamities.

To some extent these developments resulted from a growth in literacy and, at least in the main urban centers, from the considerable presence of cultural brokers. In general, the widespread networks of the written texts' diffusion and distribution mirrored an audience that had been growing from at least the sixteenth century onwards. But literacy rates may have been of secondary importance, if we consider that the complementarity of sight and hearing ensured that in a domestic or neighborhood group only one person needed to be able to read, so that a much higher number of people could hear the text. Within the cities such complementarity extended well beyond the family group due to such places of sociability as squares, taverns, workshops, or the first coffee and tea houses.[7] In the process, reading in common changed into a mostly desacralized social practice, more habitual than ritual, and also enhanced the possibilities for appropriating a text independent from the author's intentions. These were perhaps the first beginnings of that "reading revolution," which some scholars believe allowed an urban audience to emancipate itself from political and religious authority. They may reflect the birth of the bourgeois public space (Bödeker 1995; Wittmann 1999).

The oral transmission of news was in fact common practice: like sermons, stories, songs, and so on, gazettes, reports, and newspapers were read aloud in places frequented by people from all social ranks, and one could hear them discussed at length. Most of the news was spread through an oral mediation that incremented a single copy's chances to reach a potentially high number of listeners, even if they were illiterate. For example, in Venice, one of the chief centers in the production and consumption of European information, children often went "crying stories and reports around [St. Mark's] Square." In general, the sheets were sold at stalls or by going around and "crying them in the Square and at Rialto." In the event that a piece of news turned *rancide*, that is, was superseded by events or publicly contradicted, so that the value of the printed sheets diminished, the seller did not stop; instead the unsold copies were usually distributed among the "lads" who sold them around town by "crying them" (Barbierato 2012: 132).

Information professionals were well aware of the opportunities to extend the news far beyond the page. The compilers of gazettes, reports, and stories in general belonged to both the worlds of oral and written culture and they knew as much as songwriters or the composers of satirical poems that their work was channeled into a communication system relying both on orality and writing (Dooley 1999: 15). Often an interesting circular path was activated, when the rumors originating from discussions and picked up in public spaces became part of new written reports, which in their turn could again affect the

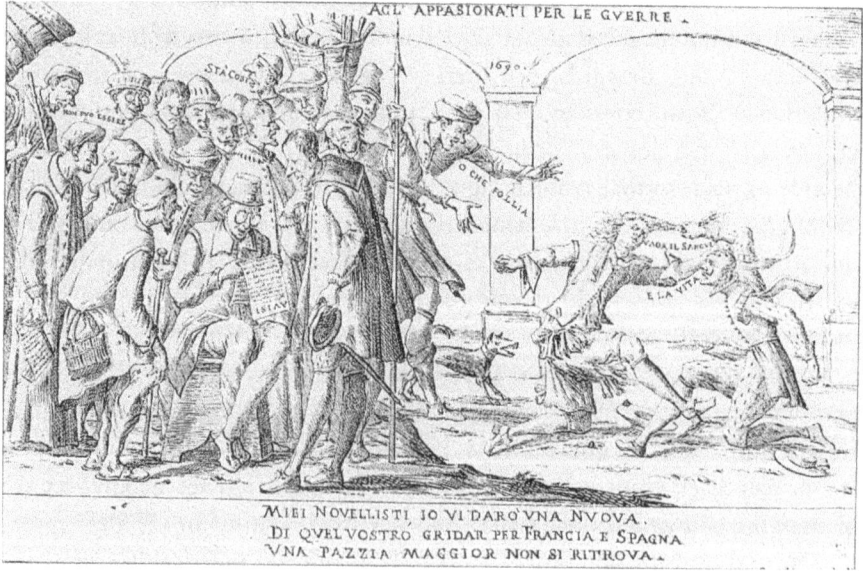

FIGURE 9.1: Giuseppe Maria Mitelli, *Agl'appassionati per le guerre*, etched engraving. Bononia, Biblioteca dell Archiginnasio.

oral channels. Similarly, in hearing an interlocutor bringing news, everybody could assess its reliability by judging his gestures, facial expression, or tone of voice. "It is no wonder, then, that early modern people long preferred to have their news by mouth when possible" (Woolf 2001: 92).[8] The thirst for news was quenched through a variety of sources, among them conversations, official communications, eavesdropping, public debates, acting, private correspondence, and, of course, the printed and written word: "All human faculties were involved in the absorption and digestion of news" (Dooley and Baron 2001: 17).

In these cases reading was often practiced with a precise scope: in view of an exchange, a discussion, or the exhibition of an idea. Here, reading was strictly bound to a type of thought that had to be expressed and was therefore intrinsically public. Texts were searched for doctrines, formulations, or discourses to be appropriated and exposed. At the same time, through texts one tried to filter, interpret, or finally challenge what was orally captured from others. To this end, readers often went back to the same works, in an attempt to get a better hold on the images and thoughts recorded, until they became their own.

What observers noted and satirized was the "confusion of the senses" that such mindless passion for discussion and reading could wreck (Infelise 2002). Folly as a result of reading was a common literary topos we do not need to revisit here. But it is interesting to note that the effects of reading could be devastating and hit all the senses: it might hamper the reader's sight, make him utter sounds and non-existing words, or make him undergo contrasting physical sensations.

Books may drive you mad, as happened to Don Quixote, and become the object of censorship by an improvised and grotesque inquisition tribunal: a priest, a barber, Don Quixote's niece, and a servant. They enter the library, and find "over a hundred large volumes very well bound and others of smaller size." Seeing this, the servant runs out to fetch "a bowl of holy water and a bunch of hyssop, saying: 'Take this, your reverence, and sprinkle the room, for fear that one of the many enchanters from those books might cast a spell on us to punish us for our intention to cast them out of the world'." Nevertheless, the curate tries to find "some that did not deserve the fire penalty." And yet, "No," cried the niece, "there is no reason why you should pardon any of them, for they have all been offenders. Better throw them in a heap, set fire to the lot; or else, take them into the backyard and let the bonfire be lit there, and the smoke will not trouble anyone" (Cervantes 2003: 85).

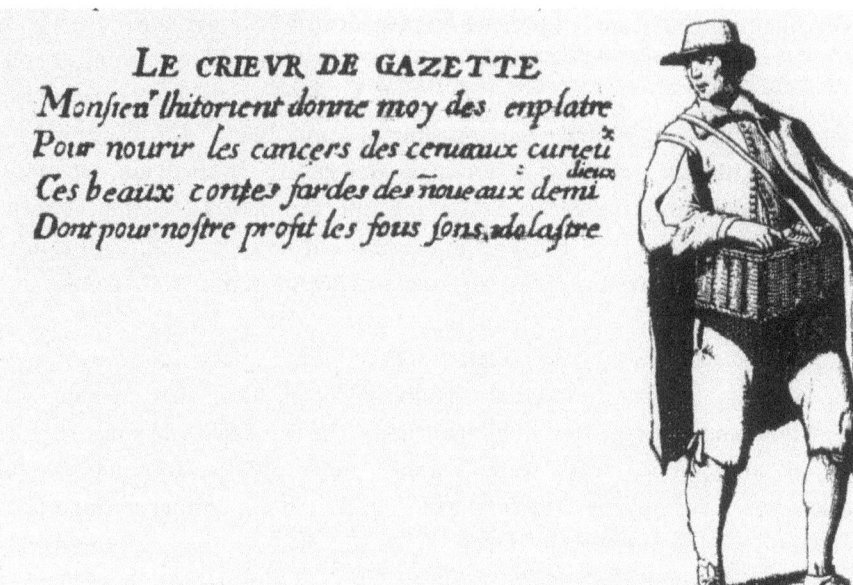

FIGURE 9.2: *Le crieur de gazette*, engraving. Paris, Bibliothèque des Arts Décoratifs.

In everyday imagery as much as in literary topoi, books could be magical, powerful objects, themselves dangerous, and capable of somehow disregarding reading itself. Danger resided not so much in the telling of the stories that had driven Don Quixote mad or in the description of a magical rite, but rather in the fact that the books, once opened, could activate dark forces, let magicians escape, or reveal deep mysteries. Michael Scot (*c.* 1175–1234) knew books of magic inhabited by spirits directly asking those who opened them to mention their name and address and voice their wishes (Klaniczay and Kristof 2001). Only the stake could banish such presences. In the fifteenth century, during the canonization proceedings of Antoninus of Florence, one witness to the sanctification reported how the air darkened and clouded after Antoninus threw a book of magic into the flames, a sure sign that it had been inhabited by demons (Kieckhefer 1997: 4–6).

Similarly, books could be used as tools for divination or be carried around as relics, and also used to protect oneself against illnesses and accidents. Like religious images, they could be touched, kissed, or even digested. Generally, texts and books had a holy and ritual dimension, more related to the spheres of touch and taste than to that of reading (Barbierato 2002; Niccoli 2011: 45–6; Watson 2007).

Such powers, like anything related to the numinous, could perturb and cause ominous concerns fitting a wider context in which even the authorities entrusted with overseeing the circulation of books could explicitly voice their mistrust of them. In 1565, in Laon, a by-law was issued ordering the inhabitants to fill up any crack in the walls facing the streets. Rumors circulated that nighttime emissaries from Calvinist Geneva had been throwing pamphlets into the houses. According to a chronicler, many citizens, infected by the pamphlets, had already abandoned the true religion to convert to the Reformation. Heretics were thus acting almost as spreaders of the plague or other contagious diseases (Higman 1990: 146).

In this respect, Renaissance texts of magic are a particularly interesting genre, capable of provoking multiple sensorial involvement. For centuries the book had formed the principal means for the implementation of religious and political rites, and the attribution of power. Therefore, anybody enacting a magical rite would use some sort of writing. But the book of magic as an object was regarded as already powerful, magic and dangerous in itself, and could be used independently of reading its contents. Having this twofold function, such texts were severely prosecuted by both the secular and the religious authorities from the fourteenth century on (Cohn 2000).

With books of magic, the appropriation of the text tended not so much to intellectual comprehension as to using its formulae, signs, and words with a very specific goal. Magic books ranked among the most widespread genres at the time, precisely because they could be used directly. Transcribing a book of magic was both an investment and a practical act, because it consisted in literally following a course of action that, according to contemporary expectations, would bring astonishing results.

At the same time, despite its prescriptive nature and its typical set of instructions to be followed, the magical text did not fully determine its reading. In translating the text into practice, readers had to perform a series of mental operations. They dissected it, filtered its information, accepted some elements while refusing others, and all this not so much based on socially determined general knowledge as on the magical insights proper to each individual and gathered through personal experience. In addition, such individual ways of reading, characterized by ritual elements and practiced during the magical evocation or experiment, were always accompanied by particular odors and particular body movements, postures, and gestures. One had to prepare physically for such practices. They were not merely mental practices but rather true performances (Barbierato 2002).

In other words, as for instance manuals of civility or *artes moriendi*, these texts "had the precise function of disappearing as discourse" (Chartier 1987: 6). At the moment the formulae were pronounced and turned into sound they were translated into actions, often encompassing all the senses. It might be required to abstain from consuming some types of food or to consume others, either of a ritual nature or not, or to wrap oneself, use perfumes, touch particular objects, and so on. Accordingly, the way a text became a magical text could be utterly accidental and unpredictable. On March 27, 1641, the gentleman Giovanni Semitecolo told the Venetian inquisitor that the year before, when visiting the nearby town of Rovigo, he had received two "secrets" from a certain Antonio Milani. This man, in turn, had learnt the "secrets" from his brother Giovan Battista, officer of the Holy Office, who owned the copy of a witch trial. Having seen the copy, Antonio extracted "some experiments *ad amorem*," which he started to circulate and also gave to the gentleman.[9]

Again, we see a gap between the intentions behind a text offered to the public and the forms of its actual reception. We also recognize the work of decontextualization, at both the material level and that of meaning. First, the supports changed: from the oral pronunciation of a deposition to a sheet of paper, from this sheet again to another sheet and then turned again into an oral form. Second, the meanings changed: the text was transformed into something else. From a judicial document on a case of witchcraft it became a repertory of some magical formulae. Such selection and subsequent codification of magic rituals was common practice, and their potential sources were infinite. Importantly, only part of these sources were books or written documents. The compiling was only partially based on pre-existing texts. Discourses or just words overheard could be selected and codified as well: the work of contamination was endless. Semitecolo's declaration reveals the liveliness and originality of communication in the Renaissance, a world in which an unclassifiable quantity of texts profiting from the interstices in censorship came to be inserted in public discourse, bringing ideas or fragments of ideas, stories or instruction, to a vast audience. Transcriptions of teachings, sermons, or speeches regarded as magically effective and fixed *pro memoria* on paper circulated in large quantities and gave writing and orality a new dimension.

As Jack Goody has argued, writing is not only a central tool for transporting and transmitting oral speech, it is also a key instrument in transforming it (Goody 1977). In the sphere of magic in particular, writing and orality constituted two cooperating systems, coordinated with the sole aim of increasing one's chances to foretell and control the world. Writing and orality were integrated, standing in a circular relation to one another. Especially in urban environments, the contrast between a popular culture (for a long time defined as oral and unchanging) and an elite culture (defined as literate and comparatively recent) should be softened. The forms of contact (and osmosis) were so many that any sharp distinctions along these lines are inadequate.

Even if the genre was widespread it was not the kind of popular literature we know, for example, from the French *Bibliothèque Bleue*, in which an editor used to revise and adapt non-popular texts to make them accessible and affordable for the lower strata of society (Chartier 1987). In the sorcery texts it was the readers who directly intervened, manipulated, and adapted the contents according to their needs, thus offering historians information on their hopes and wishes, and ultimately on themselves. There was no cultural politics here, implemented through books, only a wealth of pamphlets, manuscripts, and booklets reporting on experiments of all sorts and through their codification putting different and heterogeneous audiences in touch with one another. As Idries Shah claimed, "The fact is that every extant book of spells, charms, divination or magical conjuration … is a work which has gone through innumerable hands, been edited and re-edited, and translated in many cases two to three times between different languages" (Shah 1970: 75). In a way, every magical text was a new text, resembling in its processes of transmission that of ancient myth. As Jean-Pierre Vernant has written, Greek myth is polysemous and never fixed in a definitive form: "It always contains variants, many versions available to the storyteller, from which he selects according to the circumstances of his audience or of his own preferences, and which he can strike out, add to, or change as he likes" (Vernant 2001: xi).

But if myth traveled through predominantly oral channels, the magical knowledge of the Renaissance moved through a multiplicity of media, relying on heterogeneous codes and on a partial knowledge often selected or challenged by the variable results of tests and performances. To put it differently, many Renaissance texts were, like the magical texts, composed for ritual use, to be read aloud before an audience interested in their translation into a form of representation. Such texts were performative: they were meant to do things (Austin 1975), to arouse emotion and praise, or to work death or healing.

Many other genres recall such features, and theater is probably the most evident. In the editions of dramatic texts—for instance, the works of William Shakespeare—actual performances left their mark. One may find the traces left by a spectator or actor who watched or took part in the plays. Though condemned by playwrights as acts of intellectual piracy, practices of "copying by ear" were common. Many works were transcribed on the basis of a performance watched by a member of the audience. He may have memorized the lines by repeatedly going to the theater or else transcribed them by relying on rules of contemporary stenography to which people had access thanks to many works on the subject (Davidson 1996: 422). The next step was publication—in manuscript form or, more often, in print—of an unauthorized version of the play, sometimes quite different from the choices of the playwright. Such customs of transcribing texts were widespread and are attested particularly in Spain, France, and England (Chartier 1999: 28–47). Of course, the path could also be followed the other way round: the reading aloud of theatrical texts, involving both the eye and the ear, was the principal method for appropriating the lines. By recourse to such graphic conventions as punctuation, printed editions of this literary genre informed the reader how to "represent" the text according to the rhythm characteristic of conversations and monologues (Nelson 1977; Parkes 1993).

Another interesting genre is that of the popular songs, playing such a prominent role in the period's forms of entertainment while diffusing information and cultural codes. Countless mountebanks traveled through the towns and countryside of Europe, singing songs, sometimes to the accompaniment of a guitar, and selling the texts but also other texts or such goods as soaps, medicines, and so on (Carnelos 2012; Gentilcore 2006). In some cases police reports may become valuable allies allowing us, as they allowed Robert Darnton studying the eighteenth century, to identify circuits of writing and the performing of songs, by tracing their texts and conjecturing their musical accompaniment in an experiment of multisensory historical research (Darnton 2010; Salzberg 2010; Watt 1991).

Often songwriters ventured into productions regarded as dangerous by both secular and ecclesiastical authorities. If according to Plato poetry "paralyzed" the mind of listeners (Havelock 1986), Renaissance authorities had learnt to mistrust the square and public spaces in general. Poetry performed at such places, reaching a high number of listeners, could persuade more than a written text. At the same time, the songs could maintain their impact through time thanks to their codification in writing and their distribution. Usually, to ease the texts' memorization and reproduction, they were grafted onto melodies well-known among the audiences, the so-called mechanism of the "contrafact" (Grijp 1994).

Conversely, well-known texts, not conceived for musical or public diffusion, could be adopted by the singers. From Bernardo Tasso's *Amadigi* up to Philip Sidney's *Arcadia* and *Don Quixote*, many texts lent themselves to oral performances of various kinds (Nelson 1977). Pietro Aretino, for example, delighted in the fact that his texts were sung by mountebanks and charlatans. He thanked them "of the reputation you acquire for me everywhere; and I pray you ever so much that, with your natural eloquence, you trumpet my name well" (Aretino 1999, III: 325–7). For authors it became a form of publicity and fame. While only a limited number of people could access the written text, the public performance could reach everyone, certainly when a text's power of expression was emphasized by the skills of the orator or singer, and by the music and the public setting of the square.

Renaissance media and communication, then, appear as complex and changeable sets of practices which encompassed various senses and suggest a continuous oscillation between orality and writing, between aural and visual codes. Such codes responded to rules and alphabets, to a rhetoric and praxis that will continue into the modern world: "For it must be remembered that the arrival of a new means of communication does not replace the earlier (except in certain limited spheres), it adds to it and alters it. Speech adds to gesture, writing to speech, the electronic media to writing" (Goody 2010: 155).

NOTES

Introduction

1. In a similar vein Barbara Rosenwein (2002) already dismissed the "grand narratives" of Huizinga, Febvre, and Elias from her own perspective, that of the history of emotions. The sensory historian Mark Smith speaks ironically of the "great divide" (Rosenwein 2002; M. Smith 2007b: 8–13).

Chapter One

1. I would like to thank Iva Olah, whose discussion of ornament in Chapter 2 of her doctoral dissertation led me to this important attribute of Alberti's aesthetics.

Chapter Five

1. Although one can argue that what sight grasps for Aristotle is really just the form of the accidents inhering in the surface of a substance, not the essences themselves, which would be a more Neoplatonic reading. (Thanks to Tawrin Baker for this suggestion.)
2. See Hedwig (1972), Blumenberg (1993), and Ottaviani's (n.d.) useful lectures on medieval metaphysics of light.
3. Lev. 13:45: Vows; Deut. 22:5, Prohibitions (Idolatry). "Commandments, The 613" (1971: 766, 772).
4. Kuchta (1993: 235–6). Note that transvestite conventions of the Elizabethan drama, allowing for a gender shift, are unique within early modern European acting conventions and codes of appearance (Orgel 1996: 2).
5. Descartes, *Dioptrique* (1637), AT VI: 141, 81 / CSM I: 152. Descartes is also part of the mechanist program to reduce all contact senses to touch, in Stephen

Gaukroger's terms (introduction to Arnauld 1990: 17). See Descartes, *Replies to Fourth Objections*, AT VII: 251 / CSM II: 174; *Rules* # 12, AT X: 412 / CSM I: 40.

6. Today, neural plasticity research indicates that a blind person can use the sight area of the brain to deal with tangible information (although see also Held *et al.* 2011; thanks to Benny Goldberg for this reference).

7. Descartes, *Dioptrique*, 1er Discours (AT VI: 84 / CSM I: 153). For a comparison of the blind man in Descartes and in Diderot, see Le Ru (2000). For Lindberg it was a very old analogy, "already old in the ninth century" (Lindberg 1976: 39).

8. Gilman further notes that emblem books of the late Renaissance mostly represent touch "by an image of a woman touched or pierced by a wild animal" (1993: 206).

9. Thanks to Evan Ragland for his suggestions here.

10. Ross (1651, II.xxi: 110); Willis (1683, X ("Of the Sense in General"): 57, a point arguably going back to Aristotle's *De anima* II.2–3). Giglioni (2013: 19) cites Fernel and Ficino as holding this view.

11. Willis (1683, XI ("Of the Senses in Particular, and first of the touch"): 60); however (like Diderot later in his *Paradoxe sur le comédien*, 1769–78), Willis warns of the weakness of someone whose physiology would be constantly at the mercy of their sensitivity. (For a brilliant and evocative discussion in contemporary neurobiological terms of why "it would not be a good idea" to perceive in total, synesthetic and hallucinatory terms, see Freeman 1991.)

12. Kant also discusses Cheselden's cataract experiments in his anthropology lectures.

13. Diogenes Laertius 1959, X. 32; Epicurus, *Principal Doctrines* 23, in Long (1986: 21) (further elaborated in Cicero, *De natura deorum*, I. 70 and *De finibus*, I.30.64).

14. *Le pour et le contre*, III, in Diderot (1975–, XV: 9). Shaftesbury described our sensations as real regardless of the status of the objects in his *Inquiry Concerning Virtue or Merit* (which Diderot translated): "For let us carry scepticism ever so far, let us doubt, if we can, of everything about us, we cannot doubt of what passes within ourselves. Our passions and affections are known to us. They are certain, whatever the objects may be on which they are employed" (Shaftesbury 1964, I: 336–7).

15. *Enc.*, art. "Epicuréisme," V: 782a; *Éléments de physiologie*, in Diderot (1975–, XVII: 457); *Lettre sur les sourds et muets*, in Diderot (1975–, IV: 140).

16. We have in mind thinkers as diverse as late Husserl, Merleau-Ponty, Didier Anzieu and his notion of the "Moi-Peau" ("I-skin"), and Jean-Luc Nancy, with his "secularized Christian" fascination with embodiment *qua* incarnation. They seem to repeat the powerful mystical utterances of figures such as the twelfth-century nun Hildegard of Bingen and the thirteenth-century Flemish poet and Beguine, Hadewijch. Of course, one need not have a hyper-transcendentalized self, I, or body to arrive at a rich concept of embodiment and touch: consider J.J. Gibson's "rich" or "thick" account of perception, in which touch is not a mere contact sense but something more dynamic, involving more "intentionality" (Gibson 1966: 102, 132ff.), which partly resonates with Alois Riegl's notion of a "haptic" dimension of art (i.e., based on touch), versus its optic dimension (Riegl [1901] 1985).

Chapter Nine

1. Archivio di Stato di Venezia, *Sant'Uffizio*, busta 119, trial against Giovanni Zucco, statement by Teodoro Paganin, June 16, 1676.
2. The issue of the ways in which readers appropriated texts is now felt to be a central element of studies of the history of books, reading, and culture in general. For a primer, see the essays in Cavallo and Chartier (1995) and Chartier (1995). For further readings: Chartier (1987, 1994); Darnton (1984, 1990); Ginzburg (1980). On reader response and reception theory, see the essays collected in Holub (1989, 1992). See also Iser (1974, 1978); Rose (1992); and critical remarks in Raymond (2003).
3. The traditional point of reference for the gap between text and understanding is naturally Ginzburg (1980), who speaks of the "aggressive originality of [Menocchio's] reading." Similarly, "if there is always a gap between the content of a text and how and to what extent it is understood, this gap tends to increase considerably in the case of less informed readers, in whom the written word induces unexpected associations of ideas"; Infelise (1999: 52).
4. This is one of the main investigative areas of analytical bibliographies. Cf. Darnton (1990); Chartier (1995); McKenzie (1999); McKenzie (2002).
5. *De Anima*, 2.l.14, n. 19.
6. Before the Scientific Revolution such positive ideas that solid knowledge could be based on sight were already challenged. On these aspects, see Scribner (1994, 2001); Belting (2011); Clark (2007); Freedberg (2003). On the role of sight as mnemonic aid, Yates (1966) remains essential.
7. The possibilities for the illiterate to have access to writing are now well known, above all thanks to Roger Chartier and Donald McKenzie. For some important comments, see also Levi (1988: 181).
8. On rumors and "popular" public opinion, see Fox (1997, 2002).
9. Archivio di Stato di Venezia, *Sant'Uffizio*, busta 97, trial against Giovanni Semitecolo, deposition by Giovanni, March 27, 1641.

BIBLIOGRAPHY

à Kempis, T., 1997, *Imitation of Christ*, ed. B. J. H. Biggs, Oxford: Oxford University Press.
A Reformation Debate: Karlstadt, Emser and Eck on Sacred Images. Three treatises in translation, 1991, trans. B. D. Mangrum and G. Scavizzi, Ottawa: Dovhouse Editions.
"Alius Medicus," 1674, *Animadversions on the Medicinal Observations, of ... Frederick Loss*, London.
Addison, J., 1891, *The Spectator: a new edition, reproducing the original text both as first issued and as corrected by its authors*, ed. H. Morley, London: George Routledge & Sons.
Agnew, J.-C., 1988, *World's Apart: the market and the theatre in Anglo-American thought, 1550–1750*, Cambridge: Cambridge University Press.
Agulhon, M., 1979, *La république au village. Les populations du Var de la Révolution à la 2me République*, Paris: Seuil.
Alazard, F., 2013, "'Ogni luoco ribombava': la ville italienne de la Renaissance, un écrin et un instrument sonore," in U. Krampl and R. Beck (eds), *Les cinq sens de la ville du Moyen Âge à nos jours*, Tours: Presses Universitaires François-Rabelais.
Alberti, L. B., [c. 1441] 1987, *Dinner Pieces: a translation of the 'Intercenales'*, trans. D. Marsh, Binghamton, NY: Medieval and Renaissance Texts and Studies and the Renaissance Society of America.
Alberti, L. B., [1452] 1988, *On the Art of Building in Ten Books*, trans. J. Rykwert, N. Leach, and R. Tavernor. Cambridge, MA: MIT Press.
Alberti, L. B., 1956, *On Painting* [1435 6], trans. J. R. Spencer, New Haven, CT: Yale University Press.
Albott, R., 1599, *Wits theater of the little world*, London: Wertheim & MacIntosh.
Alexander, G., 2006, *Writing After Sidney: the literary response to Sir Philip Sidney, 1586–1640*, Oxford: Oxford University Press.

An Ease for the Overseers of the Poor, 1601, London.
Anthropologie Abstracted: or the Idea of Humane Nature Reflected in Briefe Philosophicall, and Anatomicall Collections, 1655, London.
Antoninus of Florence, 1582, *Summae Sacrae Theologiae*, Venice.
A Pleasant Conceited History Called the Taming of A Shrew, 1594, London: imprinted by Peter Short and sold by Cuthbert Barbie at his shop in the Royal Exchange.
Aretino, P., [1525] 2008, "Cortigiana," in D. Beecher (ed.), *Renaissance Comedy: The Italian Masters*, Toronto: University of Toronto Press.
Aretino, P., [1534/1536], 2005, *Dialogues*, trans. Raymond Rosenthal, Toronto: University of Toronto Press.
Aretino, P., 1538, *Delle Lettere di M. Pietro Aretino. Libro primo*, Venice: Marcolini.
Aretino, P., 1999, *Lettere*, a cura di P. Procaccioli, Roma: Salerno.
Ariosto, L., [1516] 1607, *Orlando Furioso*, trans. J. Harrington, London: imprinted by Richard Field for John Norton and Richard Waterson.
Aristotle (ed.), 1907, *De Anima, with Translation, Introduction and Notes by Robert Drew Hicks*, Cambridge: Cambridge University Press).
Aristole, 1975, *On the Soul: Parva naturalia. On breath*, trans. W. Stanley Hett, Cambridge MA: Harvard University Press.
Armas, F. A. de, 2005, "Simple magic: ekphrasis from antiquity to the age of Cervantes," in F. A. de Armas (ed.), *Ekphrasis in the Age of Cervantes*, Cranbury: Bucknell University Press.
Arnauld, A., 1990, *On True and False Ideas* [1683], Manchester: Manchester University Press.
Assaf, S., 2005, "The ambivalence of the sense of touch in Early Modern prints," *Renaissance and Reformation*, 29(1), 75–98.
Aston, M., 1988, *England's Iconoclasts: Volume I, Laws Against Images*, Oxford: Clarendon Press.
Atkinson, N., 2012, "Sonic armatures: constructing an acoustic regime in Renaissance Florence," *The Senses & Society*, 7(1), 39–52.
Augustine, 1563, *Opera Omnia*, ed. Juan Vives.
Austin, J. L., 1975, *How to do Things with Words*, Cambridge, MA: Harvard University Press.
Aziz-Zadeh, L. and Damasio, A., 2008, "Embodied semantics for actions: findings from functional brain imaging," *Journal of Physiology Paris*, 102(1–3), 35–9.
Aziz-Zadeh, L., Wilson, S., Rizzolatti, G., and Iacoboni, M., 2006, "Congruent embodied representations for visually presented actions and linguistic phrases describing actions," *Current Biology*, 12, 1818–23.
B[ulwer], J., 1644, *Chirologia; or, The Naturall Language of the Hand*, London.
Bacon, F., [1620] 2000, *The New Organon*, ed. L. Jardine and M. Silverthorne, Cambridge: Cambridge University Press.
Bacon, F., 1857–74, *The Works of Francis Bacon*, ed. J. Spedding *et al.*, 12 vols, London: Longman.
Baer, W. C., 2007, "Early retailing: London's shopping exchanges, 1550–1700," *Business History*, 49: 29–51.

Baker, D., 2005, "The allegory of a china shop: Jonson's *Entertainment at Britain's Burse*," *English Literary History*, 72, 159–80.
Bakhtin, M., 1984, *Rabelais and his World* [1965], trans. H. Iswolsky, Bloomington, IN: Indiana University Press.
Barbierato, F., 2002, *Nella stanza dei circoli. Clavicula Salomonis e libri di magia a Venezia*, Milano: Sylvestre Bonnard.
Barbierato, F., 2012, *The Inquisitor in the Hat Shop: inquisition, forbidden books, and unbelief in early modern Venice*, Farnham: Ashgate.
Bargrave, R., 1999, *The Travel Diary of Robert Bargrave, Levant merchant (1647–1656)*. ed. M. G. Brennan, London: Hakluyt Society.
Bates, C., 2007, *Masculinity, Gender, and Identity in the English Renaissance Lyric*, Cambridge: Cambridge University Press.
Baum, J. M., 2013, "From incense to idolatry: the reformation of olfaction in late medieval German ritual," *Sixteenth Century Journal*, 44(2), 323–44.
Baxandall, M., 1972, *Painting and Experience in Fifteenth-Century Italy: a primer in the social history of pictorial style*, Oxford: Oxford University Press.
Baxandall, M., 1980, *The Limewood Sculptors of Renaissance Germany*, New Haven, CT: Yale University Press.
Bayley, E., 2009, "Raising the mind to God: the sensual journey of Giovanni Morelli (1371–1444) via devotional images," *Speculum* 84(4), 984–1008.
Bearden, E., 2011, *Emblematics of the Self: ekphrasis and identity in Renaissance imitations of Greek romance*, Toronto: University of Toronto Press.
Beck, R. and Krampl, U. (eds), 2013, *Les cinq sens de la ville du Moyen Âge à nos jours*, Tours: PUFR.
Becker, A. S., 1995, *The Shield of Achilles and the Poetry of Ekphrasis*, Lanham, MD: Rowman & Littlefield.
Becon, T., 1844, *Prayers and Other Pieces of Thomas Becon*, ed. J. Ayre, Cambridge: Cambridge University Press.
Behringer, W., 2007, "Demonology, 1500–1660," in R. Po-Chia Hsia (ed.), *The Cambridge History of Christianity: reform and expansion 1500–1660*, Cambridge: Cambridge University Press.
Bellis, D., 2010, "Le visible et l'invisible dans la pensée cartésienne: figuration, imagination et vision dans la philosophie naturelle de René Descartes," PhD dissertation, Université Paris-Sorbonne/Radboud Universiteit Nijmegen.
Belting, H., 2011, *An Anthropology of Images: picture, medium, body*, Princeton, NJ: Princeton University Press.
Benedict, P., 2002, *Christ's Churches Purely Reformed: a social history of Calvinism*, New Haven, CT: Yale University Press.
Benjamin, W., 1968, "The work of art in the age of mechanical reproduction" [1936], in H. Arendt (ed.), *Illuminations*, trans. H. Zohn, New York: Schocken Books.
Bennett, J., 1971, *Locke, Berkeley, Hume. Central Themes*, Oxford: Oxford University Press.
Bensimon, M., 1974, "Modes of perception of reality in the Renaissance," in R. S. Kinsman (ed.), *The Darker Vision of the Renaissance*, Berkeley, CA: University of California Press.

Béranger, J., 1969, "Latin et langues vernaculaires dans la Hongrie du 17e siècle," *Revue Historique*, 242, 5–28.
Berarducci, M. A., 1586, *Somma corona de confessori*, Venice: Giovanni Battista Uscio.
Berkley, G., 1732, *An Essay Towards a New Theory of Vision*, London.
Bernardino da Siena, 1934, *Le prediche volgari. Firenze 1424*, ed. C. Cannarozzi, Pistoia: Pacinotti.
Bestul, T., 1996, *Texts of the Passion. Latin devotional literature and medieval society*, Philadelphia, PA: University of Pennsylvania Press.
Bethencourt, F., 2009, *The Inquisition: a global history, 1478–1834*, Cambridge: Cambridge University Press.
Biernoff, S., 2002, *Sight and Embodiment in the Middle Ages*, Basingstoke: Palgrave Macmillan.
Biow, D., 2010, *In Your Face: professional improprieties and the art of being conspicuous in sixteenth-century Italy*, Stanford, CA: Stanford University Press.
Blackman, L., 2012, *Immaterial Bodies*, London: Sage.
Blok, F. F., 1976, *Caspar Barlaeus: from the correspondence of a melancholic*, Amsterdam: Van Gorcum.
Bloom, G., 2007, *Voice in Motion: staging gender, shaping sound in early modern England*, Philadelphia, PA: University of Pennsylvania Press.
Blumenberg, H., 1983, *The Legitimacy of the Modern Age*, trans. R. M. Wallace, Cambridge, MA: MIT Press
Blumenberg, H., 1993, "Light as a metaphor for truth" [1957], in D. M. Levin (ed.), *Modernity and the Hegemony of Vision*, Berkeley, CA: University of California Press.
Boaistuau, P., 1598, *Histoires prodigieuses et memorables*, Paris.
Bober, P. and Rubinstein, R., 2010, *Renaissance Artists and Antique Sculpture: a handbook of sources*, London: Harvey Miller.
Bronzino, A., 1988, *Rime in Burla*, ed. F. Petrucci Nardelli, Rome: Istituto della Enciclopedia Italiana.
Boccaccio, G., [1353] 1993, *The Decameron*, trans. G. Waldman, Oxford: Oxford University Press.
Boccaccio, G., 1562, *L'amorosa Fiammetta di Giovanni Boccaccio*, Venice: Giolito de' Ferrari.
Bödeker, H. E., 1995, "D'une 'histoire littéraire du lecteur' à 'l'histoire du lecteur': bilan et perspectives," in R. Chartier (ed.), *Histoires de la lecture. Un bilan de recherches*, Paris: Imec.
Bono, J. J., 1995, *The Word of God and the Languages of Man: interpreting nature in early modern science and medicine, Ficino to Descartes*, Madison, WI: University of Wisconsin Press.
Botrel, J-F., 1973, "Les aveugles colporteurs d'imprimés en Espagne," *Mélanges de la Casa de Velázquez*, 9, 417–82.
Botrel, J-F., 1993, *Libros, prensa y lectura en la España del siglo XIX*, Madrid: Fundación Germán Sánchez Ruipérez.
Boulton, R., 1698, *A Treatise Concerning the Heat of the Blood*, London.
Bouwsma, W. J., 1980, "Anxiety and the formation of early modern culture," in B. C. Malament (ed.), *After the Reformation*, Manchester: University of Manchester Press.

Boyat, E. and Fleet, K., 2010, *A Social History of Ottoman Istanbul*, Cambridge: Cambridge University Press.
Boyle, R., 1772, *The Works of the Honourable Robert Boyle*, 6 vols., ed. T. Birch, London: Rivington; reprinted 1965, Hildesheim: Georg Olms.
Bradford, J., 1561, *The hurte of Hearing Mass*.
Braekman, W. L., 1999, "De 'Antwerpschen Roep' en andere straatroepen," *Volkskunde*, 100(1), 27–72.
Brant, S., 1517, *The Shyppe of Fooles*, London.
Braudel, F., 1982, *Civilisation and Capitalism: Volume 2: the wheels of commerce*, London: Collins.
Braunfels, W., 1959, *Mittelalterliche Stadtbaukunst in der Toskana*, Berlin: Mann.
Braunstein, P., 1988, "Toward intimacy: the fourteenth and fifteenth centuries," in P. Ariès and G. Duby (eds), *A History of Private Life*, Vol. 2, *Revelations of the Medieval World*, Cambridge, MA: Belknap Press.
Bredekamp, H., 2005, "Denkende Hände. Überlegungen zur Bildkunst der Naturwissenschaften," in M. Lessl and J. Mittelstrass (ed.), *Von der Wahrnehmung zur Erkenntnis*, Berlin: Springer.
Bredekamp, H., 2010, *Theorie des Bildakts: Frankfurter Adorno-Vorlesungen 2007*, Berlin: Suhrkamp.
Brendel, O., 1946, "The interpretation of the Holkham Venus," *The Art Bulletin*, 28(2).
Brereton, W., 1844, *Travels in Holland, the United Provinces, England, Scotland and Ireland M.DC.XXXIV.–M.DC.XXXV*, Manchester: Chetham Society.
Bright, T., 1586, *A Treatise of Melancholie*, London: Thomas Vautrolier.
Briost, P. *et al.*, 2002, *Croiser le fer. Violence et culture de l'escrime du XVIe au XVIIIe siècle*, Seyssel: Champvallon.
Brockliss, L. W. B., 1987, *French Higher Education in the Seventeenth and Eighteenth Centuries: a cultural history*, Oxford: Clarendon Press.
Brown, H. M., 1975, "In Onore Di Nino Pirrotta: a cook's tour of Ferrara in 1529," *Rivista Italiana di Musicologia*, 10, 216–41.
Browne, J., 1957, *The Marchant's Avizo. Verie necessarie for their sonnes and servants when they first send them beyond the seas*, ed. P. McGrath, Boston, MA: Baker Library, Harvard Graduate School of Business Administration.
Bruni, L., 2000, *Laudatio Florentine Urbis*, ed. S. U. Baldassarri, Florence, SISMEL.
Brunschwig, H., [1497] 1525, *The Noble Experyence of the Vertuous Handy Warke of Surgeri*, London.
Bucer, M., 1535, *A Treatise Declaryng and Shewing Dyvers causes that Pyctures and Other Ymages*, London: T. Godfray for W. Marshall.
Buijnsters-Smets, L., 2012, *Straatverkopers in beeld: tekeningen en prenten van Nederlandse kunstenaars ca 1540–1850*, Nijmegen: Vantilt.
Bulwer, J., 1649, *Pathomyotomia, or a Dissection of the Significative Muscles of the Affections of the Minde*, London.
Burke, P., 1995, *The Fortunes of the Courtier: the European reception of Castiglione's "Cortegiano"*, Cambridge: Polity Press.
Burke, P., 2006, "Imagining identity in the early modern city," in C. Emden *et al.* (eds), *Imagining the City*, Vol. I: *The Art of Urban Living*, Frankfurt am Main: Peter Lang.

Burke, P., 1978, *Popular Culture in Early Modern Europe*, 3rd edn, Farnham: Ashgate.

Burton, R., [1621] 1927, *The Anatomy of Melancholy*, ed. F. Dell and P. Jordan-Smith, New York: Tudor.

Butler, T., 2009, "Power in smoke: the language of tobacco and authority in Caroline England," *Studies in Philology*, 106, 100–18.

Bylebyl, J., 1993, "The manifest and the hidden in the Renaissance clinic," in W. F. Bynum and R. Porter (eds), *Medicine and the Five Senses*, Cambridge and New York: Cambridge University Press.

Bynum, C. W., 1995, "Why all the fuss about the body? A medievalist's perspective," *Critical Inquiry*, 22: 1–33.

Bynum, C. W., 2011, *Christian Materiality: an essay on religion in late medieval Europe*, New York: Zone Books.

Bynum, W. and Porter, R. (eds), 1993, *Medicine and the Five Senses*, Cambridge: Cambridge University Press.

Caffero, W., 2011, *Contesting the Renaissance*, Malden, MA: Wiley-Blackwell.

Cahill, P. A., 2009, "Renaissance literature and the study of the senses," *Literature Compass*, 6, 1014–30.

Calabi, D., 2004, *The Market and the City: square, street and architecture in Early Modern Europe*, Harmondsworth: Ashgate.

Calendar of State Papers Domestic: Elizabeth, 1591–94, 1867, 266–77, www.british-history.ac.uk.

Calvin, J., 1543, *Petit traicté monstrant que c'est que doit faire un homme fidele congnoissant la verité de l'Evangile*, Geneva.

Calvin, J., 1561, *The Institution of Christian Religion*, London.

Calvin, J., 1567, *A little booke of Iohn Caluines concernynge offences whereby at this daye diuers are feared*, London: William Seres.

Calvin, J., 1609, *A Commentary upon the Prophecie of Isaiah*, London: Felix Kyngston.

Cameron, E., 2012, *The European Reformation*, 2nd edn, Oxford: Oxford University Press.

Canisius, P., [1592] 1781, *Catechismus Minor*, Augsburg.

Cannon, J., 2010, "Kissing the Virgin's foot: *adoratio* before the Madonna and Child enacted, depicted, imagined," *Studies in Iconography*, 31, 1–50.

Carlin, M., 2008, "'What say you to a piece of beef and mustard': the evolution of public dining in medieval and Tudor London," *Huntington Library Quarterly*, 71, 199–217.

Carman, C., 2009, "Faith and vision in Leon Battista Alberti and Nicholas Cusanus: reality and rhetoric in sacred space," in O. Z. Pugliese and E. M. Kavaler (eds), *Faith and Fantasy in the Renaissance: texts, images, and religious practices*, Toronto: University of Toronto Press.

Carnelos, L., 2012, *"Con libri alla mano". L'editoria di larga diffusione a Venezia tra Sei e Settecento*, Milano: Edizioni Unicopli.

Casas Homs, J. M., 1948, "Un catecismo hispano-latino medieval," *Hispania sacra*, 1(1), 113–26.

Casola, P., 1494, *Pilgrimage to Jerusalem*, English translation, Manchester: Manchester University Press, 1907.

Castello, A. da, 1541, *Rosario Della Gloriosa Vergine*, Venice: Vittor della Serena.
Castells, R., 2000, *Fernando De Rojas and the Renaissance Vision: phantasm, melancholy, and didacticism in the Celestina*, State College, PA: Penn State University.
Castiglione, B., [1528] 1959, *The Courtier*, trans. C. S. Singleton, Garden City, NY: Anchor Books.
Castiglione, B., [1528] 1976, *The Book of the Courtier*, trans. G. Bull, 2nd edn, New York: Penguin.
Cavallo, G. and Chartier, R. (eds), 1999, *A History of Reading in the West*, Cambridge: Polity Press.
Cervantes, M. de, 1605, *El ingenioso hidalgo don Quijote de la Mancha*, Madrid: imprinted by Juan de la Cuesta for Francisco de Robles.
Cervantes, M. de, 2003, *Don Quixote*, New York: Signet.
Chambers, D., Pullan, B. S., and Fletcher, J., 1992, *Venice: a documentary history, 1450–1630*, Oxford: Blackwell.
Charleton, W., 1674, *Natural History of the Passions*, London.
Charleton, W., 1966, *Physiologia Epicuro-Gassendo-Charletoniana* . . . [1654], New York: Johnson Reprint.
Charron, P., n.d. [c. 1606], *Of Wisdome*, trans. S. Lennard, London.
Chartier, R., 1987, *The Cultural Uses of Print in Early Modern France*, Princeton, NJ: Princeton University Press.
Chartier, R., 1990, "Loisir et sociabilité: lire à haute voix dans l'Europe moderne," *Littératures Classiques*, 12, 127–47.
Chartier, R., 1991, *The Cultural Origins of the French Revolution*, Durham, NC: Duke University Press.
Chartier, R., 1994, *The Order of Books: readers, authors, and libraries in Europe between the fourteenth and eighteenth centuries*, Cambridge: Polity Press.
Chartier, R., 1995, *Forms and Meanings: texts, performances, and audiences from codex to computer*, Philadelphia, PA: University of Pennsylvania Press.
Chartier, R., 1999, *Publishing Drama in Early Modern Europe*, London: British Library.
Christin, O., 1991, *Une révolution symbolique: l'iconoclasme huguenot et la reconstruction catholique*, Paris: Minuit.
Clark, S., 1997, *Thinking with Demons: the idea of witchcraft in Early Modern Europe*, New York: Oxford University Press.
Clark, S., 2002, "Demons, natural magic and the virtually real: visual paradox in early modern Europe," in C. D. Gunnoe and G. S. Williams (eds), *Paracelsian Moments: science, medicine and astrology in early modern Europe*, Kirksville, MO: Truman State University Press.
Clark, S., 2007, *Vanities of the Eye: vision in Early Modern European culture*, Oxford: Oxford University Press.
Classen, C., 2005, "The witch's senses: sensory ideologies and transgressive femininities from the Renaissance to Modernity," in D. Howes (ed.), *Empire of the Senses: the sensual culture reader*, Oxford: Berg.
Classen, C., 2012, *The Deepest Sense: a cultural history of touch*, Urbana, IL: University of Illinois Press.

Classen, C., Howes, D., and Synnott, S., 1994, *Aroma: the cultural history of smell*, London: Routledge.

Claxton, J., 2013, "Translucent as Amber, and Subtler then Christall: The cultural context of porcelain in Early Modern England, 1588–1700," unpublished PhD, Queen Mary University of London.

Cochlaeus, J., 1572, *Speculum Missae*, ed. N. Bonfigli, Venice.

Cockayne, E., 2002, "Bad music in Early Modern English towns," *Urban History*, 29, 35–47.

Cockayne, E., 2007, *Filth, Noise and Stench in England, 1600–1700*, New Haven, CT and London: Yale University Press.

Cohen, E., 2011, "Can Colophons Be Trusted? Insights from Decorated Manuscripts Produced for Women in Renaissance Italy," in *The Hebrew Book in Early Modern Italy*, Philadelphia, PA: University of Pennsylvania Press.

Cohn, N., 2000, *Europe's Inner Demons. The demonization of Christians in medieval Christendom*, Chicago: Chicago University Press.

Colonna, F., [1499] 1999, *Hypnerotomachia Poliphili: the strife of love in a dream*, trans. J. Godwin, London: Thames & Hudson.

"Commandments, The 613," 1971, in *Encyclopaedia Judaica*, Vol. 5, C–DH, Jerusalem.

Condillac, É. B. de., [1754] 1984, *Traité des sensations*, Paris: Fayard.

Conférences (ed.), 1996, *Les conférences de l'Académie Royale de Peinture et de Sculpture au XVIIe siècle*, Paris: École Nationale des Beaux Arts.

Cortese, I., 1604, *I secreti . . . di nuovo ristampati . . .*, Venice: Nicolò Tebaldini.

Connerton, P., 1989, *How Societies Remember*, Cambridge: Cambridge University Press.

Connor, S., 2000, "Making an issue of cultural phenomenology," *Critical Quarterly*, 42(1), 2–6.

Connor, S., 2001, "Edison's teeth: touching hearing," http://www.stevenconnor.com/edsteeth, accessed July 7, 2013.

Constable, O. R., 1999, *Trade and Traders in Muslim Spain*, New York: Cambridge University Press.

Corbin, A., 1982, *The Foul and the Fragrant: odor and the French social imagination*, English translation, Leamington Spa: Berg.

Corbin, A., 1988, *The Foul and the Fragrant: odor and the French social imagination*, trans. M. Kochan *et al.*, Cambridge, MA: Harvard University Press.

Coryat, T., [1611] 1905, *Coryat's Crudities*, rpr. 2 vols, Glasgow: MacLehose.

Coster, W. and Spicer, A. (eds), 2005, *Sacred Space in Early Modern Europe*, Cambridge: Cambridge University Press.

Cotta, J., 1612, *A Short Discoverie of the Unobserved Dangers of Severall Sorts of Ignorant and Unconsiderate Practisers of Physicke in England*, London.

Cowan, A., 2007, "Not carrying out the vile and mechanical arts: touch as a measure of social distinction in early modern Venice," in A. Cowan and J. Steward (eds), *The City and the Senses: urban culture since 1500*, Aldershot: Ashgate.

Cowan, A. and Steward, J. (eds), 2007, *The City and the Senses: urban culture since 1500*, Aldershot: Ashgate.

Coxe, D., 1669, *A Discourse, Wherein the Interest of the Patient in Reference to Physick and Physicians is Soberly Debated*, London.

Craik, K. A., 2007, *Reading Sensation in Early Modern England*, Basingstoke: Palgrave Macmillan.
Cranmer, T., 1844, *The Works of Thomas Cranmer*, ed. J. E. Cox, Cambridge: Cambridge University Press.
Crashaw, R, 1982, "The flaming heart," *Seventeenth-Century Prose and Poetry*, ed. A. Witherspoon and F. Warnke, 2nd edn, Fort Worth, TX: Harcourt Brace Jovanovich College Publishers.
Crooke, H., 1616, *Microcosmographia*, London.
Curran, K. and Kearney, J., 2012, "Introduction: Shakespeare and phenomenology," *Criticism*, 54(3), 353–64.
Cusa, N. of, 1985, *Nicholas of Cusa's Dialectical Mysticism: text, translation, and interpretive study of De Visione Dei*, ed. J. Hopkins, Minneapolis, MN: Arthur J. Banning Press.
Cusa, N. of, 1990, *Nicholas of Cusa On Learned Ignorance: a translation and an appraisal of De Docta Ignorantia*, ed. J. Hopkins, Minneapolis, MN: Arthur J. Banning Press.
D'Alembert, J., [1759] 1986, *Essai sur les Éléments de philosophie*, Paris: Fayard.
D'Alton, C., 2005, "Heresy hunting and clerical reform: William Warham, John Colet, and the Lollards of Kent, 1511–1512," in I. Hunter, J. C. Laursen, and C. J. Nederman (eds), *Heresy in Transition: transforming ideas of heresy in medieval and early modern Europe*, Aldershot: Ashgate.
da Vinci, L., [1888] 1970, *The Notebooks of Leonardo da Vinci*, vol. I, ed. and trans. J. P. Richter, New York: Dover Reprints.
Dacos, N., 1969, *La découverte de la Domus Aurea et la formation des grotesques à la Renaissance*, London: The Warburg Institute.
Dallington, R., [1604] 1936, *The View of Fraunce*, facsimile edn, London: Oxford University Press.
Damasio, A., 1994, *Descartes' Error: emotion, reason, and the human brain*, New York: Putnam.
Darnton, R., 1982, *The Literary Underground of the Old Regime*, Cambridge, MA: Harvard University Press.
Darnton, R., 1984, *The Great Cat Massacre and Other Episodes in French Cultural History*, London: Allen Lane.
Darnton, R., 1990, *The Kiss of Lamourette: reflections in cultural history*, London: Faber & Faber.
Darnton, R., 1995, *The Forbidden Best-sellers of Pre-Revolutionary France*, New York and London: Norton.
Darnton, R., 2010, *Poetry and the Police: communication networks in eighteenth-century Paris*, Cambridge, MA: Harvard University Press.
Daston, L. and Park, K. (eds), 2008, *The Cambridge History of Science: early modern science*, Cambridge: Cambridge University Press.
Davidson, A., 1996, "'Some by stenography'? Stationers, shorthand, and the early Shakespearean quartos," *Papers of the Bibliographical Society of America*, 90, 417–49.

Davies, H., 1979, *Worship and Theology in England: from Cranmer to Hooker 1534–1603*, Princeton, NJ: Princeton University Press.

Davies, J., 1599, *Nosce Teipsum. This Oracle Expounded in Two Elegies 1. Of humane knowledge. 2. Of the soule of man, and the immortalitie thereof*, London: John Standish.

Davis, N. Z., 1965, *Society and Culture in Early Modern France*, Stanford, CA: Stanford University Press.

Davis, N. Z., 1973, "The rites of violence: religious riot in sixteenth-century France," *Past & Present*, 59, 51–91.

Davis, N. Z., 1975, *Society and Culture in Early Modern France*, Stanford, CA: Stanford University Press.

Day, R., 1578, *A Booke of Christian Prayers*, London: John Daye.

de Boer, W., 2001, *The Conquest of the Soul: confession, discipline, and public order in counter-Reformation Milan*, Leiden: E. J. Brill.

de Boer, W., 2012, "A Neapolitan heaven: the sensory universe of G.B. Giustiniani," in W. de Boer and C. Gottler (eds), *Religion and the Senses in Early Modern Europe*, Leiden: E. J. Brill.

de Boer, W. and Göttler, C. (eds), 2012, *Religion and the Senses in Early Modern Europe*, Leiden: Brill.

de Granada, L., 1594, *Guia de Peccadores*, Barcelona: Iayme Centrat Año.

de la Puente, L., 1609, *Meditaciones de los mysterios de nuestra santa fe*, Barcelona: Lucas Sánchez.

De Loyola, I., [1542] 1923, *The Spiritual Exercises of St. Ignatius Loyola: Spanish and English with a continuous commentary by Joseph Rickaby, S.J.*, London: Burns, Oates & Washbourne.

De Vivo, F., 2007, *Information and Communication in Venice. Rethinking Early Modern politics*, Oxford: Oxford University Press.

De Voragine, J. (ed.), 1890, *Legenda Aurea Vulgo Historia Lombardica Dicta*, Vratislaviae: Apud G. Koebner.

Dekker, T., 1603, *The Wonderful Yeare*, London: Thomas Creed (printer).

Demaitre, L., 2003, "The art and science of prognostication in early university medicine," *Bulletin of the History of Medicine*, 77, 765–78.

Dennis, F., 2008a, "Resurrecting forgotten sound: fans and handbells in Early Modern Italy," in C. Richardson and T. Hamling (eds), *Everyday Objects: medieval and Early Modern material culture and its meanings*, Aldershot: Ashgate.

Dennis, F., 2008b, "Sound and domestic space in fifteenth- and sixteenth-century Italy," *Studies in the Decorative Arts*, 16(1), 7–19.

Descartes, R., 1972, *Treatise of Man* [c. 1632], trans. T. Steele Hall, Cambridge, MA: Harvard University Press.

Descartes, R., 1985, *The Philosophical Writings of Descartes*, ed. J. Cottingham *et al.*, 3 vols, Cambridge: Cambridge University Press.

Descartes, R., 1989, *The Passions of the Soul* [1646], trans. S. H. Voss, Indianapolis, IN: Hackett.

Descartes, R., 1991, *The Philosophical Writings*, trans. J. Cottingham *et al.*, Vol. III, Cambridge: Cambridge University Press.

Dickson, S., 1954, *Panacea or Precious Bane: tobacco in sixteenth-century literature*, New York: New York Public Library.

Diderot, D., 1975–, *Œuvres complètes*, ed. H. Dieckmann, J. Proust, and J. Varloot, Paris: Hermann.

Diethelm, O., 1971, *Medical Dissertations of Psychiatric Interest Printed Before 1750*, Basel: S. Karger.

Directoria exercitiorum spiritualium, 1540–1599, 1955, "Edidit, ex integro refecit et novis textibus auxit Ignatius Iparraguirre," Rome: Apud Monumenta historica Soc. Iesu.

Dolan, J. P. (ed.), 1983, *The Essential Erasmus*, Harmondsworth: Meridian Books.

Donkin, R. A., 1999, *Dragon's Brain Perfume: an historical geography of camphor*, Leiden: Brill.

Donnelly, J. P., 1976, *Calvinism and Scholasticism in Vermigli's Doctrine of Man and Grace*, Leiden: E. J. Brill.

Dooley, B., 1999, *The Social History of Skepticism: experience and doubt in early modern culture*, Baltimore, MD and London: Johns Hopkins University Press.

Dooley, B., 2001, "Introduction," in B. Dooley and S. A. Baron (eds), *The Politics of Information in Early Modern Europe*, London and New York: Routledge.

Dooley, B. and Baron, S. A. (eds), 2001, *The Politics of Information in Early Modern Europe*, London and New York: Routledge.

Douglas, M., 1978, *Purity and Danger: an analysis of the concepts of pollution and taboo*, London: Routledge & Kegan Paul.

Douglas, M., 1999, *Implicit Meanings: selected essays in anthropology*, London: Routledge.

Douglas, M. and Isherwood, B., 1996, *The World of Goods*, Farnham: Ashgate.

Drake, S., 1957, *Discoveries and Opinions of Galileo*, New York: Doubleday.

Drewal, H. J., 2012, "African art and the senses," www.sensorystudies.org, accessed November 21, 2012.

Du Chene, D., 2000, *Life's Form: Late Aristotelian conceptions of the soul*, Ithaca, NY: Cornell University Press.

du Laurens, A., [1594] 1599, *Discourse of the Preservation of Sight; of Melancholike Diseases; of Rheumes, and of Old Age*, trans. R. Surflet, London.

Du Laurens, A., 1597, *Discours de la conservation de la vue*, Paris: J. Mettayer.

Duerloo, L., 2012, *Dynasty and Piety: Archduke Albert (1598–1621) and Habsburg political culture in an age of religious wars*, Basingstoke: Ashgate.

Dugan, H., 2008, "Scent of a woman: performing the politics of smell in Early Modern England," *The Journal of Medieval and Early Modern Studies*, 38(2), 229–52.

Dugan, H., 2009, "Shakespeare and the senses," *Literature Compass*, 6, 726–40.

Dugan, H., 2011, *The Ephemeral History of Perfume: scent and sense in Early Modern England*, Baltimore, MD: Johns Hopkins University Press.

Dupré, S. and Lüthy, C. (eds), 2011, *Silent Messagers: the circulation of material objects in the early modern Low Countries*, Berlin: LIT Verlag.

Duval, A., 1988, "Rosaire," in *Dictionnaire de Spiritualité Ascétique et Mystique*, Vol. 13, Paris: G. Beauchesne et ses fils.

Eire, C. M. N., 1986, *War Against the Idols: the reformation of worship from Erasmus to Calvin*, Cambridge: Cambridge University Press.
Eire, C. M. N., 1990, "The Reformation critique of the image," in R. W. Scribner (ed.), *Bilder und Bildersturm im Spätmittelalter und in der frühen Neuzeit*, Wiesbaden: Harrassowitz.
Elias, N., 1994, *The Civilizing Process*, trans. E. Jephcott, Oxford: Oxford University Press.
Elvin, M., 2004, *The Retreat of the Elephants: an environmental history of China*, New Haven, CT: Yale University Press.
Elyot, T., 1539, *The Castel of Helthe*, London: Thomas Berthelet.
Elyot, T., 1595, *The Castell of Health, Corrected, and in Some Places Augmented By the First Author Thereof*, London: Matthew Lownes.
Elyot, T., c. 1549, *Of the Knowledge Which Maketh a Wise Man*, London.
Erasmus, D., [1530] 1978, "On good manners for boys (De civilitate morum puerilium)," in idem, *Literary and Educational Writings*, trans. B. McGregor, Vol. 3, Toronto: University of Toronto Press.
Erasmus, D., 1997, *The Colloquies*, trans. C. R. Thompson, *The Collected Works of Erasmus*, Vols 39–40, University of Toronto Press.
Evelyn, J., 1697, *Numismata: a discourse of medals, antient and modern*, London.
Evelyn, J., 1955, *Diary*, ed. G. De Beer, 6 vols, Oxford: Clarendon Press.
Fabri, F., [1483] 1975, *Voyage en Egypte*, ed. Jacques Masson, 3 vols, Paris: Institut français d'archéologie orientale.
Falkenburg, R. L., 1994, *The Fruit of Devotion: mysticism and the imagery of love in Flemish paintings of the Virgin and Child, 1450–1550*, Amsterdam: John Benjamins.
Falkenburg, R. L., 1999, "'Toys for the soul': prayer-nuts and pomanders in late medieval devotion," in R. Falkenburg and F. G. Scholten (eds), *A Sense of Heaven: 16th-century boxwood carvings in private devotion*, Leeds: Henry Moore Institute.
Farina, L., 2012, "Once more with feeling: tactility and cognitive alterity, medieval and modern," *Postmedieval*, 3, 290–301.
Feinberg, L. J., 2002, "The Studiolo of Francesco I reconsidered," in C. A. Luchinat et al. (eds), *The Medici, Michelangelo, and the Art of Late Renaissance Florence*, New Haven, CT: Yale University Press.
Feist, U. and Rath, M. (eds), 2012, *Et in Imagine Ego. Facetten von Bildakt und Verkörperung*, Berlin: Akademie Verlag.
Feldhay, R., 2008, "Religion," in L. Daston and K. Park (eds), *The Cambridge History of Science: Early Modern science*, Cambridge: Cambridge University Press.
Fenlon, I., 2007, *The Ceremonial City*, New Haven, CT: Yale University Press.
Ferino-Pagden, S. (ed.), 1996, *Immagini del Sentire: I cinque sensi nell'arte*, Cremona: Leonardo Arte.
Fernel, J., 2003, *The Physiologia of Jean Fernel (1567)*, trans. J. M. Forrester, Philadelphia, PA: American Philosophical Association.
Ficino, M., [1489] 1989, *Three Books on Life*, ed. C. V. Caske and J. R. Clark, Binghampton, NY: Medieval & Renaissance Texts & Studies in Conjunction with the Renaissance Society of America.

Ficino, M., [1544] 2000, *Sopra lo amore o ver' convito di Platone, Commentary on Plato's Symposium on Love*, trans. S. Jayne, Dallas, TX: Spring Publications.

Ficino, M., 2001–6, *Theologia Platonica de immortalitate animae*, ed. J. Hankins *et al.*, Cambridge, MA: Harvard University Press.

Filarete, [ca. 1464], 1965, *Treatise on Architecture: being the Treatise by Antonio di Piero Averlino, known as Filarete*, trans. and ed. J. R. Spencer, New Haven, CT: Yale University Press.

Findlen, P., 1994, *Possessing Nature: museums, collecting and scientific culture in Early Modern Italy*, Berkeley, CA: University of California Press.

Fineman, J., 1986, *Shakespeare's Perjured Eye: the invention of poetic subjectivity in the sonnets*, Berkeley, CA: University of California Press.

Fingerhut, J., 2012, "Das Bild, Dein Freund: Der fühlende und der sehende Körper in der enaktiven Bildwahrnehmung," in U. Feist and M. Rath (eds), *Et in Imagine Ego. Facetten von Bildakt und Verkörperung*, Berlin: Akademie Verlag.

Fish, S., 1981, *Is There a Text in This Class? The authority of interpretive communities*, Cambridge, MA: Harvard University Press.

Floyd-Wilson, M., 2006, *English Ethnicity and Race in Early Modern Drama*, Cambridge: Cambridge University Press.

Floyer, Sir J., 1687, *Pharmakobasanos, or the Touch-Stone of Medicines*, 2 vols., London.

Floyer, Sir J., 1696, *The Preternatural State of the Animal Humours Described*, London.

Focillon, H., 1943, "Éloge de la main" [1934], in *La Vie des formes & Éloge de la main*, Paris: PUF.

Fox, A., 1997, "Rumour, news and popular opinion in Elizabethan and Early Stuart England," *Historical Journal*, 40, 597–620.

Fox, A. and Woolf, D. (eds), 2002, *The Spoken Word: oral culture in Britain, 1500–1850*, Manchester: Manchester University Press.

Foxe, J., 1563, *Acts and Monuments*, London.

Francken, A. W., 1942, *Het Leven Onzer Voorouders in de Gouden Eeuw*, The Hague: Stols.

Frangenberg, T., 1991, "Auditus Visu Prestantior: comparisons of hearing and vision in Charles de Bovelles's Liber de Sensibus," in C. Burnett, M. Fend, and P. Gouk (eds), *The Second Sense: studies in hearing and musical judgement from antiquity to the seventeenth century*, London: Warburg Institute.

Freedberg, D., 1989, *The Power of Images: studies in the history and theory of response*, Chicago: Chicago University Press.

Freedberg, D., 2003, *The Eye of the Lynx: Galileo, his friends and the beginnings of modern natural history*, Chicago: University of Chicago Press.

Freedberg, D., 2007, "Empathy, motion and emotion," in K. Herding and A. Krause-Wahl (eds), *Wie sich Gefühle Ausdruck verschaffen. Emotionen in Nachsicht*, Berlin: Driesen.

Freedberg, D. and Gallese, V., 2007, "Motion, emotion and empathy in aesthetic experience," *Trends in Cognitive Science*, 11(5), 197–203.

Freedman, L., 2003, "Michelangelo's reflections on Bacchus," *Artibus et Historiae*, 24, 121–35.

Freeman, W. J., 1991, "The physiology of perception," *Scientific American*, 264(2), 78–85.
French, R. K., 1969, *Robert Whytt, the Soul, and Medicine*, London: Wellcome Institute.
Friedlaender, W. F., 1955, *Caravaggio Studies*, Princeton, NJ: Princeton University Press.
Friedman, L. H. 2012, "Bodies and selves: re-evaluating the *blazon* in early modern England," PhD thesis. University of Virginia.
Frommel, C. L., Caneva, G., and Angeli, A., 2003, *La Villa Farnesina a Roma = The Villa Farnesina in Rome*, Modena: Panini.
Fubini, E., 2006, "Humanism and scholasticism: towards an historical definition," in A. Mazzocco (ed.), *Interpretations of Renaissance Humanism*, Leiden: E. J. Brill.
Galen, 1963, *Galen on the Passions and Errors of the Soul*, trans. P. W. Harkins, Athens, OH: Ohio State University Press.
Galen, 1997, *Selected Works*, trans. P. Singer, Oxford: Oxford University Press.
Galilei, G., 2001, *Dialogue Concerning Two Chief World Systems: Ptolemaic and Copernican*, New York: Modern Library.
Gallagher, L. and Rankin, S. (eds), 2010, *Knowing Shakespeare: senses, embodiment, cognition*, Basingstoke: Palgrave-Macmillan.
Gambaccini, P., 2003, *Mountebanks and Medicasters: a history of Italian mountebanks from the Middle Ages to the present*, New York: Mcfarland & Co.
Garnett, H., 1593, *Whether it be lawfull for catholickes to go to hereticall churches*, London.
Garrioch, D., 2003, "Sounds of the city: the soundscape of early modern European towns," *Urban History*, 30(1), 5–25.
Gaukroger, S., 1995, *Descartes: an intellectual biography*, Oxford: Oxford University Press.
Gaukroger, S., 2002, *Descartes' System of Natural Philosophy*, Cambridge: Cambridge University Press.
Gentilcore, D., 2005, "Charlatans, the regulated marketplace and the treatment of venereal disease," in K. Siena (ed.), *Sins of the Flesh: responding to sexual disease in Early Modern Europe*, Toronto: Centre for Reformation and Renaissance Studies.
Gentilcore, D., 2006, *Medical Charlatanism in Early Modern Italy*, Oxford: Oxford University Press.
Gentilcore, D., 2008, "A tale of two tribunals," in J. Jeffries Martin (ed.), *The Renaissance World*, London: Routledge.
Gentilcore, D., 2010, *Pomodoro! A History of the Tomato in Italy*, New York: Columbia University Press.
Gershow, F., [1608] 1892, "Diary of the journey of Philip Julius through England in the year 1602," *Transactions of the Royal Historical Society*, 6, 7–53.
Getz, C. S., 2005, *Music in the Collective Experience in Sixteenth-Century Milan*, Aldershot: Ashgate.
Geurts, K., 2003, *Culture and the Senses: bodily ways of knowing in an African community*, Berkeley, CA: University of California Press.

Gibson, J. J., 1966, *The Senses Considered as Perceptual Systems*, Boston, MA: Houghton Mifflin.

Giglioni, G., 2013, "Sense: Renaissance views of sense perception," in I. MacCarthy (ed.), *Renaissance Keywords*, Oxford: Legenda.

Gilio, G. A., 1564, *Dialogo degli Errori e degli Abusi de' Pittori circa l'Istorie*, Camerino: Antonio Gioioso.

Gilman, S., 1993, "Touch, sexuality and disease," in W. F. Bynum and R. Porter (eds), *Medicine and the Five Senses*, Cambridge: Cambridge University Press.

Ginzburg, C., 1980, *The Cheese and the Worms: the cosmos of a 16th century Italian miller*, trans. J. A. Tedeschi, Baltimore, MD: Johns Hopkins University Press.

Goethe, J. W. von, 1970, *Theory of Colors*, trans. C. L. Eastlake, Cambridge, MA: MIT Press.

Goldstein, C., 2012, *Print Culture in Early Modern France: Abraham Bosse and the purposes of print*, Cambridge: Cambridge University Press.

Gombrich, E., 1969, *In Search of Cultural History: the Philip Maurice Deneke lecture 1967*, Oxford: Clarendon Press.

Góngora, L. de, 2007, *Selected Poems of Luis de Góngora: a bilingual edition*, trans. J. Dent-Young, Chicago: University of Chicago Press.

Goodman, G., 1616, *The Fall of Man, or the Corruption of Nature, Proved by the Light of our Naturall Reason*, London.

Goodman, J., 1993, *Tobacco in History: the cultures of dependence*, London: Routledge.

Goody, J., 1977, *The Domestication of the Savage Mind*, Cambridge: Cambridge University Press.

Goody, J., 1993, *The Culture of Flowers*, Cambridge: Cambridge University Press.

Goody, J., 2010, *Myth, Ritual and the Oral*, Cambridge: Cambridge University Press.

Gorski, P. S., 2003, *The Disciplinary Revolution: Calvinism and the rise of the state in Early Modern Europe*, Chicago: University of Chicago Press.

Gouk, P., 2004, "Raising spirits and restoring souls: Early Modern medical explanations for music's effects," in V. Erlmann (ed.), *Hearing Cultures: essays on sound, listening and modernity*, Oxford: Berg.

Gowing, L., 2000, "The freedom of the streets: women and social space, 1560–1640," in P. Griffiths (ed.), *Londonopolis: essays in the cultural and social history of Early Modern London*, Manchester: Manchester University Press.

Gowing, L., 2007, "Speaking and listening in Early Modern London," in A. Cowan and J. Steward (eds), *The City and the Senses. Urban culture since 1500*, Aldershot: Ashgate.

Green, G., 2011, "Sensus interiores and Sensus spirituales in Nicholas of Cusa," in S. Coakley and P. Gavrilyuk (eds), *The Spiritual Senses in Christian Tradition*, Cambridge: Cambridge University Press.

Gregory, B. S., 2007a, "Anabaptist martyrdom: imperatives, experience, and memorialization," in J. D. Roth and J. M. Stayer (eds), *A Companion to Anabaptism and Spiritualism, 1521–1700*, Leiden: E. J. Brill.

Gregory, B. S., 2007b, "Christian reform and its discontents," in J. Jeffries Martin (ed.), *The Renaissance World*, Cambridge: Cambridge University Press.

Griffiths, A., 1998, *The Print in Stuart Britain*, London: British Museum.

Grijp, L. P., 1994, "A different flavour in a psalm-minded setting: Dutch Mennonite hymns from the sixteenth and seventeenth centuries," in A. Hamilton *et al.* (eds), *From Martyr to Muppy: a historical introduction to cultural assimilation processes of a religious minority in the Netherlands—the Mennonites*, Amsterdam: Amsterdam University Press.

Guylforde, R., [1506] 1851, *Pilgrimage to the Holy Land*, ed. H. Ellis, London: Camden Society.

Habib, I., 2008, *Black Lives in the English Archives, 1500–1677*, Burlington, VT: Ashgate.

Hadjnicolau, Y., 2012, "Malen, Kratzen, Modellieren: Arent de Gelder's Farbauftrag zwischen Innovation und Tradition," in M. Rath and J. Trempler (eds), *Das haptische Bild: Körperliche Bilderfahrung in der Neuzeit*, Berlin: Akademie Verlag.

Hager, A., 1991, *The Dazzling Images: the masks of Sir Philip Sidney*, Delaware: Associated UP.

Haley, G., 1965, "The narrator in Don Quijote: Maese Pedro's puppet show," *MLN*, 80(2), 145–65.

Hall, D. D., 2008, *Ways of Writing: the practice and politics of text-making in seventeenth-century New England*, Philadelphia, PA: University of Pennsylvania Press.

Hall, E., 1548, *The Union of the Two Noble and Illustre Famelies of Lancastre [and] Yorke*, London: Richard Grafton.

Hall, K. F., 1995, *Things of Darkness: economies of race and gender in early modern England*, Ithaca, NY: Cornell University Press.

Hamburger, J. F., 1997, *Nuns as Artists: the visual culture of a medieval convent*. Berkeley, CA and Los Angeles: University of California Press.

Hamesse, J., 1999, "The scholastic model of reading," in G. Cavallo and R. Chartier (eds), *A History of Reading in the West*, Oxford: Polity Press.

Hamou, P., 2002, *Voir et connaître à l'âge classique*, Paris: PUF.

Hankins, J., 2006, "Religion and the modernity of Renaissance humanism," in A. Mazzocco (ed.), *Interpretations of Renaissance Humanism*, Leiden: E. J. Brill.

Hankinson, R. J., 2003, "Stoic epistemology," in B. Inwood (ed.), *The Cambridge Companion to Stoicism*, Cambridge: Cambridge University Press.

Harkness, D. H., 2007, *The Jewel House: Elizabethan London and the Scientific Revolution*, New Haven, CT: Yale University Press.

Harris, J. G., 2007, "The smell of Macbeth," *Shakespeare Quarterly*, 58(4), 465–86.

Harvey, E. D. (ed.), 2003, *Sensible Flesh: on touch in early modern culture*, Philadelphia, PA: University of Pennsylvania Press.

Harvey, E. D., 2011, "The portal of touch," *American Historical Review*, 116, 385–400.

Harvey, E. R., 1975, *The Inward Wits: psychological theory in the Middle Ages and the Renaissance*, London: Warburg Institute.

Harvey, W., 1653, *Anatomical Exercitations concerning the Generation of living creatures* [1651], trans. M. Llewellyn, London: Octaviani Pulleyn.

Harvey, W., 1958, "A second essay to Jean Riolan" [1649], in *De Circulatione Sanguinis*, trans. K. Franklin, Oxford: Blackwell Scientific Publications.

Harvey, W., 1965, *The Works of William Harvey*, trans. R. Willis, New York: Johnson Reprint.
Hatfield, G., 1998, "The cognitive faculties," in D. Garber *et al.* (eds), *The Cambridge History of Seventeenth Century Philosophy*, 2 vols, Cambridge: Cambridge University Press.
Havelock, E., 1986, *The Muse Learns to Write: reflections on orality and literacy from antiquity to the present*, New Haven, CT: Yale University Press.
Hedwig, K., 1972, "German idealism in the context of light metaphysics," *Idealistic Studies*, 2(1), 16–38.
Held, R. *et al.*, 2011, "The newly sighted fail to match seen with felt," *Nature Neuroscience*, 14(5).
Heller-Roazen, D., 2007, *The Inner Touch: archaeology of a sensation*, New York: Zone Books.
Helmreich, S., Paxson, H., and Zeamer, E., 2012, "Sensing the unseen: an infraduction," *Sensate*, www.sensatejournal.com, accessed November 21, 2012.
Henry, A., 2005, "*Quid ais Omnium?* Maurice Kyffin's 1588 Andria and the emergence of suspension marks in printed drama," *Renaissance Drama*, 34, 47–67.
Henry, J., 1989, "The matter of souls: medical theory and theology in seventeenth-century England," in R. French and A. Wear (eds), *The Medical Revolution of the Seventeenth Century*, Cambridge: Cambridge University Press.
Herrick, R., 1648, *Hesperides, or the Works Both Humane and Divine of Robert Herrick, Esq*, London.
Hess, V. and Mendelsohn, J. A., 2010, "Case and series: medical knowledge and paper technology, 1600–1900," *History of Science*, 48, 287–314.
Higman, F. M., 1990, "Le domain français, 1520–1562," in J. F. Gilmont (ed.), *La Réforme et le livre: l'Europe de l'imprimé (1517– v. 1570)*, Paris: Ed. du Cerf.
Hippocrates, 1923, *Hippocrates*, trans. W. H. S. Jones, 8 vols, Cambridge, MA: Harvard University Press.
Hippocrates, 1950, *Medical Works*, trans. J. C. Chadwick and W. N. Mann, Oxford: Blackwell.
Hobbes, T., 1994, *Leviathan*, ed. E. Curley, with selected Latin variants, Indianapolis, IN: Hackett.
Hogarde, M., 1556, *The Displaying of the Protestantes*, London: Robert Caly.
Holland, P., 1633, *Gutta Podagrica: a treatise of the gout*, London.
Holub, R. C. (ed.), 1989, *Reception Theory: a critical introduction*, London: Routledge.
Holub, R. C., 1992, *Crossing Borders: reception theory, Poststructuralism, Deconstruction*, Madison, WI: University of Wisconsin Press.
Honig, E., 1998, *Painting and the Market in Early Modern Antwerp*, New Haven, CT: Yale University Press.
Hooke, R., 1705, *A General Scheme, or Idea of the Present State of Natural Philosophy* . . ., in *Posthumous Works*, ed. R. Waller, London: Smith & Walford.
Howard, D. and Moretti, L., 2010, *Sound and Space in Renaissance Venice*, New Haven, CT: Yale University Press.
Howes, D., 2003, *Sensual Relations: engaging the senses in culture and social theory*, Ann Arbor, MI: The University of Michigan Press.

Howes, D., 2005a, "Introduction: empires of the senses," in D. Howes (ed.), *Empire of the Senses: the sensual culture reader*, Oxford: Berg.
Howes, D., 2005b, "Hyperesthesia, or, the sensual logic of late capitalism," in D. Howes (ed.), *Empire of the Senses: the sensual culture reader*, Oxford: Berg.
Howes, D., 2006, "Scent, sound and synesthesia: intersensoriality and material culture theory," in C. Tilley, W. Keane, S. Küchler, M. Rowlands, and P. Spyer (eds), *Handbook of Material Culture*, London: Sage.
Howes, D., 2009, "Introduction: the revolving sensorium," in D. Howes (ed.), *The Sixth Sense Reader*, Oxford and New York: Berg.
Howes, D., 2011, "Hearing scents, tasting sights: toward a cross-cultural multimodal theory of aesthetics," in F. Bacci and D. Melcher (eds), *Art and the Senses*, Oxford: Oxford University Press.
Howes, D., 2013, "The expanding field of sensory studies," www.sensorystudies.org/sensorial-investigations/the-expanding-field-of-sensory-studies, accessed September 5, 2013.
Hsy, J., 2012, "Synaesthesia is not a metaphor," paper presented at the BABEL Working Group Annual Meeting, Northeastern University, Boston, 2012.
Huarte, J., [1575] 1594, *Examen de Ingenios*.
Huarte, J., [1575] 1959, *Examen de Ingenios: the examination of mens wits (1594)*, trans. T. Carew, Gainsville, FL: Scholars' Facsimile.
Hufendiek, R., 2012, "Draw a distinction: Die vielfältigen Funktionen des Zeichnens als Formen des 'extended mind'," in U. Feist and M. Rath (eds), *Et in Imagine Ego: Facetten von Bildakt und Verkörperung*, Berlin: Akademie Verlag.
Huizinga, J., [1919] 1996, *The Autumn of the Middle Ages*, English trans., Chicago: University of Chicago Press.
Hunt, A., 2008, *The Drama of Coronation: medieval ceremony in early modern England*, Cambridge: Cambridge University Press.
Hunt, A., 2010, *The Art of Hearing: English preachers and their audiences, 1590–1640*, Aldershot: Ashgate.
Hypnerotomachia Poliphili, ubi humana omnia non nisi somnium esse docet, 1499, Venice: Aldus Manutius.
Iconoclasme: Vie et mort de l'image médiévale, 2001, exhibition catalogue, Paris: Somogy.
Immagini del Sentire. I Cinque Sensi nell'Arte, 1996, exhibition catalogue, Milan: Leonardo Arte.
Infelise, M., 1999, *I libri proibiti da Gutenberg all'Encyclopédie*, Rome and Bari: Laterza.
Infelise, M., 2002, *Prima dei giornali. Alle origini della pubblica informazione. Secoli XVI–XVII*, Rome and Bari: Laterza.
Irmscher, G., 1986, "Ministrae voluptatum: stoicizing ethics in the market and kitchen scenes of Pieter Aertsen and Joachim Beuckelaer," *Simiolus: Netherlands Quarterly for the History of Art*, 16(4), 219–32.
Iser, W., 1974, *The Implied Reader: patterns of communication in prose fiction from Bunyan to Beckett*, Baltimore, MD: Johns Hopkins University Press.
Iser, W., 1978, *The Act of Reading: a theory of aesthetic response*, London: Routledge & Kegan Paul.

Iunius, S. [Hubert Languet? Philippe de Mornay?], 1599, *Vindiciae Contra Tyrannos*.
Jay, M., 2011, "In the realm of the senses," *American Historical Review*, 116, 307–15.
Jeanneret, M., 1991, *A Feast of Words: banquets and table talk in the Renaissance*, Chicago: University of Chicago Press.
Jenner, M., 1995, "The politics of London air," *Historical Journal*, 38, 535–51.
Jenner, M., 2000, "Civilization and deodorization? Smell in Early Modern English culture," in P. Burke, B. Harrison, and P. Slack (eds), *Civil Histories: essays presented to Sir Keith Thomas*, Oxford: Oxford University Press.
Jenner, M. S. R., 2011, "Follow your nose? Smell, smelling, and their histories," *American Historical Review*, 116, 335–51.
Johnson, G., 2011, "The art of touch in early modern Italy," in F. Bacci and D. Melcher (eds), *Art and the Senses*, Oxford: Oxford University Press.
Johnson, J. H., 1995, *Listening in Paris: a cultural history*, Berkeley, CA and Los Angeles: California University Press.
Johnston, T., 2000, "The Reformation and popular culture," in A. Pettegree (ed.), *The Reformation World*, London: Routledge.
Jonas, H., 1966, "The nobility of sight: a study in the phenomenology of the senses," in H. Jonas, *The Phenomenon of Life: towards a philosophical biology*, New York: Harper & Row.
Jonson, B., [1609] 1979, *Epicoene, or the Silent Woman*, ed. R. V. Holdsworth, London: Black.
Jonson, B., [1609] 2002, *The Key Keeper: a masque for the opening of Britain's Burse, April 19, 1609*, ed. J. Knowles, Tunbridge Wells: The Foundling Press.
Jurkowlaniec, G., 2009, "Faith, paragone, and commemoration in Dürer's 'Christomorphic' self-portrait of 1500," in O. Zorzi Pugliese and E. M. Kavaler (eds), *Faith and Fantasy in the Renaissance: texts, images, and religious practices*, Toronto: University of Toronto Press.
Jütte, R., 2004, *A History of the Senses: from antiquity to cyberspace*, trans. J. Lynn, Cambridge: Polity.
Kambaskovic-Sawers, D., 2012, "Two faces of love: terror and devotion in medieval and Renaissance Europe," in S. Scollay (ed.), *Love and Devotion*, Oxford: Bodleian Library.
Kant, I., 1978, *Immanuel Kants Menschenkunde*, Hildesheim: Georg Olms.
Karant-Nunn, S., 2007, "Ritual in early modern Christianity," in R. Po-Chia Hsia (ed.), *The Cambridge History of Christianity: reform and expansion 1500–1660*, Cambridge: Cambridge University Press.
Karant-Nunn, S., 2010, *The Reformation of Feeling: shaping the religious emotions in early modern Germany*, Oxford: Oxford University Press.
Katritzky, M. A., 2001, "Marketing medicine: the image of the early modern mountebank," *Renaissance Studies*, 15, 121–53.
Kavanaugh, K., 1999, *John of the Cross: doctor of light and love*, New York: Crossroad.
Kemp, C., 2012, *Floating Gold: a natural (and unnatural) history of ambergris*, Chicago: University of Chicago Press.

Kemp, M., 1974, "Disegno. Beiträge zu einer Geschichte des Begriffs zwischen 1547 und 1607," *Marburger Jahrbuch für Kunstwissenschaft*, 19, 219–40.

Kendall, T., 1577, *Flowers of Epigrammes*, London: Ihon Shepperd.

Kendrick, R. L., 2002, *The Sounds of Milan, 1585–1650*, Oxford: Oxford University Press.

Kent, F. W. (ed.), 2000, *Street Noises, Civic Spaces and Urban Identities in Italian Renaissance Cities*, Clayton, Vic.: Dept. of History, Monash University.

Kepler, J., [1604] 1968, *Ad Vitellionem paralipomena, quibus astronomiae pars optica traditur*, reprint, Brussels: Culture et Civilisation.

Kepler, J., 1610, *Dissertatio cum nuncio sidereo nuper ad mortales misso Galilaeo Galilaeo*, Florence: J. Caneum.

Kermol, E., 1990, *La rete di Vulcano. Inquisizione, libri proibiti e libertini nel Friuli del Seicento*, Trieste: Università degli Studi di Trieste.

Kessler, E. and Park, K., 1988, "The concept of psychology," in E. Kessler, C. B. Schmitt, and Q. Skinner (eds), *The Cambridge History of Renaissance Philosophy*, Cambridge: Cambridge University Press.

Kieckhefer, R., 1997, *Forbidden Rites: a necromancer's manual in the fifteenth century*, University Park, PA: Penn State University Press.

Kimmel, S., 2012, "Writing religion: sacromonte and the literary conventions of orthodoxy," in A. Cascardi and L. Middlebrook (eds), *Poesis and Modernity in the Old and New Worlds*, Nashville, TN: Vanderbilt University Press.

King, R., 2012, "'The beads with which we pray are made from it': devotional ambers in early modern Italy," in W. de Boer and C. Göttler (eds), *Religion and the Senses in Early Modern Europe*, Leiden and Boston, MA: Brill.

Kinney, A. F., 2006, "Literary humanism in the Renaissance," in A. Mazzocco (ed.), *Interpretations of Renaissance Humanism*, Leiden: E. J. Brill.

Kirk, G. S., Raven, J. E., and Schofield, M. (eds), 1983, *The Presocratic Philosophers*, Cambridge: Cambridge University Press.

Klaniczay, G. and Kristof, I., 2001, "Écritures saintes et pactes diaboliques. Les usages religieux de l'écrit (Moyen Âge et Temps modernes)," *Annales*, 56, 947–80.

Klestinec, C., 2011, *Theaters of Anatomy: students, teachers, and traditions of dissection in Renaissance Venice*, Baltimore, MD: Johns Hopkins University Press.

Klötzer, R., 2007, "The Melchorites and Munster," in J. D. Roth and J. M. Stayer (eds), *A Companion to Anabaptism and Spiritualism, 1521–1700*, Leiden: E. J. Brill.

Knox, D., 1995, "Erasmus' *De Civilitate* and the religious origins of civility in Protestant Europe," *Archiv für Reformationsgeschichte*, 86, 21–42.

Knox, D., 2007, "Gesture and comportment: diversity and uniformity," in H. Roodenburg (ed.), *Forging European Identities, 1400–1700*, Cambridge: Cambridge University Press.

Korda, N., 2008, "Gender at work in the Cries of London," in M. E. Lamb and K. Bamford (eds), *Oral Traditions and Gender in Early Modern Literary Texts*, Aldershot: Ashgate.

Korhonen, A., 2008, "To see and be seen: beauty in the Early Modern London street," *Journal of Early Modern History*, 12, 335–60.

Korrick, L., 2003, "Lomazzo's Trattato della Pittura and Galilei's *Frononimo: picturing music and sounding images in 1584*," in K. McIver (ed.), *Art and Music in the Early Modern Period: essays in honour of Franca Trinchieri Camiz*, Aldershot: Ashgate.

Koslofsky, C., 2011, *Evening's Empire: a history of the night in Early Modern Europe*, Cambridge: Cambridge University Press.

Krampl, U. and Beck, R., 2013, "Introduction," in U. Krampl and R. Beck (eds), *Les cinq sens de la ville du Moyen Âge à nos jours*, Tours: Presses Universitaires François-Rabelais.

Kraye, J., 1988, "Moral philosophy," in E. Kessler, C. B. Schmitt, and Q. Skinner (eds), *The Cambridge History of Renaissance Philosophy*, Cambridge: Cambridge University Press.

Kritzman, L. D., 1991, *Rhetoric of Sexuality and the Literature of the French Renaissance*, New York: Columbia University Press.

Kuchta, D., 1993, "The semiotics of masculinity in Renaissance England," in J. Grantham-Turner (ed.), *Sexuality and Gender in Early Modern Europe*, Cambridge: Cambridge University Press.

Kyd, T., 1987, *The Spanish Tragedy*, ed. J. R. Mulryne, London: A. C. Black Publishers.

Lacey, S., Stilla, R., and Sathian, K., 2012, "Metaphorically feeling: comprehending textural metaphors activates somatosensory cortex," *Brain and Language*, 120(3), 416–21.

Lakoff, G. and Johnson, M., 1980, *Metaphors We Live By*, Chicago: University of Chicago Press.

Langdale, A., 1999, "Aspects of the critical reception and intellectual history of Baxandall's concept of the period eye," in A. Rifkin (ed.), *About Michael Baxandall*, Oxford: Blackwell.

Langenmantel, W. and Langenmantel, J., 1594, *De Sensibus Externis et Internis*, Ingolstadt.

Lanteri, G., 1560, *Della Economica Trattato*, Venice: Vincenzo Valgrisi.

Larivaille, P., 1997, *Pietro Aretino*, Rome: Salerno.

Le Guérer, A., 1990a, "Le déclin de l'olfactif, mythe ou réalité?" *Anthropologie et Sociétés*, 14, 115–21.

Le Guérer, A, 1990b, *The Mysterious and Essential Powers of Smell*, London: Random House.

Le Ru, V., 2000, "La *Lettre sur les aveugles* et le bâton de la raison," *Recherches sur Diderot et l'Encyclopédie*, 28, 25–41.

Lemnius, L., [1561] 1633, *The Touchstone of Complexions*, trans. T. N. London: Elizabeth Allde.

Levi, A., 2002, *Renaissance and Reformation: intellectual genesis*, New Haven, CT: Yale University Press.

Levi, G., 1988, *Inheriting Power: the story of an exorcist*, Chicago: University of Chicago Press.

Levy Peck, L., 2005, *Consuming Splendour: society and culture in seventeenth-century England*, Cambridge: Cambridge University Press.

Lindberg, D. C., 1976, *Theories of Vision from Al-Kindi to Kepler*, Chicago: University of Chicago Press.

Lindner, I., Echterhoff, G., Davidson, P. S. R., and Brand, M., 2010, "Observation inflation: your actions become mine," *Psychological Science*, 21, 129–9.

Ling, N., 1598, *Politeuphuia wits common wealth*, London: I. Roberts.

Lloyd, D., 1668, *Memoires of the Lives, Actions, Suffering, and Deaths of Those Noble Revrend and Excellent Personages*, London, printed for Samuel Speed.

Locke, J., 1707, *An Essay for the Understanding of St. Paul's Epistles, by consulting St. Paul Himself*, London: Awnsham and John Churchill.

Locke, J., 1975, *An Essay Concerning Human Understanding*, ed. P. Nidditch, Oxford: Oxford University Press.

Long, A. A., 1986, *Hellenistic Philosophy: Stoics, Epicureans, Sceptics*, Berkeley, CA: University of California Press.

Loredan, G. F., 1693, *Lettere*, I, Venice: Tivani.

Lough, J., 1985, *France Observed in the Seventeenth Century by British Travellers*, Stocksfield: Oriel Press.

Loughlin, M., Bell, S., and Brace, P. (eds), 2012, *The Broadview Anthology of Sixteenth-century Poetry and Prose*, Peterborough, ON: Broadview Press.

Loyola, I., [1542] 1923, *The Spiritual Exercises of St. Ignatius Loyola: Spanish and English with a Continuous Commentary by Joseph Rickaby, S. J.*, London: Burns, Oates & Washbourne.

Loyola, I., 1914, *The Spiritual Exercises*, Baltimore, MD: Lucas Brothers.

Luther, M., [1522] 1908–10, *D. Martin Luthers Werke*, Vol. 10, Weimar: Herman Böhlaus Nachfolger.

Luther, M., 1974. *Luther's Works*, ed. H. C. Oswald, St. Louis, MO: Concordia.

MacCulloch, D., 2010, *A History of Christianity: the first three thousand years*, New York: Penguin.

Maclean, I., 2002, *Logic, Signs, and Nature in the Renaissance: the case of learned medicine*, Cambridge: Cambridge University Press.

Maclean, I., 2008, "The medical Republic of Letters before the Thirty Years War," *Intellectual History Review*, 18, 15–30.

Mader, E. O., 2012, "Conversion concepts in early modern Germany: Protestant and Catholic," in D. M. Luebke et al. (eds), *Conversion and the Politics of Religion in Early Modern Germany*, New York: Bergman.

Maier, P. L., 1980, "Fanaticism as a theological category in the Lutheran confessions," *Concordia Theological Quarterly*, 44(2–3), 173–81.

Majeska, G. P., 1984, *Russian Travelers to Constantinople in the Fourteenth and Fifteenth Centuries*, Washington DC: Dumbarton Oaks Library.

Mandressi, R., 2003, *Le regard de l'anatomiste: dissections et invention du corps en Occident*, Paris: Seuil.

Marot, C., 2006, "Du Beau Tetin," and "Du Laid Tetin," in *Lyrics of the French Renaissance: Marot, Du Bellay, Ronsard*, ed. and trans. N. R. Shapiro, Chicago: University of Chicago Press.

Marprelate, M, 1580, *Oh Read over D. John*.

Marrow, J. H., 1979, *Passion Iconography in Northern European Art of the Late Middle Ages and Early Renaissance*, Kortrijk: Van Ghemmert.

Marshall, P., 1998, "Papist as heretic: the burning of John Forest, 1538," *The Historical Journal*, 41, 351–74.

Marshall, P., 2002, *Beliefs and the Dead in Reformation England*, Oxford: Oxford University Press.
Martin, A. L., 2010, *Alcohol, Sex, and Gender in Late Medieval and Early Modern Europe*, Basingstoke: Palgrave.
Marx, K., 1977, *Selected Writings*, ed. D. McLellan, Oxford: Oxford University Press.
Masten, J., 2004, "Toward a queer address: the taste of letters and early modern male friendship," *GLQ: A Journal of Lesbian and Gay Studies*, 10(3), 367–84.
Mayer, R., 1982, *Pontormo's Diary*, New York: Out of London Press.
Mayers, K., 2012, *Visions of Empire in Colonial Spanish American Ekphrastic Writing*, Lanham, PA: Bucknell University Press.
McCabe, I., 2008, *Orientalism in Early Modern France: Eurasian trade, exoticism and the ancien regime*, Oxford: Berg.
McGinn, B., 2011, "Late medieval mystics," in S. Coakley and P. Gavrilyuk (eds), *The Spiritual Senses in Christian Tradition*, Cambridge: Cambridge University Press.
McGrath, A. E., 2005, *Iustitia Dei: a history of the Christian doctrine of justification*, Cambridge: Cambridge University Press.
McIlvenna, U., 2010, "Considering the 'Cabal of Cuckoldry': Scandal and Reputation at the Court of Catherine de Medici", unpublished PhD, Queen Mary University of London.
McKenzie, D. F., 1985, *Oral Culture, Literacy and Print in Early New Zealand: the Treaty of Waitangi*, Wellington: Victoria University Press.
McKenzie, D. F., 1999, *Bibliography and the Sociology of Texts*, Cambridge: Cambridge University Press.
McKenzie, D. F., 2002, *Making Meaning: "Printers of the Mind" and other essays*, ed. P. D. McDonald and M. F. Suarez, Amherst, MA: University of Massachusetts Press.
McKitterick, D., 2005, *Print, Manuscript and the Search for Order, 1450–1830*, Cambridge: Cambridge University Press.
McLaughlin, R. E., 2007, "Spiritualism: Schwenkfeld and Franck and their early modern resonances," in J. D. Roth and J. M. Stayer (eds), *A Companion to Anabaptism and Spiritualism, 1521–1700*, Leiden: E. J. Brill.
McLuhan, M., 1962, *The Gutenberg Galaxy*, Toronto: Toronto University Press.
McTighe, S., 2004, "Foods and the body in Italian genre paintings, about 1580: Campi, Passarotti, Carracci," *Art Bulletin*, 86(2), 301–23.
McVaugh, M. R., 1997, "Bedside manners in the Middle Ages," *Bulletin of the History of Medicine*, 71, 209–23.
Meditations on the Life of Christ: An Illustrated Manuscript of the Fourteenth Century, 1961, ed. and trans. I. Ragusa and R. B. Green, Princeton, NJ: Princeton University Press.
Melanchthon, P., 1988, *De anima* [1553], in *A Melanchthon Reader*, trans. R. Keen, New York: Peter Lang.
Melion, W. S., 2009, " 'Quae lecta Canisius offert et spectata diu': the pictorial images in Petrus Canisius's De Maria Virgine of 1577/1583," in W. S. Melion and L. Palmer Wandel (eds), *Early Modern Eyes*, Leiden: E. J. Brill.
Menius, J., 1554, *Oeconomia Christiana*.

Merback, M., 1999, *The Thief, the Cross, and the Wheel: pain and the spectacle of punishment in medieval and Renaissance Europe*, Chicago: University of Chicago Press.
Meres, F., 1598, *Granados deuotion*, London: E. Allde for Cuthbert Burby.
Mersenne, M., 1636, *L'Harmonie Universelle, contenant la théorie et la pratique de la musique*, 3 vols, Paris: Sebastien Cramoisy.
Metcalf, A. C., 2007, "Christianity in sixteenth-century Brazil," in J. Jeffries Martin (ed.), *The Renaissance World*. London: Routledge.
Meyer, B. and Verrips, J., 2008, "Aesthetics," in D. Morgan (ed.), *Key Words in Religion, Media and Culture*, New York and London: Routledge.
Michael, E., 2000, "Renaissance theories of body, soul, and mind," in J. P. Wright and P. Potter (eds), *Psyche and Soma: physicians and metaphysicians on the mind-body problem from antiquity to Enlightenment*, Oxford: Clarendon Press.
Michalski, S., 1993, *The Reformation and the Visual Arts: the Protestant image question in Western and Eastern Europe*, London and New York: Routledge.
Milner, M., 2011, *The Senses and the English Reformation*, Aldershot: Ashgate.
Milton, J., 1991, *John Milton: Critical Edition of the Major Works*, ed. S. Orgel and J. Goldberg, Oxford: Oxford University Press.
Mintz, S., 1986, *Sweetness and Power: the place of sugar in modern history*, London: Penguin.
Missfelder, J-F., 2012, "Period ear. Perspektiven einer Klanggeschichte der Neuzeit," *Geschichte und Gesellschaft*, 38: 21–47.
Mitchell, W., 1995, *Picture Theory: essays on verbal and visual representation*, Chicago: University of Chicago Press.
Mochizuki, M. M., 2008, *The Netherlandish Image after Iconoclasm, 1566–1672: material religion in the Dutch Golden Age*, Aldershot: Ashgate.
Mola, L., 2013, *Inventori e brevetti nell'Italia del Rinascimento*, Rome: Viella Editore.
Montagu, A., 1986, *Touching: the human significance of the skin*, New York: Harper Collins.
Montaigne, M. de, [1580–8] 1962, *Essais*, ed. M. Rat, Paris: Gallimard.
Montaigne, M. de, 1957, *Complete Works: essays, travel journal, letters*, ed. and trans. D. M. Frame, Stanford, CA: Stanford University Press.
Montaigne, M. de, 1958, *The Complete Essays of Michel de Montaigne*, trans. D. M. Frame, Stanford, CA: Stanford University Press.
Montaigne, M. de, n.d., *Les Essais*, The Montaigne Project, http://www.lib.uchicago.edu/efts/ARTFL/projects/montaigne/, accessed February 10, 2012.
More, T., [1523] 1969, *Responsio ad Lutherum*, ed. J. M. Headley, New Haven, CT: Yale University Press.
Mortoft, F., [1658] 1925, *His Book, Being his Travels through France and Italy, 1658–1659*, ed. M. Letts, London: Hakluyt Society.
Moryson, F., [1617] 1907, *An Itinerary*, 4 vols, Glasgow: MacLehose.
Most, G. W., 2005, *Doubting Thomas*, Cambridge, MA.: Harvard University Press.
Moulton, I. F., 2010, "In praise of touch: Mario Equicola and the nature of love," *The Senses and Society*, 5(1), 119–30.

Moureau, F. (ed.), 1993, *De bonne main. La communication manuscrite au XVIIIe siècle*, Paris and Oxford: Universitas—Voltaire Foundation.
Muir, E., 1989, "The Virgin on the streetcorner: the place of the sacred in Italian cities," in S. E. Ozment (ed.), *Religion and Culture in the Renaissance and Reformation*, Kirksville, MO: Truman State University Press.
Mundy, P., 1907–19, *Travels*, ed. R. C. Temple, 3 vols, London: Hakluyt Society.
Navarrete, I., 1994, *Orphans of Petrarch: poetry and theory in the Spanish Renaissance*, Berkeley, CA: University of California Press.
Neill, M., 1997, *Issues of Death: mortality and identity in English Renaissance tragedy*, New York: Oxford University Press.
Nelson, W., 1977, "From 'Listen, Lordings' to 'Dear Reader'," *University of Toronto Quarterly*, 46(2), 110–24.
Nemesius, 1636, *The Nature of Man*, trans. G. Wither, London.
Nemesius, 1975, *De natura hominis*, trans. B. de Pise, ed. and comm. G. Verbeke and J. R. Moncho, Leiden: Brill.
Nervèze, de, A., 1610, *Le jardin sacre de l'âme solitaire*, Lyon.
Newhauser, R., 2010, "Foreword: the senses in medieval and Renaissance intellectual history," *The Senses and Society*, 5(1), 5–9.
Newman, K., 2007, *Cultural Capitals: early modern London and Paris*, Princeton, NJ: Princeton University Press.
Niccoli, O., 2011, *Vedere con gli occhi del cuore. Alle origini del potere delle immagini*, Rome and Bari: Laterza.
Nichols, S., 2008, "Prologue," in S. Nichols, A. Kablitz, and A. Calhoun (eds), *Rethinking the Medieval Senses: heritage, fascinations, frames*, Baltimore, MD: Johns Hopkins University Press.
Nicholson, S., 1600, *Acolastus his after-witte*, London: imprinted by Felix Kingston for John Baylie.
Nordenfalk, C., 1976, "Les cinq sens dans l'art du Moyen Age," *La Revue de l'Art*, 34, 17–28.
Nordenfalk, C., 1985, "The five senses in Flemish art before 1600," in G. Cavalli-Bjorkman (ed.), *Netherlandish Mannerism: papers given at a symposium in the Nationalmuseum Stockholm*, Stockholm: Nationalmuseum.
Norton, M., 2010, *Sacred Gifts, Profane Pleasures: chocolate and tobacco in the Atlantic world*, Ithaca, MY: Cornell University Press.
Nourse, T., 1686, *A Discourse upon the Nature and Faculties of Man*, London.
Novalis, [1798] 1987, *Vorarbeiten*, in H.-J. Mähl and R. Samuel (eds), *Werke, Tagebücher und Briefe*, 3 vols, Vol. 2, *Das philosophisch-theoretische Werk*, Munich: Carl Hanser Verlag.
Nutton, V., 1993, "Galen at the bedside," in W. F. Bynum and R. Porter (eds), *Medicine and the Five Senses*, Cambridge: Cambridge University Press.
O'Shaughnessy, B., 2000, *Consciousness and the World*, Oxford: Oxford University Press.
Ong, W. J., 1982, *Orality and Literacy: the technologizing of the word*, London: Routledge.
Ong, W. J., 2005, *The Presence of the Word*, New Haven, CT and London: Yale University Press.

Onians, J., 2008, *Neuroarthistory: from Aristotle and Pliny to Baxandall and Zeki*, New Haven, CT: Yale University Press.

Orgel, S., 1996, *Impersonations: the performance of gender in Shakespeare's England*, Cambridge: Cambridge University Press.

Ottaviani, D., n.d., *La Métaphysique de la lumière au moyen âge*, http://cerphi.net/archives/cerphi%202002-2007/hum/lumcours.htm.

Ozment, S. E., 1983, *When Fathers Ruled: family life in Reformation Europe*, Cambridge, MA: Harvard University Press.

Ozment, S. E., 1996, "The private life of an early modern teenager: a Nuremberg Lutheran visits Catholic Louvain (1577)," *Journal of Family History*, 21, 22–43.

Pallasmaa, J., 2005, *The Eyes of the Skin: architecture and the senses*, Chichester: Wiley-Academy.

Pallasmaa, J., 2009, *The Thinking Hand: existential and embodied wisdom in architecture*, Chichester: Wiley.

Palma, P., 2004, "Of courtesans, knights, cooks and writers: food in the Renaissance," *MLN*, 119, 37–51.

Palmer, R., 1993, "In bad odour," in W. F. Bynum and R. Porter (eds), *Medicine and the Five Senses*, Cambridge: Cambridge University Press.

Panofsky, E., 1969, *Problems in Titian, Mostly Iconographic*, New York: New York University Press.

Park, K., 1988. "The organic soul," in C. B. Schmitt *et al.* (eds), *The Cambridge History of Renaissance Philosophy*, Cambridge: Cambridge University Press.

Parker, C. H., 1998, *The Reformation of Community: social welfare and Calvinist charity in Holland, 1572–1620*, Cambridge: Cambridge University Press.

Parkes, M. B., 1993, *Pause and Effect: an introduction to the history of punctuation in the West*, Berkleley, CA and Los Angeles: University of California Press.

Paster, G. K., 2004, *Humoring the Body: emotions and the Shakespearean stage*, Chicago: Chicago University Press.

Pastor, L. F. von, 1977, *The History of the Popes from the Close of the Middle Ages*, Vol. 8, S. l.: Consortium Books.

Peacham, H., 1593, *The Garden of Eloquence, conteining the most excellent . . . Figures of Rhetorike*, London: H. Jackson.

Pender, S., 2002, "Essaying the body: Donne, affliction, and medicine," in D. Colclough (ed.), *John Donne's Professional Lives*, Cambridge: Brewer.

Pender, S., 2006, "Examples and experience: the uncertainty of medicine," *British Journal for the History of Science*, 39, 1–28.

Pender, S., 2010, "Subventing disease: anger, passions, and the non-naturals," in J. Vaught (ed.), *Rhetorics of Bodily Disease and Health in Medieval and Early Modern England*, Aldershot: Ashgate.

Pepys, S., 1970–83, *Diary*, ed. R. Latham and W. Matthews, 11 vols, London: Bell.

Perkins, W., 1600, *A Golden Chaine: or The description of theologie containing the order of the causes of saluation and damnation, according to Gods word*, London.

Persels, J. C., 2002, "Masculine rethoric and the French *Blason Anatomique*," in K. P. Long (ed.), *High Anxiety: masculinity in crisis in early modern France*, Kirksville, MO: Truman State University Press.

Persels, J., 1999, "Cooking with the Pope: The language of food and protest in Calvinist and Catholic polemic from the 1560s," *Mediaevalia*, 22, 29–53.
Petrarch, 1999, *Il Canzoniere*, or *Rerum vulgarium fragmenta*, ed. and trans. Mark Musa, Bloomington, IN: Indiana University Press.
Pettegree, A., 2000, "Books, pamphlets, and polemic," in A. Pettegree (ed.), *The Reformation World*, London: Routledge.
Pettegree, A., 2005, *Reformation and the Culture of Persuasion*, Cambridge: Cambridge University Press.
Pettenella, A., 2002, *Storie Euganee*, Verona: Cierre Edizioni.
Pittion, J.-P., 1987, "Scepticism and medicine in the Renaissance," in R. H. Popkin and C. B. Schmitt (eds), *Scepticism from the Renaissance to the Enlightenment*, Wiesbaden: Otto Harrasowitz.
Platina, 1998, *Platina, on right pleasure and good health: a critical edition and translation of De Honesta Voluptate et Valetudine*, ed. and trans. M. E. Milham, Tempe, AZ: Medieval & Renaissance Texts & Studies.
Platt, H., 1609, *Delightes for Ladies*, London: Humfrey Lownes.
Platt, P., 2009, *Shakespeare and the Culture of Paradox*, Farnham: Ashgate.
Platter, T., 1968, *Beschreibung der Reisen durch Frankreich, Spanien, England und die Niederlande 1595–1600*, ed. R. Keiser, Basel: Schwab.
Po-Chia Hsia, R., 1992, *Social Discipline in the Reformation: Central Europe 1550–1750*, London: Taylor & Francis.
Po-Chia Hsia, R. (ed.), 2007, *The Cambridge History of Christianity: reform and expansion 1500–1660*, Cambridge: Cambridge University Press.
Polanco, J., 1554, *Breve Directorium ad Confessarii*, Louvain.
Polska, A. M., 2008, "A married man is a woman," in S. H. Hendrix and S. S. Karant-Nunn (eds), *Masculinity in the Reformation Era*, Kirksville, MO: Truman State University Press.
Pomata, G. and Siraisi, N. G. (eds), 2005, *Historia: Empiricism and Erudition in Early Modern Europe*, Cambridge, MA: MIT Press.
Porter, R., 1993, "The rise of physical examination," in W. F. Bynum and R. Porter (eds), *Medicine and the Five Senses*, Cambridge: Cambridge University Press.
Porter, R., 2005, "A touch of danger: the bedside manners of the eighteenth-century physician." in C. Classen (ed.), *The Book of Touch*, Oxford: Berg.
Pouchelle, Marie-C., 1990, *The Body and Surgery in the Middle Ages*, trans. R. Morris, Cambridge: Polity.
Preyer, B., 2006, "The Florentine Casa," in M. Ajmar-Wollheim and F. Dennis (eds), *At Home in Renaissance Italy*, London: V&A Publications.
Principe, L. M., 2011, "Alchemy Restored," *Isis*, 102(2), 305–12.
Puente, de la, L., 1609, *Meditaciones de los mysterios de nuestra santa fe*, Barcelona: Lucas Sánchez.
Pugliese, O. Z. and Kavaler, E. M. (eds), 2009, *Faith and Fantasy in the Renaissance: texts, images, and religious practices*, Toronto: University of Toronto Press.
Quiviger, F., 2010, *The Sensory World of Italian Renaissance Art*, London: Reaktion Books.

Rabelais, F., 2006, *Gargantua and Pantagruel*, trans. M. A. Screech, London and New York: Penguin Books.

Ragland, E., 2012, "Chymistry and taste in the seventeenth century: Franciscus de le Boë Sylvius as a chymical physician between Galenism and Cartesianism," *Ambix*, 59, 1–21.

Rancière, J., 2004, *The Politics of Aesthetics: the distribution of the sensible*, London: Continuum.

Rather, L. J., 1965, *Mind and Body in Eighteenth-Century Medicine: a study based on Jerome Gaub's "De regimen mentis"*, Berkeley, CA: University of California Press.

Raymond, J., 2003, "Irrational, impractical and unprofitable: reading the news in seventeenth-century Britain," in K. Sharpe and S. N. Zwicker (eds), *Reading, Society and the Politics in Early Modern England*, Cambridge: Cambridge University Press.

Reiss, T. J., 1996, "Denying the body? Memory and the dilemma's of history in Descartes," *Journal of the History of Ideas*, 57, 587–607.

Reiss, T. J., 1997, *Knowledge, Discovery and Imagination in Early Modern Europe: the rise of aesthetic rationalism*, Cambridge: Cambridge University Press.

Rendall, S., 1996, "Reading in the French Renaissance: textual communities, boredom, privacy," in J. Hart (ed.), *Reading the Renaissance: Culture, Poetics, and Drama*, New York: Garland.

Revel, J., 1989, "The uses of civility," in R. Chartier (ed.), *A History of Private Life*, Vol. 3, Cambridge, MA: Harvard University Press.

Rey, R., 1995, "Le Cat et la théorie de la vision," in M. T. Monti (ed.), *Teorie della Visione e problemi di percezione visiva nell'età moderna*, Milan: Angeli.

Reynolds, P. L., 2005, "Efficient causality and instrumentality in Thomas Aquinas's Theology of the Sacraments," in J. R. Ginther and C. N. Still (eds), *Essays in Medieval Philosophy and Theology in Memory of Walter H. Principe, CSB: fortresses and launching pads*, Burlington, VT: Ashgate.

Ricci, M., 1953, *China in the Sixteenth Century: the journals of Matteo Ricci 1583–1610*, trans. L. J. Gallagher, New York: Random House.

Richardson, B., 2009, *Manuscript Culture in Renaissance Italy*, Cambridge: Cambridge University Press.

Richardson, C., 2011, *Shakespeare and Material Culture*, Oxford: Oxford University Press.

Riegl, A., [1901] 1985, *Late Roman Art Industry*, trans. R. Winkes, Rome: Giorgio Bretschneider.

Riskin, J., 2011, "The divine optician," *American Historical Review*, 116, 352–70.

Risse, G. B., 1987–8, "Clinical instruction in hospitals: the Boerhaavian tradition in Leyden, Edinburgh, Vienna, and Pavia," in H. Beukers and J. Moll (eds), *Clinical Teaching, Past and Present*, special issue of *Clio Medica*, 21.

Roberts, L., 1638, *The Marchant's Mapp of Commerce*, London.

Roberts, L., 1995, "The death of the sensuous chemist: the 'new' chemistry and the transformation of sensuous technology," *Studies in History and Philosophy of Science*, 26, 503–29.

Roberts, L., Schaffer, S., and Dear, P. (eds), 2007, *The Mindful Hand: inquiry and invention from the late Renaissance to the Industrial Revolution*, Amsterdam: Koninklijke Nederlandse Academie van Wetenschappen.

Robins, P. and Ayede, M. (eds), 2009, *The Cambridge Handbook of Situated Cognition*, Cambridge: Cambridge University Press.

Rodrigues, J., 2001, *Account of Sixteenth-Century Japan*, ed. M. Cooper, London: Hakluyt Society.

Roggero, M., 2007, *Le carte piene di sogni. Testi e lettori in Età moderna*, Bologna: il Mulino.

Romano, D., 1996, *Housecraft and Statecraft: domestic service in Renaissance Venice, 1400–1600*, Baltimore, MD: Johns Hopkins University Press.

Ronsard, P., 2002, *Selected Poems*, trans. M. Quainton and E. Vinestock, New York: Penguin Classics.

Roodenburg, H., 2004, *The Eloquence of the Body: studies on gesture in the Dutch Republic*, Zwolle: Waanders.

Roodenburg, H., 2011, "The visceral pleasures of looking: on iconology, anthropology and the neurosciences," in B. Baert, A-S. Lehmann, and J. van der Akkerveken (eds), *New Perspectives in Iconology: visual studies and anthropology*, Brussels: Academic and Scientific Publishers.

Roodenburg, H., 2012, "A New historical anthropology? A plea to take a fresh look at practice theory," http://hsozkult.geschichte.hu-berlin.de/forum/type=diskussionen &id=1826, accessed August 9, 2012.

Roper, L., 1991, *The Holy Household: women and morals in Reformation Augsburg*, Oxford: Clarendon Press.

Rose, J., 1992, "Rereading the English Common Reader. A preface to a history of audiences," *Journal of the History of Ideas*, 53, 47–70.

Rosenberg, C., 1982, "Courtly decorations and the decorum of interior space," in G. Papagno and A. Quondam (eds), *La Corte e lo Spazio, Ferrara Estense*, Rome: Bulzoni.

Rosenfeld, S., 2011a, *Common Sense: a political history*, Cambridge, MA and London: Harvard University Press.

Rosenfeld, S., 2011b, "On being heard: a case for paying attention to the historical ear," *American Historical Review*, 116, 316–34.

Rosenwein, B., 2002, "Worrying about emotions in history," *American Historical Review*, 107, 827–36.

Ross, A., 1651, *Arcana microcosmi, or, The hid secrets of man's body discovered; in an anatomical duel between Aristotle and Galen*, London: Newcomb.

Roth, J. D., 2007, "Marpeck and the later Swiss brethren, 1540–1700," in J. D. Roth and J. M. Stayer (eds), *A Companion to Anabaptism and Spiritualism, 1521–1700*, Leiden: E. J. Brill.

Rothkegel, M., 2007, "Anabaptism in Moravia and Silesia," in J. D. Roth and J. M. Stayer (eds), *A Companion to Anabaptism and Spiritualism, 1521–1700*, Leiden: E. J. Brill.

Rubin, M. and Simons, W. (eds), 2009, *The Cambridge History of Christianity: Christianity in Western Europe c. 1100–c.1500*, Cambridge: Cambridge University Press.

Rublack, U., 2010, *Dressing Up: cultural identity in Renaissance Europe*, Oxford: Oxford University Press.

Ruggiero, G., 1993, "Marriage, love, sex and Renaissance civic morality," in J. Grantham-Turner (ed.), *Sexuality and Gender in Early Modern Europe*, Cambridge: Cambridge University Press.

Rutherford, D., 2006, "Innovation and orthodoxy in early modern philosophy," in D. Rutherford (ed.), *The Cambridge Companion to Early Modern Philosophy*, Cambridge: Cambridge University Press, pp. 11–38.

Ryrie, A., 2003, *The Gospel and Henry VIII*, Cambridge: Cambridge University Press.

Ryu, S., 2011, "Textual folds: alphabet, pictogram, and the Christian idol in New Spain," paper presented to the Renaissance Society of America, Montreal.

Sacchetti, F., [c. 1390] 1996, *Il trecentonovelle*, ed. V. Marucci, Roma: Salerno.

Saenger, P., 1997, *Space Between Words: the origins of silent reading*, Stanford, CA: Stanford University Press.

Salkeld, D., 2012, *Shakespeare Among the Courtesans: prostitution, literature and drama: 1500–1650*, Farnham: Ashgate.

Salter, A., 2010, "Intimate converse with nature: body and touch in Harvey's way of inquiry," in P. Kelly and L. E. Semler (eds), *Word and Self Estranged in English Texts, 1550–1660*, Farnham: Ashgate.

Salter, A. and Wolfe, C. T., 2009, "Empiricism contra experiment: Harvey, Locke and the revisionist view of experimental philosophy," *Bulletin de la SHESVIE*, 16(1), 113–40.

Salzberg R. M., 2010, "In the mouth of charlatans: street performers and the dissemination of pamphlets in Renaissance Italy," *Renaissance Studies*, 24(5), 638–53.

San Juan, R. M., 2001, *Rome: a city out of print*, Minneapolis, MN: University of Minnesota Press.

Sandys, G., 1615, *A Relation of a Journey Begun an: Dom: 1610*, London: Barret.

Sanger, A. E. and Walker, S. T. K. (eds), 2012, *Sense and the Senses in Early Modern Art and Cultural Practice*, Farnham: Ashgate.

Sastrow, B., 1902, *Social Germany in Luther's Time*, English trans, London: Constable.

Sawday, J., 1995, *The Body Emblazoned: dissection and the human body in Renaissance culture*, New York: Routledge.

Scappi, B., 2008, *The Opera of Bartolomeo Scappi (1570): l'Arte et Prudenza d'un Maestro Cuoco*, trans. T. Scully, Toronto: University of Toronto Press.

Schama, S., 1988, *The Embarrassment of Riches: an interpretation of Dutch culture in the Golden Age*, Berkeley, CA: University of California Press.

Schama, S., 1999, "The city in five senses," in S. Schama, *Rembrandt's Eyes*, London: Allen Lane.

Scheer, M., 2012, "Are emotions a kind of practice (and what is that what makes them have a history)? A Bourdieuan approach to understanding emotion," *History and Theory*, 51, 193–220.

Schmidt, L. E., 2000, *Hearing Things: relgion, illusion and the American Enlightenment*, Cambridge, MA and London: Harvard University Press.

Schürmann, R., 2003, *Broken Hegemonies*, trans. R. Lilly, Bloomington, IN: Indiana University Press.
Schwartz, R. M., 2008, "Toward a sacramental poetics," in J. Jeffries Martin (ed.), *The Renaissance World*, London: Routledge.
Schwartz, S. B., 2004, *Sugar and the Making of the Atlantic World, 1450–1680*, Chapel Hill, NC: University of North Carolina Press.
Scot, R., 1584, *The Discoverie of Witchcraft*.
Scott, A., 2006, "Marketing luxury at the New Exchange: Johnson's entertainment at Britain's Burse and the rhetoric of wonder," *Early Modern Literary Studies*, 12, 1–19.
Scribner, R. W., 1994, *For the Sake of Simple Folk: popular propaganda for the German Reformation*, Oxford: Clarendon Press.
Scribner, R. W., 2001, *Religion and Culture in Germany (1400–1800)*, Leiden: Brill.
Securis, J., 1566, *A Detection and Querimonie of the Daily Enormities and Abuses Committed in Physick*, n.p.
Senlis, S. de, 1620, *La philosophie des contemplatifs*, Paris.
Sennert, D., [1611] 1656, *The Institutions or Fundamentals of the Whole Art, both of Physick and Chirurgery*, London.
Sennert, D., [1618] 1661, *Thirteen Books of Natural Philosophy*, trans. N. Culpeper and A. Cole, London.
Sextus Empiricus, 2000, *Outlines of Scepticism*, ed. J. Annas and J. Barnes, Cambridge: Cambridge University Press.
Shaftesbury, A. A. C., Earl of, 1964, *Characteristicks of Men, Manners, Opinions, Times* [1711], ed. J. M. Robertson, Indianapolis, IN: Bobbs-Merrill.
Shah, I., 1970, *The Secret Lore of Magic*, New York: Citadel Press.
Shakespeare, W., 1997, *The Sonnets*, ed. K. Duncan-Jones, London: Arden Shakespeare.
Shakespeare, W., 2008, *Norton Shakespeare Based on the Oxford Edition*, ed. S. Greenblatt *et al.*, 2nd edn, New York: W. W. Norton.
Shapiro, B. J., 1983, *Probability and Certainty in Seventeenth-Century England: a study of the relationships between natural science, religion, history, law, and literature*, Princeton, NJ: Princeton University Press.
Shapiro, J., 1996, *Shakespeare and the Jews*, New York: Columbia University Press.
Shaw, J. and Welch, E., 2011, *Making and Marketing Medicine in Renaissance Florence*, Amsterdam: Rodopi.
Sherman, W. H., 2011, "The beginning of 'the end': terminal paratext and the birth of print culture," in H. Smith and L. Wilson (eds), *Renaissance Paratexts*, Cambridge: Cambridge University Press.
Siraisi, N., 1990, *Medieval and Early Renaissance Medicine: an introduction to knowledge and practice*, Chicago: University of Chicago Press.
Siraisi, N., 1997, *The Clock and the Mirror: Girolamo Cardano and Renaissance medicine*, Princeton, NJ: Princeton University Press.
Skippon, P., 1732, "An account of a journey made thro' part of the Low-Countries, Germany, Italy and France," in A. Churchill and J. Churchill (eds), *A Collection of Voyages*, 6 vols, London: Churchill, Vol. 6.

Slack, P., 1979, "Mirrors of health and treasures of poor men: the uses of the vernacular medical literature of Tudor England," in C. Webster (ed.), *Health, Medicine, and Morality in Sixteenth-Century England*, Cambridge: Cambridge University Press.
Smith, B. R., 1999, *The Acoustic World of Early Modern England: attending to the O-factor*, Chicago and London: Chicago University Press.
Smith, B. R., 2000, "Premodern sexualities," *PMLA*, 115, 318–29.
Smith, B. R., 2007, *The Acoustic World of Early Modern England: attending to the O-factor*, Chicago: University of Chicago Press.
Smith, B. R., 2008, *The Key of Green: passion and perception in Renaissance culture*, Chicago: Chicago University Press.
Smith, B. R., 2010, *Phenomenal Shakespeare*, Malden, MA: Blackwell-Wiley.
Smith, B. R., 2012, "Afterword: phenomophobia, or who's Afraid of Merleau-Ponty?," *Criticism*, 54, 3, http://digitalcommons.wayne.edu/criticism/vol54/iss3/11.
Smith, J. C., 2002, *Sensuous Worship: Jesuits and the art of the early Catholic Reformation in Germany*, Princeton, NJ: Princeton University Press.
Smith, M., 1995, *Literary Realism and the Ekphrastic Tradition*, University Park, PA: Penn State University.
Smith, M. M., 2007a, *Sensing the Past: Seeing, hearing, smelling, tasting and touching in history*, Berkeley, CA: University of California Press.
Smith, M. M., 2007b, *Sensory History*, Oxford and New York: Berg.
Smith, M. M., 2012, "Preface: styling sensory history," *Journal for Eighteenth-Century Studies*, 35(4), 469–71.
Smith, P. H., 1994, *The Business of Alchemy: science and culture in the Holy Roman Empire*, Princeton, NJ: Princeton University Press.
Smith, P. H., 2004, *The Body of the Artisan: art and experience in the Scientific Revolution*, Chicago and London: University of Chicago Press.
Smith, P. H., 2010, "Why write a book? From lived experience to the written word in early modern Europe," *Bulletin of the German Historical Institute*, 47, 25–50, http://ghi-dc.org/bulletin, accessed June 9, 2013.
Smith, P. J., 2012, *Between Two Stools: scatology and its representations in English literature, Chaucer to Swift*, Manchester: Manchester University Press.
Somerset, C., 1993, *The Travel Diary (1611–1612) of an English Catholic*, ed. M. G. Brennan, Leeds: Leeds Philosophical and Literary Society.
Spenser, E., 1999, *Amoretti, The Shorter Poems*, ed. R. A. McCabe, London: Penguin Books.
Spierenburg, P. and Roodenburg, H. (eds), 2004, *Social Control in Europe 1500–1800*, Cleveland, OH: Ohio State University Press.
Spolsky, E., 2001, *Satisfying Scepticism: embodied knowledge in the Early Modern world*, Aldershot: Ashgate.
Spruit, L., 2008, "Renaissance views of active perception," in S. Knuuttila and P. Kärkkäinen (eds), *Theories of Perception in Medieval and Early Modern Perception*, Dordrecht: Springer.
Stallybrass, P., 2002, "Books and scrolls: navigating the Bible," in J. Anderson and E. Sauer (eds), *Books and Readers in Early Modern England*, Philadelphia, PA: University of Pennsylvania Press.

Stanbury, S., 2008, *The Visual Object of Desire in Late Medieval England*, Philadelphia, PA: University of Pennsylvania Press.

Stanev, H. A., 2012, "The city out of breath: Jacobean comedy and the odor of restraint," *Postmedieval*, 3(4), 423–35.

Starkey, T., 1871, *A Dialogue between Pole and Lupset*, London: Early English Text Society.

Steinberg, L., 1987, "'How shall this be?' Reflections on Filippo Lippi's 'Annunciation' in London, Part I," *Artibus et Historiae*, 8(16), 25–44.

Sterne, J., 2003, *The Audible Past: cultural origins of sound production*, Durham, NC: Duke University Press.

Strohm, R., 1990, *Music in Late Medieval Bruges*, 2nd edn, Oxford: Oxford University Press, 1991.

Strohmeyer, U., 2007, "Engineering vision in Early Modern Paris," in A. Cowan and J. Steward (eds), *The City and the Senses: urban culture since 1500*, Aldershot: Ashgate.

Sudnow, D., 1978, *Ways of the Hand: the organization of improvised conduct*, Cambridge, MA: MIT Press.

Summers, D., 1987, *The Judgment of Sense: Renaissance naturalism and the rise of aesthetics*, Cambridge: Cambridge University Press.

Sutton, J., 2000, "Body, mind, and order: local memory and the control of mental representations in medieval and Renaissance sciences of self," in A. Corones and G. Freeland (eds), *1543 And All That: word and image in the proto-scientific revolution*, Dordrecht: Kluwer.

Sylvius, F. de le B., 1679, *Opera medica*, Amstelodami: D. Elzevirium and A. Wolfgang.

Tafur, P., 1926, *Travels and Adventures, 1435–1439*, trans. and ed. M. Letts, London: Harpers.

Talvacchia, B., 1999, *Taking Positions: on the erotic in Renaissance culture*, Princeton, NJ: Princeton University Press.

Tanner, T., 1999, " 'Which is the Merchant Here and Which is the Jew?': The Venice of Shakespeare's *Merchant of Venice*," in M. Pfister and B. Shaff (eds), *Venetian Views, Venetian Blinds: English fantasies of Venice*, Amsterdam: Rodopi.

Taylor, L. (ed.), 2002, *Preachers and People in the Reformation and Early Modern Period*, Leiden: E. J. Brill.

Taylor, M., 1992, "Voyeurism and aposiopesis in Renaissance poetry," *Exemplaria*, 4(2), 267–94.

Tellier, M. le, 1625, *La règle des âmes devotes*, Paris.

Temkin, O., 1973, *Galenism: rise and decline of a medical concept*, Ithaca, NY: Cornell University Press.

The Catechism of the Council of Trent, 1829, Baltimore: Lucas Brothers.

Thelwall, A. S., 1850, *The Heidelberg Catechism of the Reformed Christian Religion*, London: Wertheim and Macintosh.

Temple, W., 1681, *Miscellanea*, London.

Thomas, W., 1549, *The vanitee of this world*, London.

Thompson, E. P., 1991, *Customs in Common*, London: Merlin.

Thornton, D., 1997, *The Scholar in His Study: ownership and experience in Renaissance Italy*, New Haven, CT: Yale University Press.

Tuck, R., 1988, "Optics and sceptics: the philosophical foundations of Hobbes's political thought," in E. Leites (ed.), *Conscience and Casuistry in Early Modern Europe*, Cambridge: Cambridge University Press.

Tuohy, T., 1996, *Herculean Ferrara: Ercole d'Este, 1471–1505, and the invention of a ducal capital*, Cambridge: Cambridge University Press.

Tyndale, W., 1848, "A brief declaration of the sacraments," in *Doctrinal Treatises and Introductions to Different Portions of the Holy Scriptures*, ed. H. Walter, Cambridge: Cambridge University Press.

Tyndale, W., 1854, *An Answer to Sir Thomas More's Dialogue, The Supper of the Lord After the True Meaning of John VI and 1 Cor. XI, and Wm. Tracy's Testament Expounded*, ed. H. Walter, Cambridge: Cambridge University Press.

Uppenkamp, B., 2009, "The Column of Predestination: some remarks on invention in Protestant reformed imagery," in O. Z. Pugliese and E. M. Kavaler (eds), *Faith and Fantasy in the Renaissance: texts, images, and religious practices*, Toronto: University of Toronto.

Van de Wetering, E., 2004, *Rembrandt: the painter at work*, Berkeley and Los Angeles: University of California Press.

Vasari, G., [1550] 1966–76, *Le vite de' più eccellenti pittori, scultori, e architettori*, ed. R. Bettarini and P. Barocchi, 4 vols, Florence: Sansoni.

Vernant, J-P., 2001, *The Universe, the Gods, and the Mortals*, New York: Harper Collins.

Vertova, L., 1979, "Cupid and Psyche in Renaissance painting before Raphael," *Journal of the Warburg and Courtauld Institutes*, 42, 104–21.

Vickers, N., 1985, "'The blazon of sweet beauty's best': Shakespeare's Lucrece," in P. A. Parker and G. H. Hartman (eds), *Shakespeare and the Question of Theory*, New York: Methuen.

Vinge, L., 1975, *The Five Senses: studies in a literary tradition*, Lund: Publications of the Royal Society of Letters at Lund.

Vitullo, J., 2010, "Taste and temptation in Early Modern Italy," *The Senses and Society*, 5(1), 106–18.

Wabuda, S., 2002, *Preaching during the English Reformation*, New York: Cambridge University Press.

Wainwright, W. J., 2011, "Jonathan Edwards and his Puritan predecessors," in S. Coakley and P. Gavrilyuk (eds), *The Spiritual Senses in Christian Tradition*, Cambridge: Cambridge University Press.

Waite, G. K., 1990, *David Joris and Dutch Anabaptism*, Waterloo: Wilfred Laurier University Press.

Waldron, J., 2012, "'The eye of man hath not heard': Shakespeare, synaesthesia, and post-Reformation phenomenology," *Criticism*, 54(3), 403–17.

Walkington, T., 1607, *The Opticke Glasse of Humors*, London.

Wallis, P., 2008, "Consumption, retailing, and medicine in early-modern London," *The Economic History Review*, 61, 26–53.

Walsham, A., 2008, "The Reformation and 'The disenchantment of the world' reassessed," *The Historical Journal*, 51(2), 497–528.

Walsham, A., 2012, *The Reformation of the Landscape: religion, identity, and memory in early modern Britain and Ireland*, Oxford: Oxford University Press.
Wandel, L. P., 2009, "John Calvin and Michel de Montaigne on the eye," in W. S. Melion and L. P. Wandel (eds), *Early Modern Eyes*, Leiden: E. J. Brill.
Waquet, F., 2003, *Parler comme un livre. L'oralité et le savoir (XVIe-XX siècle)*, Paris: Albin Michel.
Warley, C., 2005, *Sonnet Sequences and Social Distinction in Renaissance England*, Cambridge: Cambridge University Press.
Watson, R., 2007, "Some non-textual uses of books," in S. Eliot and J. Rose (eds), *A Companion to the History of the Book*, London: Blackwell.
Watt, T., 1991, *Cheap Print and Popular Piety, 1550–1640*, Cambridge: Cambridge University Press.
Wear, A., 1982, "Galen in the Renaissance," in V. Nutton (ed.), *Galen: problems and prospects*, London: Wellcome Institute.
Wear, A., 1995, "Epistemology and learned medicine in Early Modern England," in D. Bates (ed.), *Knowledge and the Scholarly Medical Traditions*, Cambridge: Cambridge University Press.
Wear, A., 2000, *Knowledge and Practice in English Medicine 1550–1680*, Cambridge: Cambridge University Press.
Welch, E., 2005, *Shopping in the Renaissance: consumer cultures in Italy 1400–1600*, New Haven, CT: Yale University Press.
Welch, E., 2008, "Space and spectacle in the Renaissance pharmacy," *Medicina e storia*, 15, 127–58.
Welch, E., 2011, "Sites of consumption in Early Modern Europe," in F. Trentmann (ed.), *The Oxford History of Consumption*, Oxford: Oxford University Press.
Wheatley, E., 2010, *Stumbling Blocks Before the Blind: medieval constructions of a disability*, Ann Arbor, MI: University of Michigan.
Wheeler, J., 2007, "Stench in sixteenth-century Venice," in A. Cowan and J. Steward (eds), *The City and the Senses: urban culture since 1500*, Aldershot: Ashgate.
Whitehead, N. L., 2009, "The ethnographic lens in the New World: Staden, de Bry, and the representation of the Tupi in Brazil," in W. S. Melion and L. P. Wandel (eds), *Early Modern Eyes*, Leiden: E. J.Brill.
Whitford, D. M. (ed.), 2008, *Reformation and Early Modern Europe: a guide to research*, Kirksville, MO: Truman State University Press.
Willen, D. 1995. "Communion-of-the-Saints: spiritual reciprocity and the godly community in early-modern England," *Albion*, 27(1), 19–41.
Willis, T., 1679, *Pharmaceutice rationalis*, London.
Willis, T., 1683, *Two Discourses Concerning the Soul of Brutes, Which is That of the Vital and Sensitive [Soul] of Man*, London: Dring, Harper & Leigh.
Willis, T., 1684, *Dr. Willis's Practice of Physick*, London.
Wilson, C., 1997, "Discourses of vision in seventeenth-century metaphysics," in D. M. Levin (ed.), *Sites of Vision*, Cambridge, MA: MIT Press.
Wilson, E., 1995, "Plague, fairs and street cries: sounding out society and space in early modern London," *Modern Language Studies*, 25, 1–42.

Wittmann, R., 1999, "Was there a reading revolution at the end of the eighteenth century?" in G. Cavallo and R. Chartier (eds), *A History of Reading in the West*, Cambridge: Polity Press.

Wolfe, C. T., 2012, "Forms of materialist embodiment," in M. Landers and B. Muñoz (eds), *Anatomy and the Organization of Knowledge, 1500–1850*, London: Pickering & Chatto.

Wolfson, H. A., 1935, "The internal senses in Latin, Arabic, and Hebrew Philosophic Texts," *Harvard Theological Review*, 28, 69–133.

Woodbridge, L., 2006, "The pedlar and the pawn: Why did Tudor England consider pedlars to be rogues?" in C. Dionne and S. Mentz (eds), *Rogues and Early Modern English Culture*, Ann Arbor, MI: University of Michigan Press.

Woolf, D., 1986, "Speech, text, and time: the sense of hearing and the sense of the past in Renaissance England," *Albion: A Quarterly Journal Concerned with British Studies*, 18(2), 159–93.

Woolf, D., 2001, "News, history and the construction of the present in Early Modern England," in B. Dooley and S. A. Baron (eds), *The Politics of Information in Early Modern Europe*, London and New York: Routledge.

Woolgar, C. M., 2007, *The Senses in Late Medieval England*, London: Yale University Press.

Woudhuysen, H., 2004, "The dash—a short but quite dramatic account," paper given at Jacobean Printed Book Conference, Queen Mary, University of London, September.

Wright, A. D., 2005, *The Counter-Reformation: Catholic Europe and the non-Christian world*, Aldershot: Ashgate.

Wright, J. P. and Potter, P. (eds), 2000, *Psyche and Soma: physicians and metaphysicians on the mind-body problem from antiquity to the Enlightenment*, Oxford: Clarendon Press.

Wright, L., 2007, "Speaking and listening in Early Modern London," in A. Cowan and J. Steward (eds), *The City and the Senses: urban culture since 1500*, Aldershot: Ashgate.

Wroth, M., 1983, *Poems of Lady Mary Wroth*, ed. J. A. Roberts, Baton Rouge, LA: Louisiana State University.

Yandell, C., 2002, *Carpe Corpus: time and gender in Early Modern France*, Newark, DE: University of Delaware Press.

Yates, F., 1966, *The Art of Memory*, London: Routledge & Kegan Paul.

Yrjönsuuri, M., 2008, "Perceiving one's own body," in S. Knuuttila and P. Kärkkäinen (eds), *Theories of Perception in Medieval and Early Modern Perception*, Dordrecht: Springer.

Zahediah, N., 2010, *The Capital and the Colonies: London and the Atlantic economy, 1660–1700*, Cambridge: Cambridge University Press.

NOTES ON CONTRIBUTORS

Niall Atkinson is Neubauer Family Assistant Professor of Art History, University of Chicago. His research focuses on the sensorial experience of urban space and architecture within the social dimensions of the Italian Renaissance. He is the author of several articles on the soundscapes of Renaissance Florence and has just completed a monograph on the intersection of sound, architecture, and urban life in that city. Currently he is embarking on a project concerning the experience of travel and movement in relation to knowledge and representation of the early modern Italian city.

Federico Barbierato is lecturer in Early Modern History at the University of Verona, Italy. He has studied, in particular, religious dissent, unbelief, censorship, and the circulation of forbidden books between the sixteenth and eighteenth centuries. Among his books are *The Inquisitor in the Hat Shop* (2012); *Nella stanza dei circoli, Clavicula Salomonis e libri di magia a Venezia, Secoli xvii–xviii* (2002). He is coordinator of EmoDiR (International Research Group in Early Modern Religious Dissents and Radicalism).

Peter Burke studied at Oxford and taught at the new University of Sussex before moving to Cambridge, where he became Professor of Cultural History. He retired from the Chair in 2004 but remains a Life Fellow of Emmanuel College. He has published twenty-six books and his work has been translated into thirty-one languages. For most of his career he has worked on the cultural and social history of early modern Europe, with some incursions into the nineteenth and twentieth centuries.

Holly Dugan is the author of *The Ephemeral History of Perfume: scent and sense in early modern England* (2011) and numerous articles on early modern olfaction. She is the co-editor with Lara Farina of *Intimate Senses*, a special issue of the journal *Postmedieval* (2012). Her research and teaching interests center on the relationship between history, literature, and material culture, particularly the role of the senses in late medieval and early modern English literature.

Danijela Kambaskovic is Honorary Research Fellow, School of English, and Associate Investigator, Australian Research Centre of Excellence for the History of Emotions, University of Western Australia. She has published two scholarly books and numerous articles on the cultural history of love and courtship in early modern Europe. Her edited collection, *Body and Mind in Medieval and Renaissance Europe*, is awaiting publication with Springer. She is also an award-winning poet.

Matthew Milner is a Research Associate at McGill University. He is the author of *The Senses and the English Reformation* (2011) and has published related essays in *Religion and the Senses in Early Modern Europe* (2012), and the *Journal of Medieval and Early Modern Studies*. His work focuses on the relationship between religious practices and sensory culture, in particular Aristotelian natural philosophy and theology, in Reformation England. He is also an avid digital humanist.

Stephen Pender is an Associate Professor in English at the University of Windsor. He has published in *Early Science and Medicine*, the *British Journal for the History of Science*, *Rhetorica*, and *Philosophy and Rhetoric*, as well as in several collections of essays and *Rhetoric and Medicine in Early Modern Europe*, co-edited with Nancy Struever which was pubished in 2012. He is at work on a monograph exploring the passions, therapy, and counsel in early modern England.

François Quiviger obtained his Ph.D. from the Warburg Institute, London, where he works as curator of digital resources, librarian, and researcher. He has written, taught and curated projects on early modern European academies, on mythology, and on Renaissance material culture, art, and art theory. His recent book *The Sensory World of Italian Renaissance Art* (2010) explores the presence and function of sensation in Renaissance ideas and practices.

Herman Roodenburg is Professor of Historical Anthropology at the Free University of Amsterdam and a Senior Researcher at the Meertens Institute, also in Amsterdam. A cultural historian, he often cooperates with cultural anthropologists and art historians. Among his English publications are *The Eloquence of the Body* (2004) and *Forging European Identities, 1400–1700* (2007). He is currently finishing an emotional and sensory history of the Dutch (provisionally called *The Crying Dutchman*).

Evelyn Welch is author of *Making and Marketing Medicine in Renaissance Florence* (2011), *Shopping in the Renaissance* (2007), and *Art and Authority in Renaissance Italy* (2000). She has been a fellow at the Victoria and Albert Museum and is now (as of 2013) a Trustee of the Museum. Professor Welch ran a number of UK and European grants which have resulted in outputs such as *The Material Renaissance* (2007) and *Fashioning the Early Modern: Dress, Textiles and Innovation in Europe, 1500–1800*, forthcoming from Oxford University Press.

Charles T. Wolfe is a Research Fellow, Department of Philosophy and Moral Sciences and Sarton Centre for History of Science, Ghent University. His edited volumes include *Monsters and Philosophy* (2005), *The Body as Object and Instrument of Knowledge* (2010, with O. Gal), *Vitalism and the Scientific Image in Post-Enlightenment Life-Science, 1800–2010* (2013, with S. Normandin), and *Brain Theory* (forthcoming). His current project is a monograph on the conceptual foundations of Enlightenment vitalism.

INDEX

Aertsen, Pieter 32
aisthesis, Aristotelian (and Hieroclean) notion of 6, 14–17, 110
  see also sensory knowing
Alberti, Leone Battista 5, 24, 40–1, 55, 113
Albot, Richard 90
Antoninus of Florence 88–9
Aretino, Pietro 29–31, 34, 40–1, 191, 218–19
Ariosto, Ludovico 161, 166
Aristotle 20, 40–1, 110, 132, 138, 144, 153 172–3
Armenini, Giovan Battista 194
Assaf, Sharon 121
Atkinson, Niall 12, 15
Avicenna 5, 120
Augustine 153
Avila, Theresa of 100

Bacon, Francis 12, 85
Badius, Jodocus Ascensius 121–2
Bakhtin, Mikhail 29, 109
Barbicrato, Federico 12
Barclay, John 130
Bargrave, Robert 52, 54–5
Barlaeus, Caspar 143–4
Baxandall, Michael 7–8, 12, 14, 58

Bearden, Elizabeth B. 163
Behringer, Wolfgang 94
Bellay, Joachim du 157
Benjamin, Walter 109
Bennett, Jonathan 109
Berkeley, George 123
Bernini, Gian Lorenzo 100, 181, 201
Berthaud, Claude-Louis 62–4
Berckheyde, Gerrit Adriaensz 59
Beuckelaer, Joachim 73
Biernoff, Suzannah 9
Biow, Stephen 30
Boccaccio, Giovanni 22, 118, 162
body and mind (and/or "soul") 1–2, 7, 16–17, 38–9, 41, 100, 105, 108–9, 112–13, 130–3, 135–6, 146–7, 153, 173
Borchardt, Ludwig 110
Borstius, Jacobus 51
Bosse, Abraham 63, 71–2
Botticelli, Sandro 8, 196
Boulton, Richard 127, 144
Bourdieu, Pierre 7, 14–15
Bouvelles, Charles de 89
Boyle, Robert 14, 112, 120
brain
  anatomy of 146, 173–4
  areas of 154–5

perceives odors, unlike the nose 139
supporting the internal senses 136–7, 173–4
tasting of 127
touching of 127
Brant, Sebastian 89
Bravo, Juan 139
Bredekamp, Horst 16–17
Brereton, William 45–6, 54–5
Bright, Timothy 117
Bronzino, Agnolo 188–90
Brouwer, Adriaen 13, 191
Browne, John 66
Brunelleschi, Filippo 55
Bruni, Leonardo 45, 55
Bruno, Giordano 111
Brunschwig, Hieronymus 127
Buffalmacco, Buonamico 19–20
Bugenhagen, Johannes 91
Bulwer, John 108, 120, 130
Burke, Peter 4, 12, 15
Burton, Robert 117, 136–8
Bynum, Caroline Walker 8, 10, 12–13, 16

Calvin, John 9, 91, 100, 105, 119, 184
Camoes, Luis de 157
Canaletto 59
Canisius, Petrus 91, 100, 102
Caravaggio 47, 91, 200–1
Carpaccio, Vittore 52
Carracci Brothers 201
Casola, Pietro 46, 53
Castiglione, Baldassare 15, 25–8, 30, 41, 156
Cavalieri, Emilio de' 98
Cecil, Robert 61
Cellini, Benvenuto 14
Celsus 128
Cennini, Cennino 14
Cervantes, Miguel de 163
Charles V, Emperor 57
Charleton, Walter 112, 128, 146
Charron, Pierre 133–5
Chartier, Roger 206
Chigi, Agostino 34

Chrysippus 110
Cicero 33, 128
Cisneros, Francisco Jiménez de 94–5, 100
Claessens, Pieter 53
Clark, Stuart 11–12, 95, 129
Classen, Constance 8, 20, 29, 58
cognition, situated 17
    see also sensory knowing
Colet, John 94–5
Collaert, Adriaen 170
Comenius (Jan Komenský) 51
common sense (Aristotle's *koine aisthesis*; Lat. *sensus communis*), as one of the internal senses 5–7, 64, 88, 123, 130, 136–7, 173
    see also imagination; memory
common sensibles (Aristotle), encompassing figure, size, movement, and rest 173–4
    Renaissance art to be envisaged in terms of 173–4
Connerton, Paul 14
Connor, Stephen 152–3
Corbin, Alain 3, 44–5, 109
Corneille, Pierre 72
Cort, Cornelis 170
Coryate, Thomas 44, 54–5, 76, 78
Cosimo, Piero di 49
Cotta, John 137
Crashaw, Richard 162, 164
Cureau de la Chambre, Marin 130
Cusa, Nicholas of 89, 93

D'Alembert, Jean de Rond 123
Dallington, Robert 55
Dante 49
Darnton, Robert 206, 208, 218
Da Vinci, Leonardo 114
Davis, John 84
Davis, Natalie Zemon 207–208
Davies, John 121
Day, Richard 90
De Hooch, Pieter 191
Dekker, Thomas 49, 155
Del Piombo, Sebastiano 179
Del Vaga, Perino 193

Della Porta, Giambattista 114
Dering, Richard 75
Descartes, René 1–2, 6, 11, 15–16, 109, 112, 114–16, 120–1, 123–4, 136, 144, 146–7, 173
  and the "disembodied eye" 3
Desprez, Josquin 93
Diderot, Denis 124
Doni, Anton Francesco 7, 23, 193
Duffy, Eamon 90
Dugan, Holly 6, 16
Du Laurens, André 111, 124, 138
Dyck, Anthony van 201

Egregis, Guglielmo de 203–4
El Greco 200
Elias, Norbert 3, 25
Elisabeth, Princess of Bohemia 147
Elizabeth I, Queen of England 61
Elyot, Thomas 89, 130–1, 134, 137
embodiment 1–2, 6–8, 14–17, 115–19, 123–4, 149, 151–3, 155–6, 158, 160, 162, 165–6, 205
Epicurus 124
Equicola, Mario 40
Erasmus, Desiderius 15, 25–8, 33, 94, 99
D'Este, Duke Ercole 35
D'Este, Duchess Isabella 40
Evelyn, John 45–6, 48, 53–6

Faber, Zachäeus 101
Fabri, Felix 58
Farel, Guillaume 181
Febvre, Lucien 3, 110
Fernel, Jean 120, 137
Ficino, Marsilio 89, 93, 117, 198–9
Filarete (Antonio di Pietro Averlino) 24
Fioravanti, Leonardo 76
Fish, Stanley 206
Floyer, John 127
Focillon, Henri 125
Foxe, John 96, 103–4
Foucault, Michel 7
Frederic Henry, Prince of Orange 9
Freedberg, David 16

Galen 5–6, 120, 127–8, 131–2, 134–5, 137, 139–40, 143, 145, 173
Galilei, Galileo 11, 66–7, 105, 111–12, 124, 210
Gallese, Vittorio 16
Gassendi, Pierre 112, 124, 128
Gell, Alfred 10
Ghirlandaio, Domenico 93
Ghirlandaio, Rodolfo 192
Gibbons, Orlando 75
Giles of Viterbo 95
Gilio, Andrea 178–9
Ginzburg, Carlo 206
Giotto 176
Goethe, Johann Wolfgang von 124
Gongora, Luis de 157
Gonzaga, Federico II 40
Goody, Jack 209, 216
Goyen, Jan van 7
Granada, Luis de 91
Grebel, Conrad 98
Gregory I the Great, Pope 174–5
Grosseteste, Robert 124
Grote, Geert 93
Guilpin, Edward 49
Guylforde, Richard 58

Hals, Frans 7
Hamburger, Jeffrey 8
Hamou, Philippe 115
Harvey, Elizabeth 108, 133
Harvey, William 108, 113, 120–1, 124, 144–5
Haley, George 163
Heylyn, Peter 48
hearing
  and bells and clocks 50
  central to the circular paths between orality and writing 205–9
  and church music 52, 93, 97–8, 104
  and crowded housing 19–21, 23
  hearing or not hearing the Gospel 51, 101
  importance to Catholic piety 88
  and the market place 72–8

and the oral transmission of news 211–13
privileged over the other senses 108–9, 207
as a privileged and a distrusted sense 117–18
and public performances 51–2, 57–8
and reading aloud 75–6, 203–4, 208, 210–11
and rough music 52
and street cries 47–8, 50–1, 72–5, 79
and urban noise 23–4, 48–50, 72–3
and urban quiet 23, 50
Helmont, Jan Baptist van 128
Henri III, King of France 57
Henri IV, King of France 111
Henry VIII, King of England 58, 102
Herbert, George 100
Herrick, Robert 159, 161
Hierocles 110
historical cognitive science 16, 109–10
historical phenomenology 16, 151–4
Hobbes, Thomas 11, 115, 124
Homer 161, 209
Hoogstraten, Samuel van 7
Hooke, Robert 112
Hooker, Richard 97
Howell, James 45
Howes, David 153
Huarte, Juan 131, 141–3, 145–6
Huizinga, Johan 3
Huygens, Constantijn 9, 15, 55–6, 144

images
  animated nature of 181–4
  awaken our multisensory experience of the world 169
  detached from the hand 173
  as didactic tools for the illiterate 96
  as idols 96
  and mental visualization 8–9, 210
  see also matter, animated nature of; sight
imagination, as one of the internal senses 5, 64, 88, 100, 136–7, 143, 173–4

intersensoriality 4–5, 6–10, 20
  see also kinaesthesia
Irmscher, Günther 33

Janequin, Clément 75
Jay, Martin 3
Joan of Arc 90
Jonas, Hans 110
Jonson, Ben 49, 62
Joris, David 100

Kambaskovich, Danijela 16
Kant, Immanuel 123
Karant-Nunn, Susan 9, 104
Karlstadt, Andreas Bodenstein von 96, 181, 183
Kearney, James 153
Kempis, Thomas à 93
Kepler, Johannes 111–12, 114
kinaesthesia 5, 8, 58, 123
  see also intersensoriality
Knipbergen, François 7
knowledge, artisanal, bodily, or sensory 4, 13–14, 110, 124, 153–4, 162
  see also embodiment
Kyd, Thomas 117

La Mettrie, Julien Offray de 112, 113
Labé, Louise 160
Lamy, Guillaume 113
Lanteri, Giacomo 23–4
Latini, Brunetto 53
La Puente, Luis de 91
Lassels, Richard 56
Latour, Bruno 10
Lefevre d'Etaples, Jacques 89, 94
Lemnius, Levinus 131
Lentes, Thomas 9
Le Cat, Claude-Nicolas 112
L'Etoile, Pierre de 75
Leo X, Pope 34
Leyden, Jan van 103
Linacre, Thomas 131
Lippi, Filippino 192
Locke, John 116, 124, 206
Lomazzo, Giovan Paolo 193–4

Loredan, Giovan Francesco 209
Loyola, Ignatius of 100, 175–6
Lucretius 124
Luther, Martin 12, 90–1, 95–7, 99,
    101–2, 108–9, 207

Magdalene Master 176
Maillard, Olivier 51
Margaret of Austria, Archduchess 57
markets 12, 61–86
    as a model for corrupting the senses 85
    and multisensory observation 12, 66,
        71–2, 76
Marot, Clément 159
matter, animated nature of 10, 13–14, 16
    see also images, animated nature of
Mauss, Marcel 14
Mayer, Eric D. 163
Mayers, Kathryn 162
McKenzie, Donald 205
McLuhan, Marshall 3–4, 27
McTighe, Sheila 31–2
Medici, Fernando de', Grand Duke of
    Tuscany 85–6
Melanchton, Philipp 105
memory, as one of the internal senses 64,
    88, 136–7
Menocchio 10
Merleau-Ponty, Maurice 152
Mersenne, Marin 1, 109
metaphor, intrinsic part of sensation 150,
    159–66
Meyssonnier, Lazare 1
Michelangelo 92, 179, 188, 191, 200
Milani, Antonio 216
Milani, Giovan Battista 216
Milner, Matthew 5, 8, 11–12, 64
Milton, John 7, 158, 161
Modena, Nicoletto da 194
Montaigne, Michel de 6, 38–41, 45, 105,
    133, 153
Monte, Giovanni Battista da 143
Montgomery, Hugh 108
More, Thomas 12, 94, 100
Mortoft, Francis 46, 53
Moryson, Fynes 46, 54–5, 68

Moulton, Ian Frederick 41
Mundy, Peter 46–47, 57

Nashe, Thomas 72
Nero, Emperor 192
Noë, Alva 17
Nemesius, Bishop of Emesa 134
neuroscience 2, 16, 154, 173, 200
Newton, Isaac 14
North, Dudley 45
Novalis 124

Obrecht, Jacob 93
Ong, Walter 3–4, 27
Ostade, Adriaen van 191
Ovid 194–5
Osuna, Francisco de 100

Pacher, Michael 178, 201
Paganin, Teodoro 203–4
Palissy, Bernard 14
Pallavicino, Ferrante 203
Paracelsus 14
Peacham, Henry 164
Pencz, Georg 122, 170
Pender, Stephen 5
Pepys, Samuel 54–5, 58, 141
Perkins, William 100
Petrarch 122
Petrobonelli, Santo 75
Philip II, King of Spain 102
picture act theory 16–17
piety, affective and imaginative 8–9, 11,
    93, 95, 175–81
    and artificial memory 175–6
    and Catholic distrust of sensory
        delusion 94
    Catholic and Protestant piety both
        multisensory 97, 184–5
    Catholic and Protestant sensory
        practices of discernment 11 12,
        94–6
    inner sensory piety, both Catholic and
        Protestant 27, 100–1
    and the Passion of Christ 8–10, 89–90,
        172, 174–81

and Protestant distrust of sensory
  delusion 96–7
scriptural piety 96–9, 101
transformative potential to the arts 92
  and to believers 100
see also sensory anxiety
Pinder, Ulrich 99–100
Pinturicchio 192
Pisanelli, Baldassare 15, 30–1
Platina, Bartolomeo 41
Plato 20, 109–10, 117, 124, 218
Platt, Hugh 155
Platter (the Younger), Thomas 53–4
Plotinus 111
Pontormo, Jacopo 37–8
Porcellis, Jan 7
Porter, Roy 142
Pouchelle, Marie-Christine 120
Poussin, Nicolas 201
Principe, Lawrence 14
Priscianese, Francesco 37, 41
Proust, Marcel 1, 154
Puttenham, George 164–5

Quiviger, François 5, 21, 34, 98

Rabelais, François 28–30, 112, 199
Ragland, Evan 127–8
Raphael 34, 93, 192–3
Reisch, Georg 88
Reiss, Timothy 2
Rembrandt 5, 9, 201
Richardson, Catherine 163
Ricci, Matteo 45, 48
Rizzolatti, Giacomo 16
Roberts, Lewes 64
Rodrigues, Joao 54
Romano, Giulio 193
Ronsard, Pierre de 157
Roodenburg, Herman 58
Rosenfeld, Sophia 6
Ross, Alexander 122, 125
Rosselli, Stefano 85
Rudolf II, Emperor 86
Rubens, Peter Paul 16, 201
Rublack, Ulinka 13

St. Antoninus of Florence 214
St. Bernardino of Siena 40, 51, 210
St. John of the Cross 100
St. Paul 207
Sacchetti, Franco 19
Sachsen, Ludolph von 8
Sadeler the Elder, Raphael 170
Sales, François de 100
Sanctorius, Santorio 147
Sangallo, Giuliano da 191
Sandys, George 48
Sastrow, Bartholomäus 52
Scappi, Bartolomeo 34
Schama, Simon 45
Scheer, Monique 17
Schlüsselburg, Konrad 96
Schwenkfeld, Caspar 98–9
Scientific Revolution 13–14
Scot, Michael 214
Semitecolo, Giovanni 216
Seneca 39
Sennert, Daniel 129, 136, 138–9
senses
  aestheticizing of 21, 25–8, 177–81
  allegories of 170–2
  at the heart of the religious upheavals
    88
  and circularity between orality and
    writing 205–9, 216–17
  cross-modality of 4–5
  see also intersensoriality
  disciplining of 12, 25–8, 36–7, 89–92,
    94, 102–3, 134–5
  disputed role in salvation 91, 95, 99,
    101
  distrust of 10–14, 90–1
  see also sensory anxiety
  and early modern physiology 130
  essential component of religious
    learning 88–9
  ethical ambiguity of 109, 118, 121
    satirizing their disciplining 28–30
  filter the world through prior cultural
    meanings 3
  and housing 19–21, 22–5
  infallibility of 124

instrumental in discerning vice from virtue 87, 94
instrumental in shaping confessional cultures 104
internal and external senses 130, 136–7
and literary studies 151–2
and literary tropes (*blazon, ekphrasis, aposiopesis*) 118–19, 159–66
and Mannerism 188
and manners 25–8
and melancholy 6–7, 11, 118–19, 151, 143–4
number and ranking of 2–3, 5–6, 20–2, 30, 65, 107–10, 120, 125, 172–3
permeability of 119–20
and physicians' bedside examinations 140–4
and the Plague 22, 45–6, 84
and print culture, 4, 27, 205, 207–210
and reading practices 154–5, 205, 216
and social distinctions 15–16, 20–1, 30–1, 39, 65–6, 19–41, 56, 150
and urban neighbourhoods 12
universalizing theories of 16, 154, 156
see also piety, affective and imaginative
sensescapes, refers to *what* and *how* people sense 2–3
sensory anxiety 10–14
and books 213–15
and living matter 10, 13–14
and magic 11
and markets 64–8, 218
and medicine 132–3
and religion 11, 94–5
sensory excitements
hyper-stimulation of 56
increased desirability and availability of 62
and marketplaces 62
and the new global trade 62–4
sensory knowing
and aisthesis 6
of alchemists 14
of artisans 13–14
of painters 7
of physicians 127–8, 140–4
both visceral and constructed 158
see also aisthesis
sensory memory (Proust) 2, 5, 154
sensory shifts, as observed by the field's pioneers 3–4, 11, 27, 88, 205, 208
Sermisy, Claude de 75
Sextus Empiricus 128
Shah, Idries 217
Shakespeare, William 113–14, 117, 149–50, 157–60, 217
Shapiro, Barbara 128
sight
and alchemy 14
and appearance of squares and streets 52–6, 59
and day and night 56–7
and haptic visuality 7–9
importance to Protestant piety 88
inversion of the privilege of sight into a materialism of touch 125
and markets 68–72
and new technologies of vision 28, 114–16, 200
and the "period eye" 7–8, 14, 58
privileged over the other senses 2, 107, 110–12, 207
as a privileged and a distrusted sense 113–14, 116, 129
and public performances 51–2, 57–8
and street culture 53
see also images
Signorelli, Luca 192
Sixtus IV, Pope 192
Skippon, Philip 59
smell 9
and affective piety 176
alchemy 14
associated with our animal nature 109
and bath houses 48
bodily smells 38
and the brain 139
fragrant smells (ambergris, civet, musk, roses) 38, 44–6, 61–2, 184–5
and intuition 119

and market smells 78–84
and Montaigne 38
and moral judgement 119
odours conceived of as particles in the air 139
and pomanders 46, 161, 185
and rosaries 99, 184–5
and stench 23, 45–6, 68–9
Smith, Bruce R. 16, 49, 152
Smith, Mark M. 3
Smith, Pamela H. 13–16
Sodoma 178–9
Somerset, Charles 54–5
Spenser, Edmund 118, 122, 161
Spinoza, Baruch de 116
Starkey, Thomas 58
Stow, John 49
Stuckius, Johann Wilhelm 22–3
Sutton, John 16
Sydenham, Thomas 116
Sydney, Philip 119, 157, 165, 218
Sylvius, Franciscus de le Boë 113, 120–1, 127–8
synaesthesia 6
  both a neurological condition and a literary device 155–6
  see also intersensoriality

Tafur, Pero 48–9, 53
Tasso, Bernardo 218
taste
  and affective piety 176
  in alchemy 14
  associated with animal nature 109
  and banquets 21–3, 26, 28–37
  least represented in the Renaissance 196
  as marker of social status 31
  and markets 78–84
  and sweetness 80
  and tobacco 82–4
  visualized 31–4
tasting, investigative 127–8
Ter Borch, Gerard 191
Thévenot, Jean de 48
Thomas Aquinas 207

Titian 37
touch
  and affective piety 176
  alchemy 14
  and Aretino 40
  bridging mind and body 1–2, 40–1, 108
  and crowded streets 47
  and day and night 56–7
  encompassing other senses, such as thermoception, alloception and proprioception 122–3, 153, 172
  and haptic visuality 7–9
  importance to Protestant piety 88
  "inner touch" and body image 5
  inversion of the privilege of sight into a materialism of touch 125
  and manual occupations 20–1, 65
  and the market place 68–78
  massively appealed to in medical tradition 120
  and the practice of painting 7, 20–1
  privileged over the other senses 112–13, 120–1, 124
  privileged and downgraded 117, 122
  and rosaries 99, 184–5
  and sensory knowing 108
  and sight 4, 6–8, 114–17, 120–1
  situated in the "noble hand" 108, 118
  "a touchable God" 8, 20–1
  ubiquity of 7, 108, 122–3
  urban life 47–8
Tyndale, William 95–6, 100

Udine, Giovanni da 193
Urban VIII, Pope 203
Utrecht Caravaggists 191

Vasari, Georgio 187–8, 200
Vega, Carcilaso de la 157
Vega, Joseph de la 71
Velasquez, Diego 180, 201
Veneziano, Agostino 191
Vermeer, Johannes 191, 201
Vernant, Jean-Pierre 217
Vickers, Nancy 166

Vico, Enea 194
Viret, Pierre 100
Vitruvius 193
Vitullo, Juliann 40
Vives, Juan 94
Voragine, Jacobus de 175
Vos, Maerten de 170, 172

Walkington, Thomas 131
Welch, Evelyn 11–12
Welser, Sebald 104
Wey, William 47
Wiericx, Anton 170

Wither, George 134
Willemsz, Arendt 52
Willis, Thomas 111–12, 122–5, 128, 136, 173
Williams, Henry 210
Wilson, Catherine 115–16
Wolfe, Charles T. 16
Woolf, D. R. 27

Xie, Zhaozhe 45

Zuccaro, Federico 194
Zwingli, Ulrich 181

www.ingramcontent.com/pod-product-compliance
Ingram Content Group UK Ltd.
Pitfield, Milton Keynes, MK11 3LW, UK
UKHW050024200326
469166UK00009B/171